Injury & Trauma Sourcebook

Learning Disabilities Sourcebook, 4th Edition

Leukemia Sourcebook

Liver Disorders Sourcebook

Medical Tests Sourcebook, 4th Edition

Men's Health Concerns Sourcebook, 4th Edition

Mental Health Disorders Sourcebo

Mental Retardation Sourcebook

Movement Disorders Sourcebook,

Multiple Sclerosis Sourcebook

Muscular Dystrophy Sourcebook

Obesity Sourcebook

Osteoporosis Sourcebook

Pain Sourcebook, 4th Edition

Pediatric Cancer Sourcebook

Physical & Mental Issues in Aging Sourcebook

Podiatry Sourcebook, 2nd Edition

Pregnancy & Birth Sourcebook, 3rd Edition

Prostate & Urological Disorders Sourcebook

Prostate Cancer Sourcebook

Rehabilitation Sourcebook

Respiratory Disorders Sourcebook, 3rd Edition

Sexually Transmitted Diseases Sourcebook,
    5th Edition

Sleep Disorders Sourcebook, 3rd Edition

Smoking Concerns Sourcebook

Sports Injuries Sourcebook, 4th Edition

Stress-Related Disorders Sourcebook, 3rd Edition

Stroke Sourcebook, 3rd Edition

Surgery Sourcebook, 3rd Edition

Thyroid Disorders Sourcebook

Transplantation Sourcebook

Traveler's Health Sourcebook

Urinary Tract & Kidney Diseases & Disorders
    Sourcebook, 2nd Edition

Vegetarian Sourcebook

Women's Health Concerns Sourcebook, 4th Edition

Workplace Health & Safety Sourcebook

Worldwide Health Sourcebook

Teen Health Series

Abuse & Violence Information for Teens

Accident & Safety Information for Teens

Alcohol Information for Teens,
    3rd Edition

Asthma Information for Teens,
    2nd Edition

Body Information for Teens

Cancer Information for Teens,
    3rd Edition

Complementary & Alternative
    Medicine Information for Teens,
    2nd Edition

Diabetes Information for Teens,
    2nd Edition

Diet Information for Teens, 3rd Edition

Drug Information for Teens, 3rd Edition

Eating Disorders Information for Teens,
    3rd Edition

Fitness Information for Teens,
    3rd Edition

Learning Disabilities Information for
    Teens

Mental Health Information for Teens,
    4th Edition

Pregnancy Information for Teens,
    2nd Edition

Sexual Health Information for Teens,
    3rd Edition

Skin Health Information for Teens,
    3rd Edition

Sleep Information for Teens

Sports Injuries Information for Teens,
    3rd Edition

Stress Information for Teens,
    2nd Edition

Suicide Information for Teens,
    2nd Edition

Tobacco Information for Teens,
    2nd Edition

Stroke

SOURCEBOOK

Third Edition

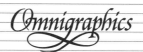

Bibliographic Note

Because this page cannot legibly accommodate all the copyright notices, the Bibliographic Note portion of the Preface constitutes an extension of the copyright notice.

Edited by Amy L. Sutton

Health Reference Series
Karen Bellenir, *Managing Editor*
David A. Cooke, MD, FACP, *Medical Consultant*
Elizabeth Collins, *Research and Permissions Coordinator*
EdIndex, Services for Publishers, *Indexers*

* * *

Omnigraphics, Inc.
Matthew P. Barbour, *Senior Vice President*
Kevin M. Hayes, *Operations Manager*

* * *

Peter E. Ruffner, *Publisher*
Copyright © 2013 Omnigraphics, Inc.
ISBN 978-0-7808-1297-0
E-ISBN 978-0-7808-1298-7

Library of Congress Cataloging-in-Publication Data

Stroke sourcebook : basic consumer health information about ischemic stroke, hemorrhagic stroke, transient ischemic attack, and other forms of brain attack, with information about stroke risk factors and prevention, diagnostic tests, post-stroke complications, and acute and rehabilitative treatments, such as stroke medications, surgeries, and therapies; along with tips on regaining independence, restoring cognitive function, and dealing with depression after stroke, a glossary of related medical terms, and a directory of resources for further help and information / edited by Amy L. Sutton. -- Third edition.
    pages cm
  Summary: "Provides basic consumer health information about stroke prevention, diagnosis, treatment, complications, and rehabilitation strategies, along with tips for coping after a stroke. Includes index, glossary of related terms, and other resources"-- Provided by publisher.
  Includes bibliographical references and index.
  ISBN 978-0-7808-1297-0 (hardcover : alk. paper) 1. Cerebrovascular disease--Popular works. I. Sutton, Amy L.
  RC388.5.S8566 2013
  616.8'1--dc23
                                                                    2013007205

Table of Contents

Visit www.healthreferenceseries.com to view *A Contents Guide to the Health Reference Series*, a listing of more than 16,000 topics and the volumes in which they are covered.

Part II: Types of Stroke

Part III: Stroke Risk Factors and Prevention

Part IV: Diagnosis and Treatment of Stroke

Part V: Post-Stroke Complications and Rehabilitation

Part VI: Life after Stroke

Part VII: Additional Help and Information

Preface

About This Book

According to the Centers for Disease Control and Prevention (CDC), stroke kills nearly 130,000 Americans each year—one out of every 18 deaths—making stroke the fourth leading cause of death in the United States. Stroke is also a leading cause of serious, long-term disability. Its effects include a broad range of cognitive and physical problems, such as speech and communication difficulties, dementia, muscle spasticity and weakness, balance problems, and incontinence. Early recognition of stroke symptoms and prompt medical attention can help patients achieve better outcomes. In addition, many strokes can be prevented through lifestyle changes that address underlying risk factors.

Stroke Sourcebook, Third Edition provides updated information about the causes, diagnosis, treatment, and prevention of stroke. Readers will learn about ischemic stroke, hemorrhagic stroke, and transient ischemic attacks (TIAs, also known as mini strokes), as well as stroke risk factors. Stroke risk factors include atherosclerosis, diabetes, heart disease, blood disorders, high cholesterol, high blood pressure, and obesity. Information on stroke diagnosis, acute and rehabilitative treatment, and post-stroke complications is also included, along with tips for living with post-stroke challenges, a glossary of related terms, and a directory of organizations that provide information to stroke patients and their caregivers.

How to Use This Book

This book is divided into parts and chapters. Parts focus on broad areas of interest. Chapters are devoted to single topics within a part.

Part I: Introduction to Stroke identifies the symptoms of stroke and discusses the incidence of stroke in children, men, women, and older adults. It also examines the impact of stroke in specific geographic regions and stroke-related health disparities among racial and ethnic populations. The part concludes with statistical information on stroke in the United States and recent findings in stroke research.

Part II: Types of Stroke discusses the two major types of stroke, ischemic and hemorrhagic. It also describes transient ischemic attacks, which are often called mini strokes, and it addresses concerns about risk factors for recurrent strokes.

Part III: Stroke Risk Factors and Prevention provides information about conditions that predispose a person to having a stroke, including atherosclerosis, carotid artery disease, atrial fibrillation, and peripheral artery disease. It also discusses the role that diabetes, high blood pressure, high cholesterol, obesity, inactivity, stress, smoking, and substance abuse play in stroke risk, and it offers strategies for stroke prevention through lifestyle changes.

Part IV: Diagnosis and Treatment of Stroke offers information about common medical tests used to identify stroke. This part also explains stroke treatments that are instrumental in saving lives, including angioplasty, stent placement, carotid endarterectomy, and medications such as tissue plasminogen activator (tPA).

Part V: Post-Stroke Complications and Rehabilitation discusses the numerous cognitive and physical problems that stroke often causes, including brain damage, dementia, and difficulties with speech and communication. It also provides information about post-stroke rehabilitation for physical disabilities, including swallowing problems, muscle spasticity and weakness, balance problems, pain, bowel and continence issues, and vision problems. The part concludes with facts about therapies used to help patients with activities of daily living during the post-stroke period.

Part VI: Life after Stroke identifies common concerns of stroke patients and their families after hospitalization or rehabilitation, such as kitchen, bathroom, and living room modifications that can improve home safety and mobility. The part also examines skin care, sleep, and sexuality issues often experienced after stroke. It concludes with a discussion about choosing long-term care facilities and finding emotional support after a stroke.

Part VII: Additional Help and Information provides a glossary of important terms related to stroke and a directory of organizations that offer information to stroke patients and their families and caregivers.

Bibliographic Note

This volume contains documents and excerpts from publications issued by the following U.S. government agencies: Centers for Disease Control and Prevention (CDC); Centers for Medicare and Medicaid Services; National Center for Complementary and Alternative Medicine (NCCAM); National Heart, Lung, and Blood Institute (NHLBI); National Institute of Child Health and Human Development (NICHD); National Institute of Diabetes and Digestive and Kidney Diseases (NIDDK); National Institute of Neurological Disorders and Stroke (NINDS); National Institute on Aging (NIA); National Institutes of Health (NIH); National Library of Medicine (NLM); Office on Minority Health (OMH); Office on Women's Health (OWH); U.S. Department of Health and Human Services (HHS); U.S. Department of Veterans Affairs (VA); and the U.S. Food and Drug Administration (FDA).

In addition, this volume contains copyrighted documents from the following organizations: A.D.A.M., Inc.; American Academy of Neurology; American Heart Association, Inc.; American Psychological Association; American Speech-Language-Hearing Association; Assisted Living Federation of America; Brain Aneurysm Foundation; Caring, Inc.; Cleveland Clinic Foundation; Hazel K. Goddess Fund for Stroke Research in Women; Internet Stroke Center; National Stroke Association; Rehabilitation Institute of Chicago; Stroke Association; and the University of Texas Southwestern Medical Center.

Full citation information is provided on the first page of each chapter or section. Every effort has been made to secure all necessary rights to reprint the copyrighted material. If any omissions have been made, please contact Omnigraphics to make corrections for future editions.

Acknowledgements

Thanks go to the many organizations, agencies, and individuals who have contributed materials for this *Sourcebook* and to medical consultant Dr. David Cooke and prepress service provider WhimsyInk.

Special thanks go to managing editor Karen Bellenir and research and permissions coordinator Liz Collins for their help and support.

About the Health Reference Series

The *Health Reference Series* is designed to provide basic medical information for patients, families, caregivers, and the general public. Each volume takes a particular topic and provides comprehensive coverage. This is especially important for people who may be dealing with a newly diagnosed disease or a chronic disorder in themselves or in a family member. People looking for preventive guidance, information about disease warning signs, medical statistics, and risk factors for health problems will also find answers to their questions in the *Health Reference Series*. The *Series*, however, is not intended to serve as a tool for diagnosing illness, in prescribing treatments, or as a substitute for the physician/patient relationship. All people concerned about medical symptoms or the possibility of disease are encouraged to seek professional care from an appropriate health care provider.

A Note about Spelling and Style

Health Reference Series editors use *Stedman's Medical Dictionary* as an authority for questions related to the spelling of medical terms and the *Chicago Manual of Style* for questions related to grammatical structures, punctuation, and other editorial concerns. Consistent adherence is not always possible, however, because the individual volumes within the *Series* include many documents from a wide variety of different producers and copyright holders, and the editor's primary goal is to present material from each source as accurately as is possible following the terms specified by each document's producer. This sometimes means that information in different chapters or sections may follow other guidelines and alternate spelling authorities. For example, occasionally a copyright holder may require that eponymous terms be shown in possessive forms (Crohn's disease *vs.* Crohn disease) or that British spelling norms be retained (leukaemia *vs.* leukemia).

Locating Information within the Health Reference Series

The *Health Reference Series* contains a wealth of information about a wide variety of medical topics. Ensuring easy access to all the fact sheets, research reports, in-depth discussions, and other material contained within the individual books of the *Series* remains one of our highest priorities. As the *Series* continues to grow in size and scope, however, locating the precise information needed by a reader may become more challenging.

A Contents Guide to the Health Reference Series was developed to direct readers to the specific volumes that address their concerns. It presents an extensive list of diseases, treatments, and other topics of general interest compiled from the Tables of Contents and major index headings. To access *A Contents Guide to the Health Reference Series*, visit www.healthreferenceseries.com.

Medical Consultant

Medical consultation services are provided to the *Health Reference Series* editors by David A. Cooke, MD, FACP. Dr. Cooke is a graduate of Brandeis University, and he received his M.D. degree from the University of Michigan. He completed residency training at the University of Wisconsin Hospital and Clinics. He is board-certified in Internal Medicine. Dr. Cooke currently works as part of the University of Michigan Health System and practices in Ann Arbor, MI. In his free time, he enjoys writing, science fiction, and spending time with his family.

Our Advisory Board

We would like to thank the following board members for providing guidance to the development of this *Series*:

- Dr. Lynda Baker, Associate Professor of Library and Information Science, Wayne State University, Detroit, MI
- Nancy Bulgarelli, William Beaumont Hospital Library, Royal Oak, MI
- Karen Imarisio, Bloomfield Township Public Library, Bloomfield Township, MI
- Karen Morgan, Mardigian Library, University of Michigan-Dearborn, Dearborn, MI
- Rosemary Orlando, St. Clair Shores Public Library, St. Clair Shores, MI

Health Reference Series *Update Policy*

The inaugural book in the *Health Reference Series* was the first edition of *Cancer Sourcebook* published in 1989. Since then, the

Series has been enthusiastically received by librarians and in the medical community. In order to maintain the standard of providing high-quality health information for the layperson the editorial staff at Omnigraphics felt it was necessary to implement a policy of updating volumes when warranted.

Medical researchers have been making tremendous strides, and it is the purpose of the *Health Reference Series* to stay current with the most recent advances. Each decision to update a volume is made on an individual basis. Some of the considerations include how much new information is available and the feedback we receive from people who use the books. If there is a topic you would like to see added to the update list, or an area of medical concern you feel has not been adequately addressed, please write to:

Editor
Health Reference Series
Omnigraphics, Inc.
155 W. Congress, Suite 200
Detroit, MI 48226
E-mail: editorial@omnigraphics.com

Part One

Introduction to Stroke

Chapter 1

What Is Stroke?

A stroke occurs when the blood supply to part of the brain is suddenly interrupted or when a blood vessel in the brain bursts, spilling blood into the spaces surrounding brain cells. In the same way that a person suffering a loss of blood flow to the heart is said to be having a heart attack, a person with a loss of blood flow to the brain or sudden bleeding in the brain can be said to be having a brain attack.

Brain cells die when they no longer receive oxygen and nutrients from the blood or when they are damaged by sudden bleeding into or around the brain. Ischemia is the term used to describe the loss of oxygen and nutrients for brain cells when there is inadequate blood flow. Ischemia ultimately leads to infarction, the death of brain cells which are eventually replaced by a fluid-filled cavity (or infarct) in the injured brain.

When blood flow to the brain is interrupted, some brain cells die immediately, while others remain at risk for death. These damaged cells make up the ischemic penumbra and can linger in a compromised state for several hours. With timely treatment these cells can be saved.

Even though a stroke occurs in the unseen reaches of the brain, the symptoms of a stroke are easy to spot. They include sudden numbness or weakness, especially on one side of the body; sudden confusion or trouble speaking or understanding speech; sudden trouble seeing in

Excerpted from "Stroke: Hope through Research," by the National Institute of Neurological Disorders and Stroke (NINDS, www.ninds.nih.gov), part of the National Institutes of Health, October 15, 2012.

3

one or both eyes; sudden trouble walking, dizziness, or loss of balance or coordination; or sudden severe headache with no known cause. All of the symptoms of stroke appear suddenly, and often there is more than one symptom at the same time. Therefore stroke can usually be distinguished from other causes of dizziness or headache. These symptoms may indicate that a stroke has occurred and that medical attention is needed immediately.

There are two forms of stroke: ischemic—blockage of a blood vessel supplying the brain, and hemorrhagic—bleeding into or around the brain.

What Is Ischemic Stroke?

An ischemic stroke occurs when an artery supplying the brain with blood becomes blocked, suddenly decreasing or stopping blood flow and ultimately causing a brain infarction. This type of stroke accounts for approximately 80 percent of all strokes. Blood clots are the most common cause of artery blockage and brain infarction. The process of clotting is necessary and beneficial throughout the body because it stops bleeding and allows repair of damaged areas of arteries or veins. However, when blood clots develop in the wrong place within an artery they can cause devastating injury by interfering with the normal flow of blood. Problems with clotting become more frequent as people age.

Blood clots can cause ischemia and infarction in two ways. A clot that forms in a part of the body other than the brain can travel through blood vessels and become wedged in a brain artery. This free-roaming clot is called an embolus and often forms in the heart. A stroke caused by an embolus is called an embolic stroke. The second kind of ischemic stroke, called a thrombotic stroke, is caused by thrombosis, the formation of a blood clot in one of the cerebral arteries that stays attached to the artery wall until it grows large enough to block blood flow.

Ischemic strokes can also be caused by stenosis, or a narrowing of the artery due to the buildup of plaque (a mixture of fatty substances, including cholesterol and other lipids) and blood clots along the artery wall. Stenosis can occur in large arteries and small arteries and is therefore called large vessel disease or small vessel disease, respectively. When a stroke occurs due to small vessel disease, a very small infarction results, sometimes called a lacunar infarction.

The most common blood vessel disease that causes stenosis is atherosclerosis. In atherosclerosis, deposits of plaque buildup along the inner walls of large and medium-sized arteries, causing thickening, hardening, and loss of elasticity of artery walls and decreased blood flow.

What Is Hemorrhagic Stroke?

In a healthy, functioning brain, neurons do not come into direct contact with blood. The vital oxygen and nutrients the neurons need from the blood come to the neurons across the thin walls of the cerebral capillaries. The glia (nervous system cells that support and protect neurons) form a blood-brain barrier, an elaborate meshwork that surrounds blood vessels and capillaries and regulates which elements of the blood can pass through to the neurons.

When an artery in the brain bursts, blood spews out into the surrounding tissue and upsets not only the blood supply but the delicate chemical balance neurons require to function. This is called a hemorrhagic stroke. Such strokes account for approximately 20 percent of all strokes.

Hemorrhage can occur in several ways. One common cause is a bleeding aneurysm, a weak or thin spot on an artery wall. Over time, these weak spots stretch or balloon out under high arterial pressure. The thin walls of these ballooning aneurysms can rupture and spill blood into the space surrounding brain cells.

Hemorrhage also occurs when arterial walls break open. Plaque-encrusted artery walls eventually lose their elasticity and become brittle and thin, prone to cracking. Hypertension, or high blood pressure, increases the risk that a brittle artery wall will give way and release blood into the surrounding brain tissue.

A person with an arteriovenous malformation (AVM) also has an increased risk of hemorrhagic stroke. AVMs are a tangle of defective blood vessels and capillaries within the brain that have thin walls and can therefore rupture.

Bleeding from ruptured brain arteries can either go into the substance of the brain or into the various spaces surrounding the brain. Intracerebral hemorrhage occurs when a vessel within the brain leaks blood into the brain itself. Subarachnoid hemorrhage is bleeding under the meninges, or outer membranes, of the brain into the thin fluid-filled space that surrounds the brain.

The subarachnoid space separates the arachnoid membrane from the underlying pia mater membrane. It contains a clear fluid (cerebrospinal fluid or CSF) as well as the small blood vessels that supply the outer surface of the brain. In a subarachnoid hemorrhage, one of the small arteries within the subarachnoid space bursts, flooding the area with blood and contaminating the cerebrospinal fluid. Since the CSF flows throughout the cranium, within the spaces of the brain, subarachnoid hemorrhage can lead to extensive damage throughout the brain. In fact, subarachnoid hemorrhage is the most deadly of all strokes.

Transient Ischemic Attacks

A transient ischemic attack (TIA), sometimes called a mini-stroke, starts just like a stroke but then resolves leaving no noticeable symptoms or deficits. The occurrence of a TIA is a warning that the person is at risk for a more serious and debilitating stroke. Of the approximately 50,000 Americans who have a TIA each year, about one-third will have an acute stroke sometime in the future. The addition of other risk factors compounds a person's risk for a recurrent stroke. The average duration of a TIA is a few minutes. For almost all TIAs, the symptoms go away within an hour. There is no way to tell whether symptoms will be just a TIA or persist and lead to death or disability. The patient should assume that all stroke symptoms signal an emergency and should not wait to see if they go away.

Recurrent Stroke

Recurrent stroke is frequent; about 25 percent of people who recover from their first stroke will have another stroke within 5 years. Recurrent stroke is a major contributor to stroke disability and death, with the risk of severe disability or death from stroke increasing with each stroke recurrence. The risk of a recurrent stroke is greatest right after a stroke, with the risk decreasing with time. About 3 percent of stroke patients will have another stroke within 30 days of their first stroke and one-third of recurrent strokes take place within 2 years of the first stroke.

How Do You Recognize Stroke?

Symptoms of stroke appear suddenly. Watch for these symptoms and be prepared to act quickly for yourself or on behalf of someone you are with:

- Sudden numbness or weakness of the face, arm, or leg, especially on one side of the body
- Sudden confusion, trouble talking, or understanding speech
- Sudden trouble seeing in one or both eyes
- Sudden trouble walking, dizziness, or loss of balance or coordination
- Sudden severe headache with no known cause

If you suspect you or someone you know is experiencing any of these symptoms indicative of a stroke, do not wait. Call 911 emergency immediately. There are now effective therapies for stroke that must be administered at a hospital, but they lose their effectiveness if not given within the first three hours after stroke symptoms appear. Every minute counts.

How Is the Cause of Stroke Determined?

Physicians have several diagnostic techniques and imaging tools to help diagnose the cause of stroke quickly and accurately. The first step in diagnosis is a short neurological examination. When a possible stroke patient arrives at a hospital, a health care professional, usually a doctor or nurse, will ask the patient or a companion what happened and when the symptoms began. Blood tests, an electrocardiogram, and a brain scan, such CT [computed tomography] or MRI [magnetic resonance imaging], will often be done. One test that helps doctors judge the severity of a stroke is the standardized NIH Stroke Scale, developed by the NINDS. Health care professionals use the NIH Stroke Scale to measure a patient's neurological deficits by asking the patient to answer questions and to perform several physical and mental tests. Other scales include the Glasgow Coma Scale, the Hunt and Hess Scale, the Modified Rankin Scale, and the Barthel Index.

Who Is at Risk for Stroke?

Some people are at a higher risk for stroke than others. Unmodifiable risk factors include age, gender, race/ethnicity, and stroke family history. In contrast, other risk factors for stroke, like high blood pressure or cigarette smoking, can be changed or controlled by the person at risk.

Unmodifiable Risk Factors

It is a myth that stroke occurs only in elderly adults. In actuality, stroke strikes all age groups, from fetuses still in the womb to centenarians. It is true, however, that older people have a higher risk for stroke than the general population and that the risk for stroke increases with age. For every decade after the age of 55, the risk of stroke doubles, and two-thirds of all strokes occur in people over 65 years old. People over 65 also have a seven-fold greater risk of dying from stroke than the general population. And the incidence of stroke is increasing proportionately with the increase in the elderly population. When the baby boomers move into the over-65 age group, stroke and other diseases will take on even greater significance in the health care field.

Gender also plays a role in risk for stroke. Men have a higher risk for stroke, but more women die from stroke. The stroke risk for men is 1.25 times that for women. But men do not live as long as women, so men are usually younger when they have their strokes and therefore have a higher rate of survival than women. In other words, even though women have fewer strokes than men, women are generally older when they have their strokes and are more likely to die from them.

Stroke seems to run in some families. Several factors might contribute to familial stroke risk. Members of a family might have a genetic tendency for stroke risk factors, such as an inherited predisposition for hypertension or diabetes. The influence of a common lifestyle among family members could also contribute to familial stroke.

The risk for stroke varies among different ethnic and racial groups. The incidence of stroke among African Americans is almost double that of white Americans, and twice as many African Americans who have a stroke die from the event compared to white Americans. African Americans between the ages of 45 and 55 have four to five times the stroke death rate of whites. After age 55 the stroke mortality rate for whites increases and is equal to that of African Americans.

Compared to white Americans, African Americans have a higher incidence of stroke risk factors, including high blood pressure and cigarette smoking. African Americans also have a higher incidence and prevalence of some genetic diseases, such as diabetes and sickle cell anemia, that predispose them to stroke.

Hispanics and Native Americans have stroke incidence and mortality rates more similar to those of white Americans. In Asian Americans stroke incidence and mortality rates are also similar to those in white Americans, even though Asians in Japan, China, and other countries of the Far East have significantly higher stroke incidence and mortality rates than white Americans. This suggests that environment and lifestyle factors play a large role in stroke risk.

The Stroke Belt

Several decades ago, scientists and statisticians noticed that people in the southeastern United States had the highest stroke mortality rate in the country. They named this region the stroke belt. For many years, researchers believed that the increased risk was due to the higher percentage of African Americans and an overall lower socio-economic status (SES) in the southern states. A low SES is associated with an overall lower standard of living, leading to a lower standard of health care and therefore an increased risk of stroke. But researchers now know that the higher percentage of African-Americans and the overall lower SES in the southern states does not adequately account for the higher incidence of, and mortality from, stroke in those states. This means that other factors must be contributing to the higher incidence of and mortality from stroke in this region.

Recent studies have also shown that there is a stroke buckle in the stroke belt. Three southeastern states, North Carolina, South Carolina, and Georgia, have an extremely high stroke mortality rate, higher than the rate in other stroke belt states and up to two times the stroke mortality rate of the United States overall. The increased risk could be due to geographic or environmental factors or to regional differences in lifestyle, including higher rates of cigarette smoking and a regional preference for salty, high-fat foods.

Other Risk Factors

The most important risk factors for stroke are hypertension, heart disease, diabetes, and cigarette smoking. Others include heavy alcohol consumption, high blood cholesterol levels, illicit drug use, and genetic or congenital conditions, particularly vascular abnormalities. People with more than one risk factor have what is called amplification of risk. This means that the multiple risk factors compound their destructive effects and create an overall risk greater than the simple cumulative effect of the individual risk factors.

Hypertension: Of all the risk factors that contribute to stroke, the most powerful is hypertension, or high blood pressure. People with hypertension have a risk for stroke that is four to six times higher than the risk for those without hypertension. One-third of the adult U.S. population, about 50 million people (including 40–70 percent of those over age 65) have high blood pressure. Forty to 90 percent of stroke patients have high blood pressure before their stroke event.

A systolic pressure of 120 mm of Hg over a diastolic pressure of 80 mm of Hg is generally considered normal. Persistently high blood pressure greater than 140 over 90 leads to the diagnosis of the disease called hypertension. The impact of hypertension on the total risk for stroke decreases with increasing age, therefore factors other than hypertension play a greater role in the overall stroke risk in elderly adults. For people without hypertension, the absolute risk of stroke increases over time until around the age of 90, when the absolute risk becomes the same as that for people with hypertension.

Like stroke, there is a gender difference in the prevalence of hypertension. In younger people, hypertension is more common among men than among women. With increasing age, however, more women than men have hypertension. This hypertension gender-age difference probably has an impact on the incidence and prevalence of stroke in these populations.

Antihypertensive medication can decrease a person's risk for stroke. Recent studies suggest that treatment can decrease the stroke incidence rate by 38 percent and decrease the stroke fatality rate by 40 percent. Common hypertensive agents include adrenergic agents, beta-blockers, angiotensin converting enzyme inhibitors, calcium channel blockers, diuretics, and vasodilators.

Heart disease: After hypertension, the second most powerful risk factor for stroke is heart disease, especially a condition known as atrial fibrillation. Atrial fibrillation is irregular beating of the left atrium, or left upper chamber, of the heart. In people with atrial fibrillation, the left atrium beats up to four times faster than the rest of the heart. This leads to an irregular flow of blood and the occasional formation of blood clots that can leave the heart and travel to the brain, causing a stroke.

Atrial fibrillation, which affects as many as 2.2 million Americans, increases an individual's risk of stroke by 4 to 6 percent, and about 15 percent of stroke patients have atrial fibrillation before they experience a stroke. The condition is more prevalent in the upper age groups, which means that the prevalence of atrial fibrillation in the United States will increase proportionately with the growth of the elderly population. Unlike hypertension and other risk factors that have a lesser impact on the ever-rising absolute risk of stroke that comes with advancing age, the influence of atrial fibrillation on total risk for stroke increases powerfully with age. In people over 80 years old, atrial fibrillation is the direct cause of one in four strokes.

Other forms of heart disease that increase stroke risk include malformations of the heart valves or the heart muscle. Some valve diseases, like mitral valve stenosis or mitral annular calcification, can double the risk for stroke, independent of other risk factors.

Heart muscle malformations can also increase the risk for stroke. Patent foramen ovale (PFO) is a passage or a hole (sometimes called a shunt) in the heart wall separating the two atria, or upper chambers, of the heart. Clots in the blood are usually filtered out by the lungs, but PFO could allow emboli or blood clots to bypass the lungs and go directly through the arteries to the brain, potentially causing a stroke. Research is currently under way to determine how important PFO is as a cause for stroke. Atrial septal aneurysm (ASA), a congenital (present from birth) malformation of the heart tissue, is a bulging of the septum or heart wall into one of the atria of the heart. Researchers do not know why this malformation increases the risk for stroke. PFO and ASA frequently occur together and therefore amplify the risk for stroke. Two other heart malformations that seem to increase the risk for stroke for unknown reasons are left atrial enlargement and left ventricular hypertrophy. People with left atrial enlargement have a larger than normal left atrium of the heart; those with left ventricular hypertrophy have a thickening of the wall of the left ventricle.

Another risk factor for stroke is cardiac surgery to correct heart malformations or reverse the effects of heart disease. Strokes occurring in this situation are usually the result of surgically dislodged plaques from the aorta that travel through the bloodstream to the arteries in the neck and head, causing stroke. Cardiac surgery increases a person's risk of stroke by about 1 percent. Other types of surgery can also increase the risk of stroke.

Blood cholesterol levels: Most people know that high cholesterol levels contribute to heart disease. But many don't realize that a high cholesterol level also contributes to stroke risk. Cholesterol, a waxy substance produced by the liver, is a vital body product. It contributes to the production of hormones and vitamin D and is an integral component of cell membranes. The liver makes enough cholesterol to fuel the body's needs and this natural production of cholesterol alone is not a large contributing factor to atherosclerosis, heart disease, and stroke. Research has shown that the danger from cholesterol comes from a dietary intake of foods that contain high levels of cholesterol. Foods high in saturated fat and cholesterol, like meats, eggs, and dairy products, can increase the amount of total cholesterol in the body to alarming levels, contributing to the risk of atherosclerosis and thickening of the arteries.

Cholesterol is classified as a lipid, meaning that it is fat-soluble rather than water-soluble. Other lipids include fatty acids, glycerides, alcohol, waxes, steroids, and fat-soluble vitamins A, D, and E. Lipids and water, like oil and water, do not mix. Blood is a water-based liquid, therefore cholesterol does not mix with blood. In order to travel through the blood without clumping together, cholesterol needs to be covered by a layer of protein. The cholesterol and protein together are called a lipoprotein.

There are two kinds of cholesterol, commonly called the good and the bad. Good cholesterol is high-density lipoprotein, or HDL; bad cholesterol is low-density lipoprotein, or LDL. Together, these two forms of cholesterol make up a person's total serum cholesterol level. Most cholesterol tests measure the level of total cholesterol in the blood and don't distinguish between good and bad cholesterol. For these total serum cholesterol tests, a level of less than 200 mg/dL is considered safe, while a level of more than 240 is considered dangerous and places a person at risk for heart disease and stroke.

Most cholesterol in the body is in the form of LDL. LDLs circulate through the bloodstream, picking up excess cholesterol and depositing cholesterol where it is needed (for example, for the production and maintenance of cell membranes). But when too much cholesterol starts circulating in the blood, the body cannot handle the excessive LDLs, which build up along the inside of the arterial walls. The buildup of LDL coating on the inside of the artery walls hardens and turns into arterial plaque, leading to stenosis and atherosclerosis. This plaque blocks blood vessels and contributes to the formation of blood clots. A person's LDL level should be less than 130 mg/dL to be safe. LDL levels between 130 and 159 put a person at a slightly higher risk for atherosclerosis, heart disease, and stroke. A score over 160 puts a person at great risk for a heart attack or stroke.

The other form of cholesterol, HDL, is beneficial and contributes to stroke prevention. HDL carries a small percentage of the cholesterol in the blood, but instead of depositing its cholesterol on the inside of artery walls, HDL returns to the liver to unload its cholesterol. The liver then eliminates the excess cholesterol by passing it along to the kidneys. Currently, any HDL score higher than 35 is considered desirable. Recent studies have shown that high levels of HDL are associated with a reduced risk for heart disease and stroke and that low levels (less than 35 mg/dL), even in people with normal levels of LDL, lead to an increased risk for heart disease and stroke.

A person may lower his risk for atherosclerosis and stroke by improving his cholesterol levels. A healthy diet and regular exercise are the best ways to lower total cholesterol levels. In some cases, physicians may prescribe cholesterol-lowering medication, and recent studies have shown that the newest types of these drugs, called reductase inhibitors or statin drugs, significantly reduce the risk for stroke in most patients with high cholesterol. Scientists believe that statins may work by reducing the amount of bad cholesterol the body produces and by reducing the body's inflammatory immune reaction to cholesterol plaque associated with atherosclerosis and stroke.

Diabetes: Diabetes is another disease that increases a person's risk for stroke. People with diabetes have three times the risk of stroke compared to people without diabetes. The relative risk of stroke from diabetes is highest in the fifth and sixth decades of life and decreases after that. Like hypertension, the relative risk of stroke from diabetes is highest for men at an earlier age and highest for women at an older age. People with diabetes may also have other contributing risk factors that can amplify the overall risk for stroke. For example, the prevalence of hypertension is 40 percent higher in the diabetic population compared to the general population.

Modifiable Lifestyle Risk Factors

Cigarette smoking is the most powerful modifiable stroke risk factor. Smoking almost doubles a person's risk for ischemic stroke, independent of other risk factors, and it increases a person's risk for subarachnoid hemorrhage by up to 3.5 percent. Smoking is directly responsible for a greater percentage of the total number of strokes in young adults than in older adults. Risk factors other than smoking—like hypertension, heart disease, and diabetes—account for more of the total number of strokes in older adults.

Heavy smokers are at greater risk for stroke than light smokers. The relative risk of stroke decreases immediately after quitting smoking, with a major reduction of risk seen after two to four years. Unfortunately, it may take several decades for a former smoker's risk to drop to the level of someone who never smoked.

Smoking increases the risk of stroke by promoting atherosclerosis and increasing the levels of blood-clotting factors, such as fibrinogen. In addition to promoting conditions linked to stroke, smoking also increases the damage that results from stroke by weakening the endothelial wall of the cerebrovascular system. This leads to greater damage to the brain from events that occur in the secondary stage of stroke.

High alcohol consumption is another modifiable risk factor for stroke. Generally, an increase in alcohol consumption leads to an increase in blood pressure. While scientists agree that heavy drinking is a risk for both hemorrhagic and ischemic stroke, in several research studies daily consumption of smaller amounts of alcohol has been found to provide a protective influence against ischemic stroke, perhaps because alcohol decreases the clotting ability of platelets in the blood. Moderate alcohol consumption may act in the same way as aspirin to decrease blood clotting and prevent ischemic stroke. Heavy alcohol consumption, though, may seriously deplete platelet numbers and compromise blood clotting and blood viscosity, leading to hemorrhage. In addition, heavy drinking or binge drinking can lead to a rebound effect after the alcohol is purged from the body. The consequences of this rebound effect are that blood viscosity (thickness) and platelet levels skyrocket after heavy drinking, increasing the risk for ischemic stroke.

The use of illicit drugs, such as cocaine and crack cocaine, can cause stroke. Cocaine may act on other risk factors, such as hypertension, heart disease, and vascular disease, to trigger a stroke. It decreases relative cerebrovascular blood flow by up to 30 percent, causes vascular constriction, and inhibits vascular relaxation, leading to narrowing of the arteries. Cocaine also affects the heart, causing arrhythmias and rapid heart rate that can lead to the formation of blood clots.

Marijuana smoking may also be a risk factor for stroke. Marijuana decreases blood pressure and may interact with other risk factors, such as hypertension and cigarette smoking, to cause rapidly fluctuating blood pressure levels, damaging blood vessels.

Other drugs of abuse, such as amphetamines, heroin, and anabolic steroids (and even some common, legal drugs, such as caffeine and L-asparaginase and pseudoephedrine found in over-the-counter decongestants), have been suspected of increasing stroke risk. Many of these drugs are vasoconstrictors, meaning that they cause blood vessels to constrict and blood pressure to rise.

Head and Neck Injuries and Stroke

Injuries to the head or neck may damage the cerebrovascular system and cause a small number of strokes. Head injury or traumatic brain injury may cause bleeding within the brain leading to damage akin to that caused by a hemorrhagic stroke. Neck injury, when associated with spontaneous tearing of the vertebral or carotid arteries caused by sudden and severe extension of the neck, neck rotation, or pressure on the artery, is a contributing cause of stroke, especially in young adults. This type of stroke is often called beauty-parlor syndrome, which refers to the practice of extending the neck backwards over a sink for hair-washing in beauty parlors. Neck calisthenics, bottoms-up drinking, and improperly performed chiropractic manipulation of the neck can also put strain on the vertebral and carotid arteries, possibly leading to ischemic stroke.

Infections and Stroke

Recent viral and bacterial infections may act with other risk factors to add a small risk for stroke. The immune system responds to infection by increasing inflammation and increasing the infection-fighting properties of the blood. Unfortunately, this immune response increases the number of clotting factors in the blood, leading to an increased risk of embolic-ischemic stroke.

Genetic Risk Factors

Although there may not be a single genetic factor associated with stroke, genes do play a large role in the expression of stroke risk factors such as hypertension, heart disease, diabetes, and vascular malformations. It is also possible that an increased risk for stroke within a family is due to environmental factors, such as a common sedentary lifestyle or poor eating habits, rather than hereditary factors.

Vascular malformations that cause stroke may have the strongest genetic link of all stroke risk factors. A vascular malformation is an abnormally formed blood vessel or group of blood vessels. One genetic vascular disease called CADASIL, which stands for cerebral autosomal dominant arteriopathy with subcortical infarcts and leukoencephalopathy. CADASIL is a rare, genetically inherited, congenital vascular disease of the brain that causes strokes, subcortical dementia, migraine-like headaches, and psychiatric disturbances. CADASIL is very debilitating and symptoms usually surface around the age of 45. The exact incidence of CADASIL in the United States is unknown.

Medications for Stroke

Medication or drug therapy is the most common treatment for stroke. The most popular classes of drugs used to prevent or treat stroke are antithrombotics (antiplatelet agents and anticoagulants) and thrombolytics.

Antithrombotics prevent the formation of blood clots that can become lodged in a cerebral artery and cause strokes. Antiplatelet drugs prevent clotting by decreasing the activity of platelets, blood cells that contribute to the clotting property of blood. These drugs reduce the risk of blood-clot formation, thus reducing the risk of ischemic stroke. In the context of stroke, physicians prescribe antiplatelet drugs mainly for prevention. The most widely known and used antiplatelet drug is aspirin. Other antiplatelet drugs include clopidogrel, ticlopidine, and dipyridamole. The NINDS sponsors a wide range of clinical trials to determine the effectiveness of antiplatelet drugs for stroke prevention.

Anticoagulants reduce stroke risk by reducing the clotting property of the blood. The most commonly used anticoagulants include warfarin (also known as Coumadin), heparin, and enoxaparin (also known as Lovenox). The NINDS has sponsored several trials to test the efficacy of anticoagulants versus antiplatelet drugs. The Stroke Prevention in Atrial Fibrillation (SPAF) trial found that, although aspirin is an effective therapy for the prevention of a second stroke in most patients with atrial fibrillation, some patients with additional risk factors do better on warfarin therapy. Another study, the Trial of Org 10127 in Acute Stroke Treatment (TOAST), tested the effectiveness of low-molecular weight heparin (Org 10172) in stroke prevention. TOAST showed that heparin anticoagulants are not generally effective in preventing recurrent stroke or improving outcome.

Thrombolytic agents are used to treat an ongoing, acute ischemic stroke caused by an artery blockage. These drugs halt the stroke by dissolving the blood clot that is blocking blood flow to the brain. Recombinant tissue plasminogen activator (r-tPA) is a genetically engineered form of tPA, a thrombolytic substance made naturally by the body. It can be effective if given intravenously within 3 hours of stroke symptom onset, but it should be used only after a physician has confirmed that the patient has suffered an ischemic stroke. Thrombolytic agents can increase bleeding and therefore must be used only after careful patient screening. The NINDS r-tPA Stroke Study showed the efficacy of tPA and in 1996 led to the first FDA-approved treatment for acute ischemic stroke. Other thrombolytics are currently being tested in clinical trials.

Neuroprotectants are medications that protect the brain from secondary injury caused by stroke. Although no neuroprotectants are FDA [U.S. Food and Drug Administration]-approved for use in stroke at this time, many are in clinical trials. There are several different classes of neuroprotectants that show promise for future therapy, including glutamate antagonists, antioxidants, apoptosis inhibitors, and many others.

Surgery

Surgery can be used to prevent stroke, to treat acute stroke, or to repair vascular damage or malformations in and around the brain. There are two prominent types of surgery for stroke prevention and treatment: carotid endarterectomy and extracranial/intracranial (EC/IC) bypass.

Carotid endarterectomy is a surgical procedure in which a doctor removes fatty deposits (plaque) from the inside of one of the carotid arteries, which are located in the neck and are the main suppliers of blood to the brain. As mentioned earlier, the disease atherosclerosis is characterized by the buildup of plaque on the inside of large arteries, and the blockage of an artery by this fatty material is called stenosis. The NINDS has sponsored two large clinical trials to test the efficacy of carotid endarterectomy: the North American Symptomatic Carotid Endarterectomy Trial (NASCET) and the Asymptomatic Carotid Atherosclerosis Study (ACAS). These trials showed that carotid endarterectomy is a safe and effective stroke prevention therapy for most people with greater than 50 percent stenosis of the carotid arteries when performed by a qualified and experienced neurosurgeon or vascular surgeon.

Currently, the NINDS is sponsoring the Carotid Revascularization Endarterectomy vs. Stenting Trial (CREST), a large clinical trial designed to test the effectiveness of carotid endarterectomy versus a newer surgical procedure for carotid stenosis called stenting. The procedure involves inserting a long, thin catheter tube into an artery in the leg and threading the catheter through the vascular system into the narrow stenosis of the carotid artery in the neck. Once the catheter is in place in the carotid artery, the radiologist expands the stent with a balloon on the tip of the catheter. The CREST trial will test the effectiveness of the new surgical technique versus the established standard technique of carotid endarterectomy surgery.

EC/IC bypass surgery is a procedure that restores blood flow to a blood-deprived area of brain tissue by rerouting a healthy artery in the scalp to the area of brain tissue affected by a blocked artery. The NINDS-sponsored EC/IC Bypass Study tested the ability of this surgery to prevent recurrent strokes in stroke patients with atherosclerosis. The study showed that, in the long run, EC/IC does not seem to benefit these patients. The surgery is still performed occasionally for patients with aneurysms, some types of small artery disease, and certain vascular abnormalities.

One useful surgical procedure for treatment of brain aneurysms that cause subarachnoid hemorrhage is a technique called clipping. Clipping involves clamping off the aneurysm from the blood vessel, which reduces the chance that it will burst and bleed.

A new therapy that is gaining wide attention is the detachable coil technique for the treatment of high-risk intracranial aneurysms. A small platinum coil is inserted through an artery in the thigh and threaded through the arteries to the site of the aneurysm. The coil is then released into the aneurysm, where it evokes an immune response from the body. The body produces a blood clot inside the aneurysm, strengthening the artery walls and reducing the risk of rupture. Once the aneurysm is stabilized, a neurosurgeon can clip the aneurysm with less risk of hemorrhage and death to the patient.

Rehabilitation Therapy

Stroke is the number one cause of serious adult disability in the United States. Stroke disability is devastating to the stroke patient and family, but therapies are available to help rehabilitate post-stroke patients.

For most stroke patients, physical therapy (PT) is the cornerstone of the rehabilitation process. A physical therapist uses training, exercises, and physical manipulation of the stroke patient's body with the intent of restoring movement, balance, and coordination. The aim of PT is to have the stroke patient relearn simple motor activities such as walking, sitting, standing, lying down, and the process of switching from one type of movement to another.

Another type of therapy involving relearning daily activities is occupational therapy (OT). OT also involves exercise and training to help the stroke patient relearn everyday activities such as eating, drinking, dressing, bathing, cooking, reading and writing, and toileting. The goal of OT is to help the patient become independent or semi-independent.

Speech and language problems arise when brain damage occurs in the language centers of the brain. Due to the brain's great ability to learn and change (called brain plasticity), other areas can adapt to take over some of the lost functions. Speech-language pathologists help stroke patients relearn language and speaking skills, including swallowing, or learn other forms of communication. Speech therapy is appropriate for any patients with problems understanding speech or written words, or problems forming speech. A speech therapist helps stroke patients help themselves by working to improve language skills, develop alternative ways of communicating, and develop coping skills to deal with the frustration of not being able to communicate fully. With time and patience, a stroke survivor should be able to regain some, and sometimes all, language and speaking abilities.

Many stroke patients require psychological or psychiatric help after a stroke. Psychological problems, such as depression, anxiety, frustration, and anger, are common post-stroke disabilities. Talk therapy, along with appropriate medication, can help alleviate some of the mental and emotional problems that result from stroke. Sometimes it is also beneficial for family members of the stroke patient to seek psychological help as well.

What Disabilities Can Result from a Stroke?

Although stroke is a disease of the brain, it can affect the entire body. Some of the disabilities that can result from a stroke include paralysis, cognitive deficits, speech problems, emotional difficulties, daily living problems, and pain.

Paralysis: A common disability that results from stroke is complete paralysis on one side of the body, called hemiplegia. A related disability that is not as debilitating as paralysis is one-sided weakness or hemiparesis. The paralysis or weakness may affect only the face, an arm, or a leg or may affect one entire side of the body and face. A person who suffers a stroke in the left hemisphere of the brain will show right-sided paralysis or paresis. Conversely, a person with a stroke in the right hemisphere of the brain will show deficits on the left side of the body. A stroke patient may have problems with the simplest of daily activities, such as walking, dressing, eating, and using the bathroom. Motor deficits can result from damage to the motor cortex in the frontal lobes of the brain or from damage to the lower parts of the brain, such as the cerebellum, which controls balance and coordination. Some stroke patients also have trouble swallowing, called dysphagia.

Cognitive deficits: Stroke may cause problems with thinking, awareness, attention, learning, judgment, and memory. In some cases of stroke, the patient suffers a neglect syndrome. The neglect means that a stroke patient has no knowledge of one side of his or her body, or one side of the visual field, or is unaware of the deficit. A stroke patient may be unaware of his or her surroundings, or may be unaware of the mental deficits that resulted from the stroke.

Language deficits: Stroke victims often have problems understanding or forming speech. A deficit in understanding or forming speech is called aphasia. Aphasia usually occurs along with similar problems in reading or writing. In most people, language problems result from damage to the left hemisphere of the brain. Slurred speech due to weakness or incoordination of the muscles involved in speaking is called dysarthria, and is not a problem with language. Because it can result from any weakness or incoordination of the speech muscles, dysarthria can arise from damage to either side of the brain.

Emotional deficits: A stroke can lead to emotional problems. Stroke patients may have difficulty controlling their emotions or may express inappropriate emotions in certain situations. One common disability that occurs with many stroke patients is depression. Post-stroke depression may be more than a general sadness resulting from the stroke incident. It is a clinical behavioral problem that can hamper recovery and rehabilitation and may even lead to suicide. Post-stroke depression is treated as any depression is treated, with antidepressant medications and therapy.

Pain: Stroke patients may experience pain, uncomfortable numbness, or strange sensations after a stroke. These sensations may be due to many factors including damage to the sensory regions of the brain, stiff joints, or a disabled limb. An uncommon type of pain resulting from stroke is called central stroke pain or central pain syndrome (CPS). CPS results from damage to an area in the mid-brain called the thalamus. The pain is a mixture of sensations, including heat and cold, burning, tingling, numbness, and sharp stabbing and underlying aching pain. The pain is often worse in the extremities—the hands and feet—and is made worse by movement and temperature changes, especially cold temperatures. Unfortunately, since most pain medications provide little relief from these sensations, very few treatments or therapies exist to combat CPS.

What Special Risks Do Women Face?

Some risk factors for stroke apply only to women. Primary among these are pregnancy, childbirth, and menopause. These risk factors are tied to hormonal fluctuations and changes that affect a woman in different stages of life. Research in the past few decades has shown that high-dose oral contraceptives, the kind used in the 1960s and 1970s, can increase the risk of stroke in women. Fortunately, oral contraceptives with high doses of estrogen are no longer used and have been replaced with safer and more effective oral contraceptives with lower doses of estrogen. Some studies have shown the newer low-dose oral contraceptives may not significantly increase the risk of stroke in women.

Other studies have demonstrated that pregnancy and childbirth can put a woman at an increased risk for stroke. Pregnancy increases the risk of stroke as much as three to 13 times. Of course, the risk of stroke in young women of childbearing years is very small to begin with, so a moderate increase in risk during pregnancy is still a relatively small risk. Pregnancy and childbirth cause strokes in approximately eight in 100,000 women. Unfortunately, 25 percent of strokes during pregnancy end in death, and hemorrhagic strokes, although rare, are still the leading cause of maternal death in the United States. Subarachnoid hemorrhage, in particular, causes one to five maternal deaths per 10,000 pregnancies.

A study sponsored by the NINDS showed that the risk of stroke during pregnancy is greatest in the postpartum period—the six weeks following childbirth. The risk of ischemic stroke after pregnancy is about nine times higher and the risk of hemorrhagic stroke is more than 28 times higher for postpartum women than for women who are not pregnant or postpartum. The cause is unknown.

In the same way that the hormonal changes during pregnancy and childbirth are associated with increased risk of stroke, hormonal changes at the end of the childbearing years can increase the risk of stroke. Several studies have shown that menopause, the end of a woman's reproductive ability marked by the termination of her menstrual cycle, can increase a woman's risk of stroke. Fortunately, some studies have suggested that hormone replacement therapy can reduce some of the effects of menopause and decrease stroke risk. Currently, the NINDS is sponsoring the Women's Estrogen for Stroke Trial (WEST), a randomized, placebo-controlled, double-blind trial, to determine whether estrogen therapy can reduce the risk of death or recurrent stroke in postmenopausal women who have a history of a recent TIA or non-disabling stroke. The mechanism by which estrogen can prove beneficial to postmenopausal women could include its role in cholesterol control. Studies have shown that estrogen acts to increase levels of HDL [high-density lipoprotein] while decreasing LDL [low-density lipoprotein] levels.

Are Children at Risk for Stroke?

The young have several risk factors unique to them. Young people seem to suffer from hemorrhagic strokes more than ischemic strokes, a significant difference from older age groups where ischemic strokes make up the majority of stroke cases. Hemorrhagic strokes represent 20 percent of all strokes in the United States and young people account for many of these.

Clinicians often separate the young into two categories: Those younger than 15 years of age, and those 15 to 44 years of age. People 15 to 44 years of age are generally considered young adults and have many risk factors, such as drug use, alcohol abuse, pregnancy, head and neck injuries, heart disease or heart malformations, and infections. Some other causes of stroke in the young are linked to genetic diseases.

Medical complications that can lead to stroke in children include intracranial infection, brain injury, vascular malformations such as moyamoya syndrome, occlusive vascular disease, and genetic disorders such as sickle cell anemia, tuberous sclerosis, and Marfan syndrome.

The symptoms of stroke in children are different from those in adults and young adults. A child experiencing a stroke may have seizures, a sudden loss of speech, a loss of expressive language (including body language and gestures), hemiparesis (weakness on one side of the body), hemiplegia (paralysis on one side of the body), dysarthria (impairment of speech), convulsions, headache, or fever. It is a medical emergency when a child shows any of these symptoms.

In children with stroke the underlying conditions that led to the stroke should be determined and managed to prevent future strokes. For example, a recent clinical study sponsored by the National Heart, Lung, and Blood Institute found that giving blood transfusions to young children with sickle cell anemia greatly reduces the risk of stroke. The Institute even suggests attempting to prevent stroke in high-risk children by giving them blood transfusions before they experience a stroke.

Most children who experience a stroke will do better than most adults after treatment and rehabilitation. This is due in part to the immature brain's great plasticity, the ability to adapt to deficits and injury. Children who experience seizures along with stroke do not recover as well as children who do not have seizures. Some children may experience residual hemiplegia, though most will eventually learn how to walk.

What Research Is Being Done by the NINDS?

The NINDS is the leading supporter of stroke research in the United States and sponsors a wide range of experimental research studies, from investigations of basic biological mechanisms to studies with animal models and clinical trials.

Currently, NINDS researchers are studying the mechanisms of stroke risk factors and the process of brain damage that results from stroke. Some of this brain damage may be secondary to the initial death of brain cells caused by the lack of blood flow to the brain tissue. This secondary wave of brain injury is a result of a toxic reaction to the primary damage and mainly involves the excitatory neurochemical, glutamate. Glutamate in the normal brain functions as a chemical messenger between brain cells, allowing them to communicate. But an excess amount of glutamate in the brain causes too much activity and brain cells quickly burn out from too much excitement, releasing more toxic chemicals, such as caspases, cytokines, monocytes, and oxygen-free radicals. These substances poison the chemical environment of surrounding cells, initiating a cascade of degeneration and programmed cell death, called apoptosis. NINDS researchers are studying the mechanisms underlying this secondary insult, which consists mainly of inflammation, toxicity, and a breakdown of the blood vessels that provide blood to the brain. Researchers are also looking for ways to prevent secondary injury to the brain by providing different types of neuroprotection for salvageable cells that prevent inflammation and block some of the toxic chemicals created by dying brain cells. From this research, scientists hope to develop neuroprotective agents to prevent secondary damage.

Basic research has also focused on the genetics of stroke and stroke risk factors. One area of research involving genetics is gene therapy. Gene therapy involves putting a gene for a desired protein in certain cells of the body. The inserted gene will then program the cell to produce the desired protein. If enough cells in the right areas produce enough protein, then the protein could be therapeutic. Scientists must find ways to deliver the therapeutic DNA to the appropriate cells and must learn how to deliver enough DNA to enough cells so that the tissues produce a therapeutic amount of protein. Gene therapy is in the very early stages of development and there are many problems to overcome, including learning how to penetrate the highly impermeable blood-brain barrier and how to halt the host's immune reaction to the virus that carries the gene to the cells. Some of the proteins used for stroke therapy could include neuroprotective proteins, anti-inflammatory proteins, and DNA/cellular repair proteins, among others.

The NINDS supports and conducts a wide variety of studies in animals, from genetics research on zebrafish to rehabilitation research on primates. Much of the Institute's animal research involves rodents, specifically mice and rats. For example, one study of hypertension and stroke uses rats that have been bred to be hypertensive and therefore stroke-prone. By studying stroke in rats, scientists hope to get a better picture of what might be happening in human stroke patients. Scientists can also use animal models to test promising therapeutic interventions for stroke. If a therapy proves to be beneficial to animals, then scientists can consider testing the therapy in human subjects.

One promising area of stroke animal research involves hibernation. The dramatic decrease of blood flow to the brain in hibernating animals is extensive—extensive enough that it would kill a non-hibernating animal. During hibernation, an animal's metabolism slows down, body temperature drops, and energy and oxygen requirements of brain cells decrease. If scientists can discover how animals hibernate without experiencing brain damage, then maybe they can discover ways to stop the brain damage associated with decreased blood flow in stroke patients. Other studies are looking at the role of hypothermia, or decreased body temperature, on metabolism and neuroprotection.

Both hibernation and hypothermia have a relationship to hypoxia and edema. Hypoxia, or anoxia, occurs when there is not enough oxygen available for brain cells to function properly. Since brain cells require large amounts of oxygen for energy requirements, they are especially vulnerable to hypoxia. Edema occurs when the chemical balance of brain tissue is disturbed and water or fluids flow into the brain cells, making them swell and burst, releasing their toxic contents into the surrounding tissues. Edema is one cause of general brain tissue swelling and contributes to the secondary injury associated with stroke.

The basic and animal studies discussed above do not involve people and fall under the category of preclinical research; clinical research involves people. One area of investigation that has made the transition from animal models to clinical research is the study of the mechanisms underlying brain plasticity and the neuronal rewiring that occurs after a stroke.

New advances in imaging and rehabilitation have shown that the brain can compensate for function lost as a result of stroke. When cells in an area of the brain responsible for a particular function die after a stroke, the patient becomes unable to perform that function. For example, a stroke patient with an infarct in the area of the brain responsible for facial recognition becomes unable to recognize faces, a syndrome called facial agnosia. But, in time, the person may come to recognize faces again, even though the area of the brain originally programmed to perform that function remains dead. The plasticity of the brain and the rewiring of the neural connections make it possible for one part of the brain to change functions and take up the more important functions of a disabled part. This rewiring of the brain and restoration of function, which the brain tries to do automatically, can be helped with therapy. Scientists are working to develop new and better ways to help the brain repair itself to restore important functions to the stroke patient.

One example of a therapy resulting from this research is the use of transcranial magnetic stimulation (TMS) in stroke rehabilitation. Some evidence suggests that TMS, in which a small magnetic current is delivered to an area of the brain, may possibly increase brain plasticity and speed up recovery of function after a stroke. The TMS device is a small coil which is held outside of the head, over the part of the brain needing stimulation. Currently, several studies at the NINDS are testing whether TMS has any value in increasing motor function and improving functional recovery.

Clinical Trials

Clinical research is usually conducted in a series of trials that become progressively larger. A phase I clinical trial is directly built upon the lessons learned from basic and animal research and is used to test the safety of therapy for a particular disease and to estimate possible efficacy in a few human subjects. A phase II clinical trial usually involves many subjects at several different centers and is used to test safety and possible efficacy on a broader scale, to test different dosing for medications or to perfect techniques for surgery, and to determine the best methodology and outcome measures for the bigger phase III clinical trial to come.

A phase III clinical trial is the largest endeavor in clinical research. This type of trial often involves many centers and many subjects. The trial usually has two patient groups who receive different treatments, but all other standard care is the same and represents the best care available. The trial may compare two treatments, or, if there is only one treatment to test, patients who do not receive the test therapy receive instead a placebo. The patients are told that the additional treatment they are receiving may be either the active treatment or a placebo. Many phase III trials are called double-blind, randomized clinical trials. Double-blind means that neither the subjects nor the doctors and nurses who are treating the subjects and determining the response to the therapy know which treatment a subject receives. Randomization refers to the placing of subjects into one of the treatment groups in a way that can't be predicted by the patients or investigators. These clinical trials usually involve many investigators and take many years to complete. The hypothesis and methods of the trial are very precise and well thought out. Clinical trial designs, as well as the concepts of blinding and randomization, have developed over years of experimentation, trial, and error. At the present time, researchers are developing new designs to maximize the opportunity for all subjects to receive therapy.

Most treatments for general use come out of phase III clinical trials. After one or more phase III trials are finished, and if the results are positive for the treatment, the investigators can petition the FDA for government approval to use the drug or procedure to treat patients. Once the treatment is approved by the FDA, it can be used by qualified doctors throughout the country. The back packet of this brochure contains cards with information on some of the many stroke clinical trials the NINDS supports or has completed.

NINDS-Sponsored Stroke Clinical Trials: September 2012

Clinical trials give researchers a way to test new treatments in human subjects. Clinical trials test surgical devices and procedures, medications, rehabilitation therapies, and lifestyle and psychosocial interventions to determine how safe and effective they are and to establish the proper amount or level of treatment. Because of their scope and the need for careful analysis of data and outcomes, clinical trials are usually conducted in three phases and can take several years or more to complete.

Phase I clinical trials are small (involving fewer than 100 people) and are designed to define side effects and tolerance of the medication or therapy.

Phase II trials are conducted with a larger group of subjects and seek to measure the effects of a therapy and establish its proper dosage or level of treatment.

Phase III trials often involve hundreds (sometimes thousands) of volunteer patients who are assigned to treatment and non-treatment groups to test how well the treatment works and how safe it is at the recommended dosage or level of therapy. Many of these trials use a controlled, randomized, double-blind study design. This means that patients are randomly assigned to groups and neither the subject nor the study staff knows to which group a patient belongs. Phase III randomized clinical trials are often called the gold standard of clinical trials.

NINDS conducts clinical trials at the NIH Clinical Center and also provides funding for clinical trials at hospitals and universities across the United States and Canada. In the following text are findings from some of the largest and most significant recent clinical trials in stroke, as well as summaries of some of the most promising clinical trials in progress.

Findings From Recently Completed Clinical Trials

The Carotid Revascularization Endarterectomy vs. Stenting Trial (CREST)

The use of dilation and stenting techniques similar to those used to unclog and open heart arteries has been proposed as a less invasive alternative to carotid endarterectomy (surgery to remove the buildup of plaque within the carotid artery, which supplies blood to the head and neck). Carotid endarterectomy is considered the gold standard treatment for preventing stroke and other vascular events. Stenting is a newer, less invasive procedure in which an expandable metal stent (tube) is inserted into the carotid artery to keep it open after it has been widened with balloon dilation. The CREST study showed that the overall safety and effectiveness of the two procedures was largely the same—with equal benefits for both men and women, and for people who had previously had a stroke and for those who had not. Physicians will now have more options to tailor treatments for people at risk for stroke.

Carotid Occlusion Surgery Study (COSS)

The goal of this randomized clinical trial was to determine the preventive power of extracranial bypass surgery in a group of stroke survivors who have both a blocked carotid artery and an increased oxygen extraction fraction (or OEF, which indicates how hard the brain has to work to pull oxygen from the blood supply). An increased OEF has been shown to be a powerful and independent risk factor for subsequent stroke. Extracranial bypass surgery uses a healthy blood vessel to detour blood flow around the site of the blocked artery and results in increased blood flow to the brain. The results showed that in spite of the surgical success of improving cerebral blood flow, extracranial-intracranial bypass surgery did not demonstrate any benefit in reducing the risk of having a stroke recurrence due to the much better than expected recurrence rate in the non-surgical medical alone group.

Locomotor Experience Applied Post-Stroke (LEAPS)

Only 37 percent of stroke survivors are able to walk after the first week following their stroke. The investigators of the Locomotor Experience Applied Post-Stroke (LEAPS) trial set out to compare the effectiveness of the body-weight supported treadmill training with walking practice started at two different stages—two months post-stroke (early locomotor training) and six months post-stroke (late locomotor training). The locomotor training was also compared against a home exercise program managed by a physical therapist, aimed at enhancing patients' flexibility, range of motion, strength and balance as a way to improve their walking. The primary measure was each group's improvement in walking at one year after the stroke. The study found that stroke patients who had physical therapy at home improved their ability to walk just as well as those who were treated in a training program that requires the use of a body-weight supported treadmill device followed by walking practice. In addition, the study also found that patients continued to improve up to one year after stroke, defying conventional wisdom that recovery occurs early and tops out at six months.

Secondary Prevention of Small Subcortical Strokes (SPS3)

In this trial, investigators are testing new approaches to stroke prevention for people with a history of small subcortical strokes. The trial was designed to compare: 1) aspirin alone vs. combined antiplatelet therapy (aspirin and clopidogrel), and 2) intensive vs. standard blood pressure control. Subcortical strokes, also called lacunar strokes, occur when the thread-like arteries within cerebral tissue become blocked and halt blood flow to the brain. They account for up to one-fifth of all strokes in the United States and are especially common among people of Hispanic descent. In the antiplatelet component of SPS3, researchers have found that the combined antiplatelet therapy was about equal to aspirin in reducing stroke risk, but it almost doubled the risk of gastrointestinal bleeding. The blood pressure component of the trial is ongoing.

Stenting vs. Aggressive Medical Management for Preventing Recurrent Stroke in Intracranial Stenosis (SAMMPRIS)

The best treatment for preventing another stroke or TIA in patients with narrowing of a brain artery is uncertain. The purpose of this trial was to compare the safety and effectiveness of aggressive medical treatment (i.e., intensive management of key stroke risk factors including blood pressure, cholesterol, and lifestyle modification) alone to aggressive medical therapy plus a Food and Drug Administration (FDA)-approved intracranial stent to prevent another stroke in individuals who recently had either a transient ischemic attack or non-disabling stroke. The results of this trial, which was stopped early, showed that the group that received the intensive medical management alone had better outcomes than the group who also received the stent. This study provides an answer to a long-standing question by physicians—what to do to prevent a devastating second stroke in a high risk population.

Ongoing Clinical Trials

Albumin in Acute Ischemic Stroke (ALIAS) Trial

Human serum albumin is a protein found in human blood plasma that may have neuroprotective benefit in stroke. The Albumin in Acute Ischemic Stroke trial will compare the use of intravenous albumin administered over a two-hour period to placebo among individuals with acute ischemic stroke, beginning within five hours of stroke onset. Individuals will also receive concurrent treatment with a thrombolytic drug given either intravenously or intra-arterially when appropriate. Patients receiving either albumin or placebo will be followed for one year. The primary outcome will be an assessment of neurological function at three months post-stroke.

Antihypertensive Treatment of Acute Cerebral Hemorrhage (ATACH II)

Intensive blood pressure management following an intracerebral hemorrhage (ICH) may slow the rate and magnitude of the hemorrhage. The primary goal of the Antihypertensive Treatment of Acute Cerebral Hemorrhage trial is to determine the efficacy and safety of intensive systolic blood pressure management in ICH patients treated within three hours of symptom onset. The approach of intensive systolic blood pressure control represents a strategy that can be made widely available without the need of specialized equipment and personnel. Therefore, it has the potential to make a major impact on outcome in patients with ICH.

A Randomized Trial of Unruptured Brain Arteriovenous Malformations (ARUBA)

Arteriovenous malformations (AVMs) are defects of the circulatory system comprised of tangles of arteries and veins that are present from birth. These defects, which can occur in the brain, spinal cord, or other organs, may cause symptoms such as headaches or seizures. AVM that have not ruptured may be left untreated until they become symptomatic or may undergo surgical radiation or endovascular treatment to prevent future rupture. In A Randomized Trial of Unruptured Brain Arteriovenous Malformations (ARUBA), scientists will treat participants with unruptured brain AVMs either conservatively (medical management) or using invasive therapy (surgery, radiation, embolization) and follow their progress for at least five years to compare benefit in terms of reduced risk of subsequent stroke or AVM rupture. The outcome of this trial will indicate the best way to treat individuals with unruptured brain AVMs and offer doctors a more definitive standard of treatment.

Clot Lysis: Evaluating Accelerated Resolution of Intraventricular Hemorrhage, Phase III (CLEAR III)

The objective of the randomized Clot Lysis: Evaluating Accelerated Resolution of Intraventricular Hemorrhage III study is to determine any benefit of the use of the clot-busting drug recombinant tissue plasminogen activator (tPA) in conjunction with clot removal for intraventricular hemorrhage. The investigators will compare extraventricular draining (surgically inserting tubes that drain fluid from the brain's ventricles) plus tPA with extraventricular draining plus placebo in managing and treating individuals with small intracerebral hemorrhage and large intraventricular hemorrhage. Participants will receive either tPA or a placebo every eight hours for up to nine doses. Symptom onset must be within 24 hours prior to a diagnostic CT scan. The neurological function of the two groups will be compared at six months following treatment.

Field Administration of Stroke Therapy Magnesium Trial (FAST-MAG)

Currently, the drug tPA—the only treatment shown to be effective in treating acute ischemic stroke—must be administered after hospital arrival and within the first three hours of stroke occurrence. There is a need for new treatments that can be administered safely at an earlier time. The purpose of this multicenter, randomized, double-blind trial is to determine if paramedic initiation of the neuroprotective agent magnesium sulfate in the ambulance is an effective and safe treatment for acute stroke. This study will compare magnesium sulfate, an experimental therapy for stroke, vs. placebo among ambulance-transported patients with acute stroke. This trial will also determine if paramedics can safely, effectively and rapidly start neuroprotective therapies for stroke.

Insulin Resistance Intervention after Stroke Trial (IRIS)

The Insulin Resistance Intervention after Stroke (IRIS) trial tests a therapy based on evidence that links insulin resistance to an increased risk for stroke or heart disease. The goal of the trial is to determine if pioglitazone, a drug used to treat type 2 diabetes, is effective in lowering the risk for stroke and heart attack in a group of nondiabetic men and women who have recently had a stroke and developed insulin resistance. If this intervention is effective, it has the potential to benefit a large number of stroke survivors.

Interdisciplinary Comprehensive Arm Rehabilitation Evaluation (I-CARE)

Building on the positive outcome of the EXCITE clinical trials, investigators in the Interdisciplinary Comprehensive Arm Rehabilitation Evaluation (I-CARE) trial are testing an experimental arm therapy called Accelerated Skills Acquisition Program (ASAP). This therapy combines challenging, intensive, and meaningful practice of tasks of the participant's choice compared to two standard types of therapy (customary arm therapy totaling 30 hours, and customary arm therapy for a duration indicated on the therapy prescription). ASAP is targeted at the acute period of stroke recovery and will enroll participants who are within one to three months after their stroke. Based on compelling scientific data, this combined therapeutic approach is designed to capitalize on the brain's inherent recovery capability to improve upper limb function in people with stroke who have weakness on one side of the body.

Interventional Management of Stroke Trial (IMS III)

The Interventional Management of Stroke Trial (IMS III) is a large study that compares two different strategies for restoring blood flow to the brain in patients who have had a severe ischemic stroke. Patients are randomized to receive either the standard FDA-approved intravenous (IV) treatment of the clot-dissolving drug tPA alone or a combination approach that provides both standard IV tPA and an intra-arterial (IA) therapy using either tPA delivered into the artery directly at the site of the clot or an FDA-approved device to remove the blood clot in the brain. Therapy using both approaches will be initiated within three hours of stroke onset. The trial will measure the ability of participants to live and function independently three months after the stroke. It will also determine and compare the safety and cost effectiveness of the combined IV/IA approach to the standard IV tPA approach.

Platelet-Oriented Inhibition in New TIA and Minor Ischemic Stroke (POINT) Trial

A transient ischemic attack (TIA) is a brief episode of neurological dysfunction that often is a harbinger of disabling strokes. The primary goal of the Platelet-Oriented Inhibition in New TIA and Minor Ischemic Stroke (POINT) trial is to determine if the drug clopidogrel (used to reduce or prevent blood clots) combined with aspirin is effective in preventing ischemic stroke and myocardial infarction. Individuals over age 18 who can begin treatment within 12 hours of symptom onset will be enrolled. If trial results are positive, treatment with clopidogrel could reduce the burden of stroke in the United States and substantially reduce costs of care.

Stroke Hyperglycemia Insulin Network Effort Trial (SHINE)

Nearly 40 percent of patients who experience an ischemic stroke are hyperglycemic upon arriving at the hospital. Current research has indicated that severe or prolonged hyperglycemia is associated with poorer outcome and increased disability. At present there are no clear guidelines for treating this condition. The purpose of this clinical trial is to determine whether tight glucose control of hyperglycemia with three days of intravenous insulin therapy is superior to the standard therapy of glucose control with subcutaneous insulin. The results from this 1,400 participant clinical trial will guide clinical practice all over the nation and the world.

Chapter 2

Stroke Symptoms and What You Should Do If Someone Has Them

Stroke is the third leading cause of death in the United States and a leading cause of serious, long-term disability in adults. About 600,000 new strokes are reported in the United States each year. The good news is that treatments are available that can greatly reduce the damage caused by a stroke. However, you need to recognize the symptoms of a stroke and get to a hospital quickly. Getting treatment within 60 minutes can prevent disability.

A stroke, sometimes called a brain attack, occurs when blood flow to the brain is interrupted. When a stroke occurs, brain cells in the immediate area begin to die because they stop getting the oxygen and nutrients they need to function.

There are two major kinds of stroke. The first, called an ischemic stroke, is caused by a blood clot that blocks or plugs a blood vessel or artery in the brain. About 80 percent of all strokes are ischemic. The second, known as a hemorrhagic stroke, is caused by a blood vessel in the brain that breaks and bleeds into the brain. About 20 percent of strokes are hemorrhagic.

Although stroke is a disease of the brain, it can affect the entire body. The effects of a stroke range from mild to severe and can include paralysis, problems with thinking, problems with speaking, and emotional problems. Patients may also experience pain or numbness after a stroke.

Excerpted from "Know Stroke, Know the Signs, Act in Time," by the National Institute of Neurological Disorders and Stroke (NINDS, www.ninds.nih.gov), May 21, 2010.

Because stroke injures the brain, you may not realize that you are having a stroke. To a bystander, someone having a stroke may just look unaware or confused. Stroke victims have the best chance if someone around them recognizes the symptoms and acts quickly.

Symptoms of a Stroke

The symptoms of stroke are distinct because they happen quickly:

- Sudden numbness or weakness of the face, arm, or leg (especially on one side of the body)

- Sudden confusion, trouble speaking, or understanding speech

- Sudden trouble seeing in one or both eyes

- Sudden trouble walking, dizziness, loss of balance, or coordination

- Sudden severe headache with no known cause

What Should a Bystander Do?

If you believe someone is having a stroke—if he or she suddenly loses the ability to speak, or move an arm or leg on one side, or experiences facial paralysis on one side—call 911 immediately.

Act in Time

Stroke is a medical emergency. Every minute counts when someone is having a stroke. The longer blood flow is cut off to the brain, the greater the damage. Immediate treatment can save people's lives and enhance their chances for successful recovery.

Why is there a need to act fast? Ischemic strokes, the most common type of strokes, can be treated with a drug called tPA [tissue plasminogen activator], that dissolves blood clots obstructing blood flow to the brain. The window of opportunity to start treating stroke patients is three hours, but to be evaluated and receive treatment, patients need to get to the hospital within 60 minutes.

A five-year study by the National Institute of Neurological Disorders and Stroke (NINDS) found that some stroke patients who received tPA within three hours of the start of stroke symptoms were at least 30 percent more likely to recover with little or no disability after three months.

What Can I Do to Prevent a Stroke?

The best treatment for stroke is prevention. There are several risk factors that increase your chances of having a stroke:

- High blood pressure
- Heart disease
- Smoking
- Diabetes
- High cholesterol

If you smoke—quit. If you have high blood pressure, heart disease, diabetes, or high cholesterol, getting them under control—and keeping them under control—will greatly reduce your chances of having a stroke.

Chapter 3

Strokes in Children

Although cerebrovascular disorders occur less often in children than in adults, recognition of stroke in children has probably increased because of the widespread application of noninvasive diagnostic studies such as magnetic resonance imaging (MRI), magnetic resonance angiography (MRA), computed tomography (CT) and, in the neonate, cranial ultrasound studies. These studies allow confirmation of a diagnosis that in previous years would not have been suspected or at least not recognized as a vascular lesion. Also, the number of patients with cerebrovascular lesions from certain risk factors may have increased as more effective treatments for some causes of stroke have allowed patients to survive long enough to develop vascular complications. Patients with sickle cell disease or with leukemia, for example, now have a longer life expectancy, and during this time they may have a stroke.

Most of the pediatric cerebrovascular literature consists of single case reports or small groups of children with a common etiology. These reports offer some insight into the relative frequency of various causes of stroke and draw attention to individual risk factors, but their usefulness is otherwise limited. Larger series of children selected for a common anatomic lesion or a single cause offer additional insight into the unique features of cerebrovascular lesions in children, but patients

Excerpted from "Proceedings of a National Symposium on Rapid Identification and Treatment of Acute Stroke," by the National Institute of Neurological Disorders and Stroke (NINDS, www.ninds.nih.gov), August 1997. NIH Publication No. 97-4239. This document was updated May 17, 2011.

37

collected from large medical centers may not be representative of all children with stroke. None of these studies can accurately judge the incidence of cerebrovascular disease in children.

Schoenberg and colleagues studied cerebrovascular disease in children of Rochester, Minnesota from 1965 through 1974. Excluding strokes related to intracranial infection, trauma, or birth, they found three hemorrhagic strokes and one ischemic stroke in an average at risk population of 15,834, for an estimated average annual incidence rate of 1.89/100,000/year and 0.63/100,000/year for hemorrhagic and ischemic strokes respectively. Their overall average annual incidence rate for children through fourteen years of age was 2.52/100,000/year. In this population, hemorrhagic strokes occurred more often than ischemic strokes, while in the Mayo Clinic referral population, ischemic strokes were more common. The risk of childhood cerebrovascular disease in this study is about half the risk for neoplasms of the central nervous system of children, but neonates and children with traumatic lesions are excluded. Despite our impression that cerebrovascular disorders are recognized more often in children than in previous years, Broderick and colleagues found an incidence of 2.7 cases/100,000/year, similar to the figure reported by Schoenberg and colleagues. In the Canadian Pediatric Ischemic Stroke Registry incidence of arterial and venous occlusion is estimated to be 1.2/100,000 children/year.

The frequency of several individual risk factors for stroke in children is known, but in most instances, the occurrence of secondary cerebrovascular disease is so variable that it is difficult to assess the relative contribution of each risk factor to the problem of cerebrovascular disease as a whole. In one report which included both children and young adults, children were less likely than young adult stroke patients to have identifiable risk factors and more often fall victim to infectious or inflammatory disorders. The implication is that children may have additional, as yet unknown, risk factors.

The Origin of Stroke in Children

Probably the most fundamental difference between cerebrovascular diseases in children and adults is the wide array of risk factors seen in children versus adults. Congenital heart disease and sickle cell disease, for example, are common causes of stroke in children, while atherosclerosis is rare in children. No cause can be detected in about a fifth of the children with ischemic infarction, yet many of these children seem to do well. The recognized causes of cerebrovascular disorders in children are numerous, and the probability of identifying the cause depends on the thoroughness of the evaluation. A probable cause of cerebral infarction was identified in 184 of 228 (79%) children in the Canadian Pediatric Ischemic Stroke Registry. The source of an intracranial hemorrhage is even more likely to be found.

The most common cause of stroke in children is probably congenital or acquired heart disease. In the Canadian Pediatric Ischemic Stroke Registry, heart disease was found in 40 of 228 (19%) of the children with arterial thrombosis. Many of these children are already known to have heart disease prior to their stroke, but in other instances a less obvious cardiac lesion is discovered only after a stroke. Complex cardiac anomalies involving both the valves and chambers are collectively the biggest problem, but virtually any cardiac lesion can sometimes lead to a stroke. Of particular concern are cyanotic lesions with polycythemia, which increase the risk of both thrombosis and embolism.

Both the frequency and the cause of pediatric stroke may depend somewhat on both the geographic location and the specific hospital setting. The Canadian Pediatric Ischemic Stroke Registry, for example, lists only five children (2%) with cerebral infarction due to sickle cell anemia. A large metropolitan hospital in the United States might care for this many patients in a year, but early estimates that cerebral infarction occurred in 17% of people with sickle cell disease proved far higher than the 4–5% figure derived from more representative samples in Jamaica and in Africa.

Chapter 4

Strokes in Men and Women

Chapter Contents

Section 4.1

Men and Women
May Differ in Stroke Symptoms

It is important to recognize stroke symptoms and act quickly. Common stroke symptoms seen in both men and women:

- Sudden numbness or weakness of face, arm, or leg—especially on one side of the body

- Sudden confusion, trouble speaking, or understanding

- Sudden trouble seeing in one or both eyes

- Sudden trouble walking, dizziness, loss of balance, or coordination

- Sudden severe headache with no known cause

Women may report unique stroke symptoms:

- Sudden face and limb pain

- Sudden hiccups

- Sudden nausea

- Sudden general weakness

- Sudden chest pain

- Sudden shortness of breath

- Sudden palpitations

Call 911 immediately if you have any of these symptoms

Every minute counts for stroke patients and acting F.A.S.T. can lead patients to the stroke treatments they desperately need. The most effective stroke treatments are only available if the stroke is recognized and diagnosed within the first three hours of the first symptoms.

Actually, many Americans are not aware that stroke patients may not be eligible for stroke treatments if they arrive at the hospital after the three-hour window.

If you think someone may be having a stroke, act F.A.S.T. and do this simple test:

- **F—FACE:** Ask the person to smile. Does one side of the face droop?

- **A—ARMS:** Ask the person to raise both arms. Does one arm drift downward?

- **S—SPEECH:** Ask the person to repeat a simple phrase. Is their speech slurred or strange?

- **T—TIME:** If you observe any of these signs, call 911 immediately.

Note the time when any symptoms first appear. If given within three hours of the first symptom, there is an FDA [U.S. Food and Drug Administration]-approved clot-buster medication that may reduce long-term disability for the most common type of stroke.

Learn as many stroke symptoms as possible so you can recognize stroke as FAST as possible.

"Understanding the warning signs is important because there are treatments we can give for stroke. If you understand the warning signs and get to the hospital quickly we can even possibly reverse the stroke itself," says Dr. Dawn Kleindorfer, assistant professor of neurology at University of Cincinnati School of Medicine.

Section 4.2

Estrogen, Women, and Stroke

"Estrogen, Women, and Stroke," by Cheryl D. Bushnell, MD, MHS, Patricia
Denise Hurn, PhD, and Louise D. McCullough, MD, PhD. © The Hazel K.
Goddess Fund for Stroke Research in Women (www.thegoddessfund.org).
All rights reserved. Reprinted with permission. This document is undated.
Reviewed by David A. Cooke, MD, FACP, January 31, 2013.

The focus of this text is to inform women about estrogen and stroke.
But first, it is important to know that stroke is a common and serious disease in women. The term stroke actually refers to a group of
diseases involving the blood vessels leading to, or within, the brain.
Most commonly a blood vessel becomes occluded and a segment of the
blood supply to the brain is cut off. This results in a localized injury
within the brain.

There are nearly three-quarters of a million strokes in the United
States each year, with a third of these occurring in people under the
age of 65 years. So while many think of stroke as a disease of older
men, this is not the case. Stroke not only afflicts younger people, but
it kills more women than the number who die from breast cancer and
AIDS [acquired immunodeficiency syndrome] combined. Over half
of all strokes and 60% of all stroke-related deaths occur in women.
In fact, stroke ranks as the second leading cause of death in women
worldwide. Women of all ages should discuss their risk for stroke and
heart disease with their physicians. Women with hypertension, diabetes, abnormal lipids, cigarette smoking, or a family history of stroke
or heart attack are all at increased risk for stroke. African-American
and Hispanic-American women are also at higher risk for stroke. The
good news is that the majority of strokes that might occur in women
could be prevented if women at risk are identified and treated in time.

If a stroke does occur, it is critical to get medical attention quickly.
There are therapies that can reduce the injury associated with stroke
or decrease the complications following a stroke. Therapies such as tPA
(tissue plasminogen activator, or clot busters) can help reopen blocked
blood vessels, but most patients fail to receive this therapy in time.
Stroke is a medical emergency. Every minute counts.

Female hormones like estrogen play a role in stroke. A hormone is a chemical signal produced in one part of the body that has actions elsewhere in the body. You can think of a hormone as a messenger. Produced in the ovaries, estrogen travels the blood stream, signaling the brain, blood vessels, uterus, breasts, bones, liver, and many other organs.

Estrogen is produced throughout the first half of a woman's adult life. Production dramatically decreases at the time of menopause, in the late 40s and early 50s for most women. Decreases in estrogen have been associated with common symptoms of menopause, such as hot flashes, vaginal dryness, headaches, changes in mood and difficulty with sleeping.

Low estrogen levels have also been associated with an increased risk for heart disease, stroke, osteoporosis (thinning of the bones), cognitive changes, and dementia. Estrogen actions protect teeth, the eyes, and skin. New evidence also points to estrogen's supportive effects on immune response. These benefits decrease as estrogen levels decrease.

Women have been using hormone replacement therapy (HRT) after menopause for over 60 years. Estrogen alone is prescribed for women without a uterus, women who have had a hysterectomy. Women with a uterus take a progesterone-like hormone in addition to estrogen in order to protect the lining of the uterus, since unopposed estrogen can lead to uterine cancer. The addition of the progesterone essentially eliminates that risk. Most women use HRT for less than two years, primarily to control hormone deficiency symptoms at the time of menopause. Because symptoms usually persist for more than five years—and in about 25% of women, for more than ten years—hormone use can be prescribed for longer periods. However, some women opt to discontinue treatment because of possible negative side effects of chronic estrogen replacement, such as an increased incidence of breast cancer and stroke.

New developments in hormone replacement therapy are appealing because the doses are lower, the delivery of the hormones is better controlled and the products are purer. As a result, treatment of symptoms is more effective, side effects are reduced and concern about cancer is lessened, especially among women who use HRT for about five years. These new treatments hold the possibility of more effective prevention of disease due to hormone deficiency but many are still under investigation.

Whichever HRT is used, as with all other hormone therapies, it is important that treatment be used as directed. Missing pills or forgetting to change a hormone-containing patch can lead to irregular bleeding or induce hot flashes, headaches, and other withdrawal effects. These in turn often lead to discontinuation of treatment.

Initial epidemiological studies indicated that women who used hormone replacement therapy following menopause had lower rates of heart attack and stroke. HRT's potential benefits against stroke were also suggested by a decade of laboratory-based animal studies that repeatedly emphasized estrogen's protective actions for the heart, blood vessels, bone, and brain. In randomized clinical trials, however, it remained unclear whether to attribute the decreased disease rates to the estrogen or to the women who used the estrogen (i.e., a statistical bias). Women who use estrogen are more likely to go to their doctor, more likely to know their risk factors and have them treated and more likely to take their medications. All of these measures are associated with a lower rate of heart attack and stroke.

The best way to address the possible bias is to set up a study that randomly assigns women to hormone replacement therapy or an inactive pill (placebo). Some of these studies have now been completed. Surprising results have emerged over the past decade that have shown a possible detrimental effect of hormone replacement in both healthy women as well as women with known vascular disease. In the Women's Estrogen for Stroke Trial (WEST) Study, postmenopausal women who had a recent stroke or a transient ischemic attack (TIA) were randomly assigned to estrogen or a placebo. They were monitored for several years for the occurrence of a recurrent stroke or death. In the WEST, women who were assigned to estrogen had the same rate of a recurrent stroke as those assigned to a placebo. Additionally, women who were randomly assigned to receive estrogen therapy had a higher risk of fatal stroke, which was a concerning finding. It is possible that estrogen loses its beneficial effects if women already have established vascular disease.

It is important to note that women in the WEST trial had known vascular disease, so hormone replacement was being investigated for prevention of future events (secondary prevention). Less was known about the effect of hormone replacement in healthy women until the release of the Women's Health Initiative (WHI). In July 2002 the WHI, the largest study to date to examine the effects of hormone replacement therapy on stroke, published its findings that the combination of estrogen and a potent progestin—a drug called Prempro—caused an increase both in strokes and heart attacks in healthy postmenopausal women as compared with placebo. Initially it was thought that the progesterone may be responsible for the increased stroke risk, but in 2004, similar results were reported for women with a prior hysterectomy treated with estrogen without progesterone. The use of estrogen was found to increase the risk of stroke in postmenopausal women. While there are indications for the use of hormonal therapy, available data from the WEST study indicate that women who have had a stroke should not be started on hormonal therapy to prevent a recurrent stroke, myocardial infarction, or death. The Women's Health Initiative, moreover, cautions postmenopausal women who have never had a stroke against hormone replacement therapy use if it is solely for the prevention of stroke. Many new trials are ongoing to try to figure out why hormone therapy seems to be so beneficial in observational and experimental studies, yet does not seem to protect the women who used it in the WEST and WHI. One possibility is that hormone replacement was begun too late, as most of the women in these trials were well past (over 10 years) menopause. It is quite possible that if therapy is begun early at menopause, the beneficial effects will become apparent. Further research has never been more crucial. A woman who is considering HRT should consult her physician to determine her risk.

Among women before menopause, the use of oral contraceptives has also been associated with a small increase in the risk for stroke. This small increase appears to be lower with modern, lower dose, oral contraceptives. The risk, however, remains higher among women who also have a history of migraines and who smoke. This trial of oral contraceptives, migraines, and smoking should alert younger women, as well, to their potential risk for a stroke or related complication.

Women are living longer than ever before. As they do, it is vital that they also live healthier longer. Women need to be aware of their risk and the preventative measures they can take to protect themselves against the occurrence and effects of stroke.

Section 4.3

Contraceptive Use and Stroke Risk

Excerpted from "Stroke Fact Sheet," by the
Office on Women's Health (www.womenshealth.gov), part of the U.S.
Department of Health and Human Services, January 28, 2009.

What is a stroke?

A stroke is sometimes called a brain attack. A stroke can injure the brain like a heart attack can injure the heart. A stroke occurs when part of the brain doesn't get the blood it needs.

There are two types of stroke:

- Ischemic stroke (most common type): This type of stroke happens when blood is blocked from getting to the brain. This often happens because the artery is clogged with fatty deposits (atherosclerosis) or a blood clot.

- Hemorrhagic stroke: This type of stroke happens when a blood vessel in the brain bursts, and blood bleeds into the brain. This type of stroke can be caused by an aneurysm—a thin or weak spot in an artery that balloons out and can burst.

Both types of stroke can cause brain cells to die. This may cause a person to lose control of their speech, movement, and memory. If you think you are having a stroke, call 911.

Does taking birth control pills increase my risk for stroke?

Taking birth control pills is generally safe for young, healthy women. But birth control pills can raise the risk of stroke for some women, especially women over 35; women with high blood pressure, diabetes, or high cholesterol; and women who smoke. Talk with your doctor if you have questions about the pill.

If you are taking birth control pills, and you have any of the symptoms listed below, call 911:

- Eye problems such as blurred or double vision

- Pain in the upper body or arm

- Bad headaches

- Problems breathing

- Spitting up blood

- Swelling or pain in the leg

- Yellowing of the skin or eyes

- Breast lumps

- Unusual (not normal) heavy bleeding from your vagina

Does using the birth control patch increase my risk for stroke?

The patch is generally safe for young, healthy women. The patch can raise the risk of stroke for some women, especially women over 35; women with high blood pressure, diabetes, or high cholesterol; and women who smoke.

Recent studies show that women who use the patch may be exposed to more estrogen (the female hormone in birth control pills and the patch that keeps users from becoming pregnant) than women who use the birth control pill. Research is underway to see if the risk for blood clots (which can lead to heart attack or stroke) is higher in patch users. Talk with your doctor if you have questions about the patch.

If you are using the birth control patch, and you have any of the symptoms listed below, call 911:

- Eye problems such as blurred or double vision

- Pain in the upper body or arm

- Bad headaches

- Problems breathing

- Spitting up blood

- Swelling or pain in the leg

- Yellowing of the skin or eyes

- Breast lumps

- Unusual (not normal) heavy bleeding from your vagina

Section 4.4

Rate of Stroke Increasing in Women during and after Pregnancy

Study highlights:

- Researchers report a large increase in the number of women having strokes while pregnant and in the three months after childbirth.

- The overall rate of pregnancy-related stroke went up 54 percent between 1994–1995 and 2006–2007.

- The increase is due to women having more risk factors, including high blood pressure and obesity.

The stroke rate for pregnant women and those who recently gave birth increased alarmingly over the past dozen years, according to research reported in *Stroke: Journal of the American Heart Association*.

Researchers gathered data from a large national database of 5 to 8 million discharges from 1,000 hospitals and compared the rates of strokes from 1994–1995 to 2006–2007 in women who were pregnant, delivering a baby, and who had recently had a baby.

Pregnancy-related stroke hospitalizations increased 54 percent, from 4,085 in 1994–1995 to 6,293 in 2006–2007.

"I am surprised at the magnitude of the increase, which is substantial," said Elena V. Kuklina, MD, PhD, lead author of the study and senior service fellow and epidemiologist at the Centers for Disease Control and Prevention's Division for Heart Disease and Stroke Prevention in Atlanta, Georgia. "Our results indicate an urgent need to take a closer look. Stroke is such a debilitating condition. We need to put more effort into prevention.

"When you're relatively healthy, your stroke risk is not that high," Kuklina said. "Now more and more women entering pregnancy already have some type of risk factor for stroke, such as obesity, chronic hypertension, diabetes, or congenital heart disease. Since pregnancy by itself is a risk factor, if you have one of these other stroke risk factors, it doubles the risk."

For expectant mothers, the rate of stroke hospitalizations rose 47 percent. In pregnant women and in women who had a baby in the last 12 weeks (considered the postpartum period), the stroke rate rose 83 percent. However, the rate remained the same for stroke hospitalizations that occurred during the time immediately surrounding childbirth.

Furthermore, high blood pressure was more prevalent in pregnant women who were hospitalized because of stroke.

In 1994–1995, among pregnant women with stroke, researchers found high blood pressure in:

- 11.3 percent of the pregnant women prior to birth;

- 23.4 percent of those at or near delivery; and

- 27.8 percent of those within 12 weeks of delivery.

In 2006–2007, they discovered high blood pressure among stroke patients in:

- 17 percent of those pregnant;

- 28.5 percent of those at or near delivery; and

- 40.9 percent of women in the postpartum period.

It's best for women to enter pregnancy with ideal cardiovascular health—without additional risk factors, Kuklina said. Next, she suggests developing a comprehensive, multidisciplinary plan that gives doctors and patients guidelines for appropriate monitoring and care before, during, and after childbirth.

A major problem is that pregnant women typically aren't included in clinical trials because most drugs pose potential harm to the fetus. Therefore, doctors don't have enough guidance on which medications are best for pregnant women who have an increased risk for stroke.

"We need to do more research on pregnant women specifically," said Kuklina, who found only 11 cases of pregnancy-related stroke in her review of previously published literature.

Co-authors are: Xin Tong, MPH; Pooja Bansil, MPH; Mary G. George, MD, MSPH; and William M. Callaghan, MD, MPH. Author disclosures are on the manuscript.

The study received no outside funding.

Section 4.5

Hormone Therapy Use and Stroke

"Hormone Therapy," Office on Women's Health, U.S. Department of
Health and Human Services (www.womenshealth.gov), 2010.

What is hormone therapy?

Hormone therapy (HT), also called menopausal hormone therapy,
is a treatment for women who are going through or have gone through
menopause. The female hormone estrogen is the most common type of
hormone therapy. Because taking estrogen alone may increase the risk
of uterine cancer, it is usually combined with another type of hormone
called a progestogen. Estrogen alone is only given to women who have
had a hysterectomy (had their uterus surgically removed).

What is hormone therapy used for?

Hormone therapy is used to treat menopausal symptoms such as
hot flashes, night sweats, sleep disturbances, and vaginal dryness.

Hormone therapy has also been investigated as a way to prevent or
treat many diseases that become common after menopause—from heart
disease, stroke, and cancer to Alzheimer disease and osteoporosis—but
results have generally been disappointing so far.

What are the different kinds of hormone therapy?

There are three main types of hormone therapy:

• Estrogen-only therapy (ET)

• Progestogen-only therapy

• Combined estrogen-progestogen therapy (EPT)

There are many variations on these main themes: Hormone therapies come in different combinations of estrogens and progestogens,
with different dosing strengths and schedules. It is generally recommended that you use the lowest dose that controls your symptoms.

Hormone therapy can be applied in many ways. It is usually given as a pill, but can also be given as an injection, or absorbed through the skin as a patch, gel, cream, or spray, or as a vaginal cream, ring, or tablet.

How do my body's natural hormones affect my risk of stroke?

Women tend to develop stroke and heart disease later in life than men. This delay is thought to be largely due to the protective effects of estrogen. Estrogen alters the levels of cholesterol and fat in your blood, changes the way your blood forms clots, affects how well your blood flows though the body and how the blood vessels respond, and has an impact on many factors related to the buildup of fatty plaque in the arteries. All of these processes influence the development of heart disease and stroke.

When a woman goes through menopause, her body stops producing estrogen and these protective effects are lost. After menopause a woman's risk of heart disease and stroke begins to increase. It was therefore thought that replacing the lost estrogen might help prevent heart and blood vessel disease.

Does hormone therapy increase my risk of having a stroke?

Yes. Hormone therapy, either estrogen alone or combined with progestin, increases your risk of stroke and does not prevent you from having a heart attack or dying of heart disease. In the past, some doctors prescribed hormone therapy in an attempt to lower the risk of heart and blood vessel disease, but current guidelines state that hormone therapy should not be used to treat or prevent heart disease or stroke in women.

Early studies that compared women who chose to take hormone therapy with those who didn't showed that hormone therapy users had a lower risk of heart disease and the same risk of stroke, but that they were likely to have less severe strokes. However, when more tightly controlled experiments randomly assigned women to hormone therapy or a dummy pill, the results were not positive.

The Women's Health Initiative study of more than 16,000 healthy postmenopausal women found that a combination of estrogen and progestin provided no protection from heart attack, stroke, or heart disease. In fact, hormone therapy users had a slightly higher risk of heart disease, stroke, and blood clots. The trial was stopped early because women taking hormone therapy also began to show an increased risk of breast cancer. The Women's Health Initiative also found that estrogen alone increased the risk of stroke and blood clots and had no effect on the risk of heart disease or breast cancer. Overall, researchers decided that while the risk of harm is small from using hormone therapy to prevent heart disease and stroke, it still outweighs any potential benefits.

The increases in stroke risk when using hormone therapy to treat menopausal symptoms is relatively small. Over 1 year, if 10,000 healthy women were to take combination hormone therapy, more women would suffer a stroke compared with a group of 10,000 women not taking hormone therapy. In women with a hysterectomy who are taking estrogen-only hormone therapy, there would be 12 additional strokes per 10,000 women treated.

Most studies of hormone therapy have only looked at one type of estrogen-plus-progesterone pill, called Prempro, and one type of estrogen alone pill, called Premarin. It is not known whether other forms of hormone therapy have the same effects. Some research has shown that when hormones are imbedded in a patch and absorbed through the skin, they affect the body differently.

Do the stroke risks of hormone therapy change with age?

When women of all ages are looked at together, using hormone therapy increases the risk of stroke and heart disease. Results from the Women's Health Initiative study of hormone therapy found that younger women taking hormone therapy within five years of menopause may not be at increased risk for heart disease, and may actually have a slightly lower risk. The effects of younger age on stroke were smaller, with an increased stroke risk regardless of years since menopause. However, while stroke risk did not decrease in women of any age taking hormones, in women aged 50 to 59 there was no significant increase in risk with therapy.

For now, hormone therapy should not be taken to prevent heart disease or stroke even among very young postmenopausal women. However, the results of studies like the Women's Health Initiative should reassure younger women who want to take HT for menopausal symptoms that they need not be scared off by the possible stroke risks.

Can I take hormones for menopausal symptoms if I have a history of stroke?

No. If you have had a stroke or blood clots in the past, or have been diagnosed with heart disease, you should not take hormone therapy. A study of women who had already had a stroke or transient ischemic attack (TIA) found that estrogen-only hormone therapy did not decrease the risk of having another stroke, and actually doubled the risk of having a recurrent stroke in the first 6 months of therapy. Among women who had another stroke, those who were taking estrogen therapy were three times as likely to die; those who survived had worse mental and functional disabilities. Combination hormone therapy increases the risk of stroke and blood clots and increases the risk of heart attack in the first year of therapy.

What alternatives to hormone therapy are being studied?

Currently, researchers are looking into a group of drugs called selective estrogen-receptor modulators (SERMs), which have also been called designer estrogens. They are compounds that have beneficial effects on bone density like estrogen, but without estrogen's negative effects on the breast or lining of the uterus. The hope is that these new compounds will provide the benefits of replacement estrogen without the negative side effects, such as stroke, heart problems, and cancer. So far, most studies of SERMs have found that although they have better risk profiles for heart disease, like hormone therapy they increase the risk of stroke and blood clots.

The most studied of the four FDA-approved SERMs is raloxifene (Evista), used to prevent and treat postmenopausal osteoporosis (thinning of the bones) and to prevent breast cancer in women at high risk. In the RUTH trial, over 10,000 women with heart disease or multiple risk factors received raloxifene or a dummy pill once a day for more than 5 years. Raloxifene cut the risk of breast cancer and spine fractures, and did not increase the risk of heart attack, hospitalization for heart disease, or dying of heart disease. However, women taking raloxifene had a slightly higher risk of dying of a stroke or having blood clots in the leg veins, which can move to other parts of the body.

Current guidelines state that, like hormone therapy, SERMs should not be used for the prevention or treatment of heart disease or stroke in women.

Chapter 5

Strokes in Older Adults

A stroke is serious, just like a heart attack. Each year in the United States, there are more than 700,000 new strokes. Stroke is the third leading cause of death in the United States, after heart disease and cancer. And stroke causes more serious long-term disabilities than any other disease.

Nearly three-quarters of all strokes occur in people over the age of 65. And the risk of having a stroke more than doubles each decade between the ages of 55 and 85.

Stroke occurs in all age groups, in both sexes, and in all races in every country. It can even occur before birth, when the fetus is still in the womb.

Learning about stroke can help you act in time to save a relative, neighbor, or friend. And making changes in your lifestyle can help you prevent stroke.

What Is Stroke?

A stroke is sometimes called a "brain attack." Most often, stroke occurs when blood flow to the brain stops because it is blocked by a clot. When this happens, the brain cells in the immediate area begin to die.

Some brain cells die because they stop getting the oxygen and nutrients they need to function. Other brain cells die because they are damaged by sudden bleeding into or around the brain. The brain cells

Excerpted from "Stroke," by the National Institute on Aging (NIA, www.nia .nih.gov), part of the National Institutes of Health, June 8, 2012.

that don't die immediately remain at risk for death. These cells can linger in a compromised or weakened state for several hours. With timely treatment, these cells can be saved.

New treatments are available that greatly reduce the damage caused by a stroke. But you need to arrive at the hospital as soon as possible after symptoms start to prevent disability and to greatly improve your chances for recovery. Knowing stroke symptoms, calling 911 immediately, and getting to a hospital as quickly as possible are critical.

Ischemic Stroke

There are two kinds of stroke. The most common kind of stroke is called ischemic stroke. It accounts for approximately 80 percent of all strokes. An ischemic stroke is caused by a blood clot that blocks or plugs a blood vessel in the brain. Blockages that cause ischemic strokes stem from three conditions:

- The formation of a clot within a blood vessel of the brain or neck, called thrombosis

- The movement of a clot from another part of the body, such as from the heart to the neck or brain, called an embolism

- A severe narrowing of an artery in or leading to the brain, called stenosis

Hemorrhagic Stroke

The other kind of stroke is called hemorrhagic stroke. A hemorrhagic stroke is caused by a blood vessel that breaks and bleeds into the brain.

One common cause of a hemorrhagic stroke is a bleeding aneurysm. An aneurysm is a weak or thin spot on an artery wall. Over time, these weak spots stretch or balloon out due to high blood pressure. The thin walls of these ballooning aneurysms can rupture and spill blood into the space surrounding brain cells.

Artery walls can also break open because they become encrusted, or covered with fatty deposits called plaque, eventually lose their elasticity and become brittle, thin, and prone to cracking. Hypertension, or high blood pressure, increases the risk that a brittle artery wall will give way and release blood into the surrounding brain tissue.

Effects of a Stroke

Stroke damage in the brain can affect the entire body—resulting in mild to severe disabilities. These include paralysis, problems with thinking, trouble speaking, and emotional problems.

Movement Problems

A common disability that results from stroke is complete paralysis on one side of the body, called hemiplegia. A related disability that is not as debilitating as paralysis is one-sided weakness, or hemiparesis. The paralysis or weakness may affect only the face, an arm, or a leg, or it may affect one entire side of the body and face.

A stroke patient may have problems with the simplest of daily activities, such as walking, dressing, eating, and using the bathroom. Movement problems can result from damage to the part of the brain that controls balance and coordination. Some stroke patients also have trouble swallowing, called dysphagia.

Thinking Problems

Stroke may cause problems with thinking, awareness, attention, learning, judgment, and memory.

In some cases of stroke, the patient suffers a neglect syndrome. The neglect syndrome means that the stroke patient has no knowledge of one side of his or her body, or one side of the visual field, and is unaware of the problem. A stroke patient may be unaware of his or her surroundings, or may be unaware of the mental problems that resulted from the stroke.

Speech Problems

Stroke victims often have a problem forming or understanding speech. This problem is called aphasia. Aphasia usually occurs along with similar problems in reading and writing. In most people, language problems result from damage to the left hemisphere of the brain.

Slurred speech due to weakness or incoordination of the muscles involved in speaking is called dysarthria, and is not a problem with language. Because it can result from any weakness or incoordination of the speech muscles, dysarthria can arise from damage to either side of the brain.

Emotional Problems

A stroke can also lead to emotional problems. Stroke patients may have difficulty controlling their emotions or may express inappropriate emotions in certain situations. One common disability that occurs with many stroke patients is depression.

Post-stroke depression may be more than a general sadness resulting from the stroke incident. It is a serious behavioral problem that can hamper recovery and rehabilitation and may even lead to suicide. Post-stroke depression is treated as any depression is treated, with antidepressant medications and therapy.

Stroke patients may experience pain, uncomfortable numbness, or strange sensations after a stroke. These sensations may be due to many factors, including damage to the sensory regions of the brain, stiff joints, or a disabled limb.

Pain

An uncommon type of pain resulting from stroke is called central stroke pain or central pain syndrome or CPS. CPS results from damage to an area called the thalamus. The pain is a mixture of sensations, including heat and cold, burning, tingling, numbness, and sharp stabbing and underlying aching pain.

The pain is often worse in the hands and feet and is made worse by movement and temperature changes, especially cold temperatures. Unfortunately, since most pain medications provide little relief from these sensations, very few treatments or therapies exist to combat CPS.

Chapter 6

Racial and Ethnic Stroke Disparities

Stroke in American Indian and Alaska Natives

Stroke is the fifth leading cause of death among American Indians and Alaska Natives. In 2003, stroke caused 552 deaths among American Indians and Alaska Natives.

Heart disease and stroke are also major causes of disability and can decrease a person's quality of life.

The American Indian and Alaska Native Population

- There are approximately 4.5 million American Indians and Alaska Natives in the United States, 1.5% of the population, including those of more than one race.

- The median age of American Indians and Alaska Natives is 30.7 years, which is younger than the 36.2 years of the total U.S. population.

This chapter contains text from the following documents: Excerpted from "American Indian and Alaska Native Heart Disease and Stroke Fact Sheet," by the Centers for Disease Control and Prevention (CDC, www.cdc.gov), January 17, 2012; "Stroke and African Americans," by the Office of Minority Health (minority health.hhs.gov), part of the U.S. Department of Health and Human Services, September 5, 2012; "Stroke and Asian Americans," by the Office of Minority Health, September 5, 2012; and "Stroke and Hispanic Americans," by the Office of Minority Health, September 5, 2012.

- California has the largest population of American Indians and Alaska Natives (696,600), followed by Oklahoma (401,100), and Arizona (334,700). Alaska has the highest proportion of American Indians and Alaska Natives in its populations (20%), followed by Oklahoma and New Mexico (11% each). Los Angeles County is the county with the most American Indians and Alaska Natives (154,000).

- A language other than English is spoken at home by 25% of American Indians and Alaska Natives aged 5 years and older.

- A high school diploma is held by 76% of American Indians and Alaska Natives over age 25; 14 percent have a bachelor's degree or higher. The poverty rate of people who report American Indian and Alaska Native race only is 25%.

- Approximately 177,000 American Indians and Alaska Natives are veterans.

American Indian and Alaska Native Heart Disease and Stroke Facts

- Heart disease is the first and stroke the sixth leading cause of death Among American Indians and Alaska Natives.

- The heart disease death rate was 20 percent greater and the stroke death rate 14 percent greater among American Indians and Alaska Natives (1996–1998) than among all U.S. races (1997) after adjusting for misreporting of American Indian and Alaska Native race on state death certificates.

- The highest heart disease death rates are located primarily in South Dakota and North Dakota, Wisconsin, and Michigan.

- Counties with the highest stroke death rates are primarily in Alaska, Washington, Idaho, Montana, Wyoming, South Dakota, Wisconsin, and Minnesota.

- American Indians and Alaska Natives die from heart diseases at younger ages than other racial and ethnic groups in the United States. Thirty-six percent of those who die of heart disease die before age 65.

- Diabetes is an extremely important risk factor for cardiovascular disease among American Indians.

- Cigarette smoking, a risk factor for heart disease and stroke, is highest in the Northern Plains (44.1%) and Alaska (39.0%) and lowest in the Southwest (21.2%) among American Indians and Alaska Natives.

Stroke and African Americans

African American adults are 60 percent more likely to have a stroke than their white adult counterparts. Further, men are 60% more likely to die from a stroke than their white adult counterparts. See Tables 6.1 and 6.2.

Analysis from a Centers for Disease Control and Prevention health interview survey also reveals that African-American stroke survivors are more likely to become disabled and have difficulty with activities of daily living than their non-Hispanic white counterparts.

Table 6.1. Age-Adjusted Percentages of Stroke among Persons 18 Years of Age and over, 2010

	African American	White	African American/ White Ratio
Men and Women	3.9	2.5	1.6
Men	4.0	2.7	1.5
Women	3.9	2.3	1.7

Source: CDC 2011. Summary Health Statistics for U.S. Adults: 2010. Table 2. http://www.cdc.gov/nchs/data/series/sr_10/sr10_252.pdf

Table 6.2. Age-Adjusted Stroke Death Rates per 100,000 (2009)

	Non-Hispanic Black	Non-Hispanic White	Non-Hispanic Black/ Non-Hispanic White Ratio
Men	61.6	38.1	1.6
Women	51.2	37.0	1.4
Total	55.7	37.8	1.5

Source: CDC, 2012. National Vital Statistics Report. Vol. 60, No. 3 Table 17. http://www.cdc.gov/nchs/data/nvsr/nvsr60/nvsr60_03.pdf

Stroke and Asian Americans

Overall, Asians Americans adults are less likely than white adults to die from a stroke. In general, Asian-American adults have lower rates of being overweight or obese, lower rates of hypertension, and they are less likely to be current cigarette smokers. See Tables 6.3 and 6.4.

Table 6.3. Age-Adjusted Percentages of Stroke among Persons 18 Years of Age and over, 2010

Asian	Non-Hispanic White	Asian/Non-Hispanic White Ratio
2.0	2.5	0.8

Source: CDC 2011. Summary Health Statistics for U.S. Adults: 2010. Table 2. http://www.cdc.gov/nchs/data/series/sr_10/sr10_252.pdf

Table 6.4. Age-Adjusted Stroke Death Rates per 100,000 (2009)

	Asians/Pacific Islanders	Non-Hispanic White	Asians/Pacific Islanders/Non-Hispanic White Ratio
Men	34.1	38.1	0.9
Women	29.6	37.0	0.8
Total	31.6	37.8	0.8

Source: CDC 2012. National Vital Statistics Report. Vol.60, No. 03 Table 16–17. http://www.cdc.gov/nchs/data/nvsr/nvsr60/nvsr60_03.pdf

Table 6.5. Age-Adjusted Percentages of Stroke among Persons 18 Years of Age and over, 2010

	Hispanics/Latinos	Non-Hispanic White	Hispanic/Non-Hispanic White Ratio
Men and Women	2.6	2.5	1.0
Men	2.4	2.7	0.9
Women	2.8	2.3	1.2

Source: CDC 2011. Summary Health Statistics for U.S. Adults: 2010. Table 2. http://www.cdc.gov/nchs/data/series/sr_10/sr10_252.pdf

Table 6.6. Age-Adjusted Stroke Death Rates per 100,000 (2009)

	Hispanic	Non-Hispanic White	Hispanic/Non-Hispanic White Ratio
Men	30.9	38.1	0.8
Women	28.0	37.0	0.8
Total	29.5	37.8	0.8

Source: CDC, 2012. National Vital Statistic Report. Vol. 60, No. 03 Table 17. http://www.cdc.gov/nchs/data/nvsr/nvsr60/nvsr60_03.pdf

Stroke and Hispanic Americans

Hispanic American adults have similar risks of suffering from a stroke as their non-Hispanic White adult counterparts. They are less likely to die from a stroke and they have lower rates of hypertension and high cholesterol as non-Hispanic white adults. However, Hispanic women are 20 percent more likely to have a stroke than non-Hispanic White Women, according to one survey. See Tables 6.5 and 6.6.

Chapter 7

Geography and Stroke: The Stroke Belt

What is the stroke belt?

The stroke belt is an area of the southeastern United States where people are much more likely to die of stroke than in the rest of the country. People in the stroke belt have, on average, a 50% higher risk of dying from stroke than people who live in other regions. This trend was first noticed in the 1950s; since then the specific states have changed, but the general area has remained the same.

Some researchers have called North Carolina, South Carolina, and Georgia the "buckle" of the stroke belt: For some age groups in these states, death rates from stroke are twice as high as in the rest of the nation.

Why is the stroke rate so much higher in certain areas?

Many reasons for the existence of the stroke belt have been proposed, but so far none of these theories have been able to completely explain it. It is likely that the stroke belt is the result of a combination of genes and lifestyle factors such as smoking, lack of exercise, and diets high in saturated fat. This leads to higher rates of stroke risk factors (such as high blood pressure) and therefore strokes. It seems that the high death rates from stroke in the stroke belt are because people in these areas are more likely to have a stroke, not because they receive worse treatment.

"Geography: Stroke Belt," Office on Women's Health, U.S. Department of Health and Human Services (www.womenshealth.gov), 2010.

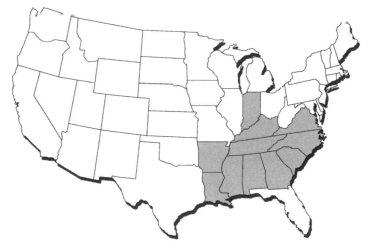

Figure 7.1. *The stroke belt states.*

It has long been thought that control of high blood pressure, one of the strongest risk factors for stroke, could be the reason the stroke belt exists. People in this region might be more likely to receive less treatment or have their blood pressure under control. However, a recent large study has cast doubt on parts of the high blood pressure theory. The REGARDS trial looked at nearly 12,000 patients (half were women) and found that in both African Americans and whites, awareness of high blood pressure in the stroke belt was the same as in other regions, and the stroke belt had better treatment and control of blood pressure. High blood pressure is more common in the south, however, (especially in African-American women) and this likely contributes to the higher stroke rates in the region.

The effects of the stroke belt on a person's risk may happen mostly in childhood: One study looked at 18,000 people (56% were women) and compared those who had lived in the stroke belt in childhood with those who had never lived there. They found that living in the stroke belt as a child was associated with a higher risk of stroke (30% higher in women), even if the person later moved away. This risk was about the same in women who had lived there during childhood and then moved away as in people who remained there all their lives, suggesting that, whatever the specific reasons for the increase in stroke risk, most of the damage is done during childhood. This may be because changes in the body caused by the stroke belt lifestyle have a permanent effect on your risk, or simply because dietary and exercise habits you acquire as a child are likely to be continued for the rest of your life, regardless of where you live.

I live in the stroke belt; what can I do to protect myself?

People living in the stroke belt need to be especially conscious of their risk factors for stroke, such as high blood pressure, high cholesterol, obesity, and smoking.

Chapter 8

Statistics on Stroke in the United States

Stroke Facts

Stroke is a leading cause of death in the United States, killing nearly 130,000 Americans each year—that's 1 of every 18 deaths.

A stroke, sometimes called a brain attack, occurs when a clot blocks the blood supply to the brain or when a blood vessel in the brain bursts.

Someone in the United States has a stroke every 40 seconds. Every four minutes, someone dies of stroke.

Every year, about 795,000 people in the United States have a stroke. About 610,000 of these are first or new strokes; 185,000 are recurrent strokes.

Stroke is an important cause of disability. Stroke reduces mobility in more than half of stroke survivors age 65 and over.

Stroke costs the nation $54 billion annually, including the cost of health care services, medications, and lost productivity.

You can't control some stroke risk factors, like heredity, age, gender, and ethnicity. Some medical conditions—including high blood pressure, high cholesterol, heart disease, diabetes, overweight or obesity, and previous stroke or transient ischemic attack (TIA)—can also raise your stroke risk. Avoiding smoking and drinking too much alcohol, eating

This chapter contains text from "Stroke Fact Sheet," by the Centers for Disease Control and Prevention (CDC, www.cdc.gov), October 17, 2012, and excerpted from "Hospitalization for Stroke in U.S. Hospitals, 1989–2009," by the National Center for Health Statistics, Centers for Disease Control and Prevention (CDC, www.cdc.gov), May 9, 2012.

a balanced diet, and getting exercise are all choices you can make to reduce your risk.

Common Stroke Warning Signs and Symptoms

- Sudden numbness or weakness of the face, arm, or leg—especially on one side of the body
- Sudden confusion, trouble speaking or understanding
- Sudden trouble seeing in one or both eyes
- Sudden trouble walking, dizziness, loss of balance or coordination
- Sudden severe headache with no known cause

Hospitalization for Stroke

An estimated 7 million Americans have had a stroke (cerebrovascular disease). In 2008, direct medical costs of stroke were about $18.8 billion, with almost half of this amount being for hospitalization. Stroke was the fourth leading U.S. cause of death in 2009 and 2010.

Numerous public health campaigns have sought to educate the public on how to lower stroke risk: for example, by increasing physical activity, controlling weight, stopping smoking, and taking medication to lower high blood pressure and high cholesterol. This text examines nationally representative data from 1989 to 2009 to see how inpatient hospital care for stroke has changed.

Has the rate of hospitalization for stroke changed from 1989 to 2009?

The rate of hospitalization for stroke increased from 32.4 to 34.9 per 10,000 population from 1989 to 1999, but by 2009 the rate had decreased to 31.8 per 10,000.

The stroke hospitalization rate increased 5% for those aged 65–74 from 1989 to 1999, and then decreased 20% from 1999 to 2009. For those aged 75 and over, the rates did not change significantly from 1989 to 1999, but from 1999 to 2009 the rate decreased 24% for those aged 75–84 and 20% for those 85 and over.

Have the characteristics of persons hospitalized for stroke changed between 1989 and 2009?

- There were close to 800,000 hospitalizations for stroke in 1989 and almost 1 million in both 1999 and 2009.

- In 1989, the proportion of those hospitalized for stroke who were male was 43%, but by 2009 the share of males and females was similar.

- The average age of stroke patients (70–71 years) was similar in 1989, 1999, and 2009.

The percentage of stroke hospitalizations with a comorbidity (secondary diagnosis) of diabetes rose from 18% in 1989 to 23% in 1999, but remained the same from 1999 to 2009. Stroke hospitalizations with a comorbidity of hypertension increased from 37% in 1989 to 55% in 1999.

In 2009 the percentage with hypertension was 58%, but this was not a significant change from1999. These conditions, as well as atrial fibrillation (which did not change over this time period), have been shown to increase the risk of stroke.

What is the relationship between age and hospitalization for stroke?

- The rate of hospitalization for stroke for the population aged 65 and over increased with age in 1989, 1999, and 2009.

- The rate of hospitalization for stroke for those aged 85 and over was three times the rate for those aged 65–74 in 1989, and in 1999 and 2009 it was more than two and one half times greater for the group aged 85 and over compared with those aged 65–74.

Did the length of hospital stay for stroke inpatients change from 1989 to 2009?

- The average length of stay for stroke patients was 10.2 days in 1989, 5.4 days in 1999, and 5.3 days in 2009.

- From 1989 to 1999, the average length of stay for stroke patients decreased 47%. During this same period, the length of stay for all hospitalizations decreased 23%.

- From 2000 to 2009, the average length of stay for all patients, as well as for stroke patients, did not change significantly.

Chapter 9

Recent Research on Stroke

Chapter Contents

Section 9.1

Researchers Investigate Genes Involved in Brain Repair after Stroke

From the National Institute of Neurological Disorders and Stroke (NINDS, www.ninds.nih.gov), part of the National Institutes of Health, January 28, 2011.

A stroke can kill millions of brain cells within minutes, leaving an area of nonviable brain tissue surrounded by a halo of surviving cells. A fraction of these surviving neurons grows vigorously, sprouting new branches (or axons), making new connections and contributing to recovery. Identifying what drives this sprouting may lead to therapies that improve recovery.

Toward that end, researchers funded by the National Institute of Neurological Disorders and Stroke (NINDS) compared the gene activity patterns of sprouting and non-sprouting neurons in rats after a stroke. They also examined how these gene activity patterns changed with age.

"We found that there are unique genetic programs associated with the growth of new axonal connections after a stroke, and that these programs change dramatically with age," said senior author S. Thomas Carmichael, MD, PhD, an associate professor of neurology at the David Geffen School of Medicine, University of California, Los Angeles.

The study was published in *Nature Neuroscience.*

Until now, researchers were unable to sort through the jumble of axons in the brain and separate the neurons that sprout after a stroke from their non-sprouting neighbors. Dr. Carmichael and his team developed a way to find newly sprouted axons by using colorful tracers that are absorbed at the axon tip. They injected one tracer into the brain at the time of stroke, followed by a distinct tracer at the same site one to three weeks later. Axons that took up both tracers must have been present at the time of stroke and persisted afterward. But axons that took up only the second tracer must have sprouted after the stroke.

Next, the researchers used a laser to extract the sprouting and non-sprouting neurons, and measured the activity of thousands of genes inside the cells. They also compared the sprouting response in rats at a few months old to rats at age two, considered elderly in rat years.

The largest changes in gene activity occurred in young animals within one week after stroke. However, at all ages and time points studied, the sprouting neurons activated or deactivated hundreds of genes, many of which have been previously implicated in brain development.

In follow-up experiments, the researchers analyzed the role of several genes whose activity increased with sprouting in the older rats. Those genes are of interest because most strokes occur in older people, with the risk doubling each decade between 55 and 85.

"We chose to focus on genes that have very different functions and seem to work at different control points in the sprouting process," Dr. Carmichael said. Three of those genes were ATRX, IGF1, and Lingo1.

ATRX: This gene is known to support neuronal survival and help neurons reach their proper locations in the developing brain. The researchers found that in the aged brain ATRX supports axon sprouting. Blocking ATRX function after a stroke blocked the sprouting response.

IGF1: This growth factor supports axon sprouting during brain development. But the researchers found that blocking IGF1 function one week after stroke not only kept neurons from sprouting, it killed them. Until now experts thought that neuronal death ended within a few days of stroke, but this shows that neurons continue to struggle for survival for at least a week, Dr. Carmichael said.

Lingo1: The Lingo1 protein inhibits neuronal growth, and in animal studies blocking Lingo1 can improve recovery from spinal cord injuries. Paradoxically, Lingo1 is one of the genes that become more active in sprouting neurons after a stroke. An antibody that blocks Lingo1 increased sprouting.

These three genes are promising targets for drug therapy, but there are challenges ahead, according to Dr. Carmichael. First, it is unclear how such drugs would be delivered. Repeated injections into the brain would be difficult and potentially harmful for stroke patients, who are often medically unstable, he said. However, the study shows that a biopolymer implant can steadily release molecules (such as the Lingo1 antibody) into the rat brain over several weeks.

Another step is to test whether changing the activity of genes like Lingo1 can restore movement, sensation, and other functions after a stroke. These experiments are underway in animal models, Dr. Carmichael said.

"We hope that if we block growth inhibitors or turn on growth promoters, the new connections that are formed will be beneficial. But that might not always be the case. The adult brain probably has systems in place to control the formation of unneeded or excessive connections," he said.

Source: Li S et al. "An age-related sprouting transcriptome provides molecular control of axonal sprouting after stroke." *Nature Neuroscience*, December 2010, Vol. 13, pp. 1496–1504.

Section 9.2

Stem Cell Therapy and Stroke

"Repairing the Nervous System with Stem Cells," by the
National Institutes of Health (NIH, www.nih.gov), March 19, 2009.

Diseases of the nervous system, including congenital disorders, cancers, and degenerative diseases, affect millions of people of all ages. Congenital disorders occur when the brain or spinal cord does not form correctly during development. Cancers of the nervous system result from the uncontrolled spread of aberrant cells. Degenerative diseases occur when the nervous system loses functioning of nerve cells. Most of the advances in stem cell research have been directed at treating degenerative diseases. While many treatments aim to limit the damage of these diseases, in some cases scientists believe that damage can be reversed by replacing lost cells with new ones derived from cells that can mature into nerve cells, called neural stem cells. Research that uses stem cells to treat nervous system disorders remains an area of great promise and challenge to demonstrate that cell-replacement therapy can restore lost function.

Strategies to Repair the Nervous System

The nervous system is a complex organ made up of nerve cells (also called neurons) and glial cells, which surround and support neurons. Neurons send signals that affect numerous functions including thought processes and movement. One type of glial cell, the oligodendrocyte, acts to speed up the signals of neurons that extend over long distances, such as in the spinal cord. The loss of any of these cell types may have catastrophic results on brain function.

Although reports dating back as early as the 1960s pointed toward the possibility that new nerve cells are formed in adult mammalian brains, this knowledge was not applied in the context of curing devastating brain diseases until the 1990s. While earlier medical research focused on limiting damage once it had occurred, in recent years researchers have been working hard to find out if the cells that can give rise to new neurons can be coaxed to restore brain function. New neurons in the adult brain arise from slowly-dividing cells that appear to be the remnants of stem cells that existed during fetal brain development. Since some of these adult cells still retain the ability to generate both neurons and glia, they are referred to as adult neural stem cells.

These findings are exciting because they suggest that the brain may contain a built-in mechanism to repair itself. Unfortunately, these new neurons are only generated in a few sites in the brain and turn into only a few specialized types of nerve cells. Although there are many different neuronal cell types in the brain, we now know that these new neurons can correctly assist brain function. The discovery of these cells has spurred further research into the characteristics of neural stem cells from the fetus and the adult, mostly using rodents and primates as model species. The hope is that these cells may be able to replenish those that are functionally lost in human degenerative diseases such as Parkinson Disease, Huntington Disease, and amyotrophic lateral sclerosis (ALS, also known as Lou Gehrig disease), as well as from brain and spinal cord injuries that result from stroke or trauma.

Scientists are applying these new stem cell discoveries in two ways in their experiments. First, they are using current knowledge of normal brain development to modulate stem cells that are harvested and grown in culture. Researchers can then transplant these cultured cells into the brain of an animal model and allow the brain's own signals to differentiate the stem cells into neurons or glia. Alternatively, the stem cells can be induced to differentiate into neurons and glia while in the culture dish, before being transplanted into the brain. Much progress has been made the last several years with human embryonic stem (ES) cells that can differentiate into all cell types in the body. While ES cells can be maintained in culture for relatively long periods of time without differentiating, they usually must be coaxed through many more steps of differentiation to produce the desired cell types. Recent studies, however, suggest that ES cells may differentiate into neurons in a more straightforward manner than many other cell types.

Second, scientists are identifying growth (trophic) factors that are normally produced and used by the developing and adult brain. They are using these factors to minimize damage to the brain and to activate the patient's own stem cells to repair damage that has occurred. Each of these strategies is being aggressively pursued to identify the most offective treatments for degenerative diseases. Most of these studies have been carried out initially with animal stem cells and recipients to determine their likelihood of success. Still, much more research is necessary to develop stem cell therapies that will be useful for treating brain and spinal cord disease in the same way that hematopoietic stem cell therapies are routinely used for immune system replacement.

The majority of stem cell studies of neurological disease have used rats and mice, since these models are convenient to use and are well-characterized biologically. If preliminary studies with rodent stem cells are successful, scientists will attempt to transplant human stem cells into rodents. Studies may then be carried out in primates (e.g., monkeys) to offer insight into how humans might respond to neurological treatment. Human studies are rarely undertaken until these other experiments have shown promising results. While human transplant studies have been carried out for decades in the case of Parkinson disease, animal research continues to provide improved strategies to generate an abundant supply of transplantable cells.

Stroke and Stem Cell Research

Stroke affects about 750,000 patients per year in the United States and is the most common cause of disability in adults. A stroke occurs when blood flow to the brain is disrupted. As a consequence, cells in affected brain regions die from insufficient amounts of oxygen. The treatment of stroke with anti-clotting drugs has dramatically improved the odds of patient recovery. However, in many patients the damage cannot be prevented, and the patient may permanently lose the functions of affected areas of the brain. For these patients, researchers are now considering stem cells as a way to repair the damaged brain regions. This problem is made more challenging because the damage in stroke may be widespread and may affect many cell types and connections.

However, researchers from Sweden recently observed that strokes in rats cause the brain's own stem cells to divide and give rise to new neurons. However, these neurons, which survived only a couple of weeks, are few in number compared to the extent of damage caused. A group from the University of Tokyo added a growth factor, bFGF, into the brains of rats after stroke and showed that the hippocampus was able to generate large numbers of new neurons. The researchers found evidence that these new neurons were actually making connections with other neurons. These and other results suggest that future stroke treatments may be able to coax the brain's own stem cells to make replacement neurons.

Taking an alternative approach, another group attempted transplantation as a means to treat the loss of brain mass after a severe stroke. By adding stem cells onto a polymer scaffold that they implanted into the stroke-damaged brains of mice, the researchers demonstrated that the seeded stem cells differentiated into neurons and that the polymer scaffold reduced scarring. Two groups transplanted human fetal stem cells in independent studies into the brains of stroke-affected rodents; these stem cells not only survived but migrated to the damaged areas of the brain. These studies increase our knowledge of how stem cells are attracted to diseased areas of the brain.

There is also increasing evidence from numerous animal disease models that stem cells are actively drawn to brain damage. Once they reach these damaged areas, they have been shown to exert beneficial effects such as reducing brain inflammation or supporting nerve cells. It is hoped that, once these mechanisms are better understood, this stem cell recruitment can potentially be exploited to mobilize a patient's own stem cells.

Similar lines of research are being considered with other disorders such as Huntington Disease and certain congenital defects. While much attention has been called to the treatment of Alzheimer disease, it is still not clear if stem cells hold the key to its treatment. But despite the fact that much basic work remains and many fundamental questions are yet to be answered, researchers are hopeful that repair for once-incurable nervous system disorders may be amenable to stem cell based therapies.

Considerable progress has been made the last few years in our understanding of stem cell biology and devising sources of cells for transplantation. New methods are also being developed for cell delivery and targeting to affected areas of the body. These advances have fueled optimism that new treatments will come for millions of persons who suffer from neurological disorders. But it is the current task of scientists to bring these methods from the laboratory bench to the clinic in a scientifically sound and ethically acceptable fashion.

Section 9.3

Technology and Its Role in Stroke Care

Excerpted from "Mind Games: Computerized Cognitive Exercise Is Big Business. But Do the Industry's Claims Stand Up?" by Amy Paturel, *Neurology Now,* July/August 2010. © 2010 American Academy of Neurology. Reprinted with permission.

Developed primarily for the aging brain, computerized brain training programs are booming, so to speak. With the first wave of baby boomers now past 60, scientists (and manufacturers) are working around the clock to come up with creative mental workouts to help keep the brain in top shape. Computerized brain workouts like Happy-Neuron, CogniFit, Lumosity, and Posit Science's Brain Fitness Program are becoming increasingly popular. According to business estimates, Americans are buying the industry's claims, to the tune of $225 million per year—a figure that is expected to grow to $2 billion by 2015.

Since there are few drug options available to protect cognition, boomers aren't the only people relying on these programs for their cognitive health. People with Alzheimer's disease and dementia, multiple sclerosis, Parkinson's disease, and other neurologic conditions—along with their caregivers—are hoping that brain training can improve cognition.

"Computer programs have been used for 25 to 30 years for people who have had strokes or other kinds of brain impairments. So it's not new," says Elizabeth Zelinski, PhD, professor of gerontology and psychology at the Leonard Davis School of Gerontology at the University of Southern California. "What you're trying to do is establish new connections in parts of the brain that haven't been injured, or in some cases, you're trying to reinforce old connections."

The goal is for people to start with activities that are mildly challenging and continually increase the level of difficulty—all while having fun. Some anecdotal and study data are encouraging, suggesting that computerized brain training can in fact improve memory and attention in older adults.

Most programs, such as Posit Science's Brain Fitness Program, are divided into time blocks so patients at all levels of cognitive function can receive tailored training.

Part Two

Types of Stroke

Chapter 10

Ischemic Stroke

Chapter Contents

Section 10.1

What Is Ischemic Stroke?

Ischemic (is-skeem-ic) stroke occurs when an artery to the brain is blocked. The brain depends on its arteries to bring fresh blood from the heart and lungs. The blood carries oxygen and nutrients to the brain, and takes away carbon dioxide and cellular waste. If an artery is blocked, the brain cells (neurons) cannot make enough energy and will eventually stop working. If the artery remains blocked for more than a few minutes, the brain cells may die. This is why immediate medical treatment is critical.

What Causes It?

Ischemic stroke can be caused by several different kinds of diseases. The most common problem is narrowing of the arteries in the neck or head. This is most often caused by atherosclerosis, or gradual cholesterol deposition. If the arteries become too narrow, blood cells may collect and form blood clots. These blood clots can block the artery where they are formed (thrombosis), or can dislodge and become trapped in arteries closer to the brain (embolism). Another cause of stroke is blood clots in the heart, which can occur as a result of irregular heartbeat (for example, atrial fibrillation), heart attack, or abnormalities of the heart valves. While these are the most common causes of ischemic stroke, there are many other possible causes. Examples include use of street drugs, traumatic injury to the blood vessels of the neck, or disorders of blood clotting.

Types of Ischemic Stroke

Ischemic stroke can be divided into two main types: Thrombotic and embolic.

A thrombotic stroke occurs when diseased or damaged cerebral arteries become blocked by the formation of a blood clot within the brain.

Clinically referred to as cerebral thrombosis or cerebral infarction, this type of event is responsible for almost 50 percent of all strokes. Cerebral thrombosis can also be divided into an additional two categories that correlate to the location of the blockage within the brain: Large-vessel thrombosis and small-vessel thrombosis. Large-vessel thrombosis is the term used when the blockage is in one of the brain's larger blood-supplying arteries such as the carotid or middle cerebral, while small-vessel thrombosis involves one (or more) of the brain's smaller, yet deeper, penetrating arteries. This latter type of stroke is also called a lacunar stroke.

An embolic stroke is also caused by a clot within an artery, but in this case the clot (or emboli) forms somewhere other than in the brain itself. Often from the heart, these emboli will travel in the bloodstream until they become lodged and cannot travel any farther. This naturally restricts the flow of blood to the brain and results in near-immediate physical and neurological deficits.

Who Gets It?

Ischemic stroke is by far the most common kind of stroke, accounting for about 88 percent of all strokes. Stroke can affect people of all ages, including children. Many people with ischemic strokes are older (60 or more years old), and the risk of stroke increases with age. Each year, about 55,000 more women than men have a stroke, and it is more common among African Americans than members of other ethnic groups. Many people with stroke have other problems or conditions which put them at higher risk for stroke, such as high blood pressure (hypertension), heart disease, smoking, or diabetes.

Section 10.2

Carotid Artery Dissection

What is carotid artery dissection?

The four carotid arteries, two on each side of the neck (an internal and an external carotid), deliver blood from the aorta (the heart's main artery) to the brain, the eyes, the face, and other structures in the head. The carotid arteries can be felt on each side of the lower neck, immediately below the angle of the jaw.

The artery walls are made up of three layers of different types of tissue, each with a specific function. Dissection occurs when a tear in the artery wall allows blood to leak between the layers and separate them. The effect has been described as what happens to a piece of plywood that gets wet.

What causes carotid artery dissection?

Certain medical conditions such as Marfan syndrome—a genetic connective tissue disease—fibromuscular dysplasia or atherosclerosis (the accumulation of fatty plaque in the artery walls) put individuals at risk for developing carotid artery dissection. Carotid artery dissection in these patients is called spontaneous, meaning that it occurs without trauma to the head or neck.

Carotid artery dissection also can occur in the general population as a result of blunt trauma injury to the neck, such as a car accident or a fall, or from hyperextension of the neck in sports or exercise. The incidence of carotid artery dissection as a result of blunt injury (mainly high-speed car accidents) ranges from less than 1 percent to 3 percent, according to a recent study.

High blood pressure and smoking increase the risk for both types of carotid artery dissection. Some cases of carotid artery dissection also have been reported after invasive diagnostic procedures.

How does carotid artery dissection develop?

Carotid artery dissection begins as a tear in one layer of the artery wall. Blood leaks through this tear and spreads between the layers of the wall. As the blood collects in the area of the dissection, it forms a clot that limits blood flow through the artery. If the clot is large enough to completely block blood flow, the result can be a stroke. Equally dangerous, pieces of the clot can break off and travel up through the bloodstream to become trapped in the smaller arteries in the brain which can limit the blood flow to a region of the brain and cause a stroke.

Depending on where the dissection occurs in the artery, it may cause the artery to bulge in the area where the blood is pooling. This bulging, blood-filled area is called a pseudoaneurysm. A pseudoaneurysm can cause symptoms of stroke by pressing on surrounding brain structures.

What are the symptoms of carotid artery dissection?

Sometimes a stroke is the first sign of carotid artery dissection and emergency treatment is required. More commonly, symptoms develop over a period of hours or days, even in patients who have traumatic injuries. Symptoms are general rather than specific and include headache, neck and face pain (especially pain around the eyes), vision disturbances such as double vision or a droopy eyelid, a sudden decrease in sense of taste, and weakness on one side of the body.

Stroke can develop hours, days, or even a week after these symptoms begin. This is the most serious risk of carotid artery dissection.

How is carotid artery dissection diagnosed?

When a patient comes to the doctor's office or the emergency room with any of the symptoms described in the preceding text, the doctor may suspect carotid artery dissection. To accurately diagnose this condition, the doctor can choose from several different imaging technologies to see how well blood is flowing through the carotid arteries.

Helical computed tomography angiography (CTA) is becoming the gold standard for use in trauma patients with symptoms of carotid artery dissection. This is a noninvasive type of imaging that uses computed tomography (CT) technology and a contrast material to provide an accurate, three-dimensional picture of the arteries on a computer screen.

Magnetic resonance angiography (MRA) or magnetic resonance imaging (MRI) are additional, very accurate, noninvasive imaging techniques that can be used for diagnosing carotid artery dissection. They use a magnetic field and radio waves to provide pictures of the carotid arteries.

In addition to blood flow, these technologies can show changes in the dimension of the carotid artery, blood in the wall of the artery, and changes to structures surrounding the blood vessel. CTA is especially useful because it can create cross-sectional images of the blood vessel that will show separation of the layers of the vessel wall that is characteristic of dissection. These studies can also assess the brain and determine if there has been damage to brain tissue as a result of the dissection.

Doppler ultrasonography (DUS) is gaining popularity as a useful tool in identifying carotid artery dissection. This technology is now widely available in the hospital setting. Doppler ultrasound can detect abnormal blood flow in a dissected artery. DUS has the advantages of being fast, noninvasive, and easy to use at the patient's bedside.

As these new technologies have developed and improved, the use of conventional angiography for diagnosing carotid artery dissection has decreased.

This type of angiography uses a contrast dye and X-ray to image the blood vessels. It is not as accurate as the newer imaging technologies, is invasive, and has a 1 percent risk of complications.

How is carotid artery dissection treated?

In some cases, carotid artery dissection is not diagnosed until after a stroke has developed. In those patients, treating stroke to prevent lasting effects is the goal.

When a patient comes into the doctor's office or the emergency room with symptoms of carotid artery dissection without stroke, preventing stroke is the primary treatment goal. Appropriate treatment for an individual patient depends on whether the patient has an underlying disorder such as Marfan syndrome or has experienced trauma, where and how the injury occurred, and where the patient has other injuries or medical conditions.

First-line treatment for carotid artery dissection usually is anticoagulation or medication to thin the blood and prevent the formation of blood clots. Heparin given intravenously (through the vein) followed by warfarin that is taken orally are the most common therapies used. These medications prevent blood clot formation and thus can help protect against stroke. They usually are prescribed for three to six months, but some patients may require longer treatment.

Anti-platelet drugs such as aspirin, ticlopidine, or clopidogrel sometimes are used in combination with or instead of warfarin. These drugs prevent blood clot formation by a different mechanism than the anticoagulants and can be equally effective. There is no scientific evidence yet that one class of drugs is better than the other for preventing clot formation in patients with carotid dissection.

Those patients who are unable to take either anticoagulants or antiplatelet agents, those who are on warfarin but continue to have symptoms such as vision disturbances or weakness, or those who have very low blood flow to the brain due to carotid artery dissection may need a procedure to try and correct the process of dissection. Normally, these are minimally invasive treatments that are performed through the blood vessels. Angioplasty (repairing the dissected section of artery) or placement of a stent (a mesh-like device that holds the artery open) are two endovascular procedures that are used to treat carotid artery dissection. They frequently are used together to provide the longest-lasting treatment. Cleveland Clinic interventional cardiologist, neurointerventionalist, and vascular surgeons perform over 200 endovascular procedures every year on patients with carotid artery disease.

What is the outlook following carotid artery dissection?

For spontaneous carotid artery dissection, the mortality is less than 5 percent. The risk for lasting neurological impairment from the disease is considerably higher. More than half of patients with spontaneous carotid artery dissection develop a stroke, sometimes delayed by hours or days. Even so, an estimated 75 percent of patients with spontaneous carotid artery dissection make a good recovery.

In patients with dissection following trauma (car accident, sports injury, etc.) the stroke rate ranges from 3 to 44 percent, depending on the severity of injury. An estimated 37 to 58 percent of patients with dissection following trauma have lasting neurological problems. They also have a higher mortality rate compared with patients who have spontaneous carotid artery dissection.

Following the first incidence of carotid artery dissection, patients have a 1 percent risk of recurrence per year over the next 10 years. Risk of recurrence is higher in younger patients than older patients, but younger patients also respond better to treatment and have a better outlook. Some patients have reported persistent headache after carotid artery dissection, lasting years after the event.

People who have had carotid artery dissection should see a vascular specialist for a CTA, DUS, or other imaging to assess the severity and extension of the dissection. This imaging is normally repeated several months later to have the dissection re-evaluated for either progression, resolution, or stability of the injury.

How can I prevent carotid artery dissection?

If you have an underlying disease that increases your risk of carotid artery dissection, it is important that you are under the care of a vascular specialist and follow your doctor's instructions. For other individuals, following the same steps that reduce your risk of heart disease—healthy eating, weight management, exercise, and smoking cessation—can reduce your risk of carotid artery dissection by improving the health of your blood vessels.

Chapter 11

Hemorrhagic Stroke

Chapter Contents

Section 11.1

Intracerebral and Subarachnoid Hemorrhagic Stroke

Intracerebral Hemorrhage

Intracerebral hemorrhage occurs when a diseased blood vessel within the brain bursts, allowing blood to leak inside the brain. (The name means within the cerebrum or brain). The sudden increase in pressure within the brain can cause damage to the brain cells surrounding the blood. If the amount of blood increases rapidly, the sudden buildup in pressure can lead to unconsciousness or death. Intracerebral hemorrhage usually occurs in selected parts of the brain, including the basal ganglia, cerebellum, brain stem, or cortex.

What Causes It?

The most common cause of intracerebral hemorrhage is high blood pressure (hypertension). Since high blood pressure by itself often causes no symptoms, many people with intracranial hemorrhage are not aware that they have high blood pressure, or that it needs to be treated. Less common causes of intracerebral hemorrhage include trauma, infections, tumors, blood clotting deficiencies, and abnormalities in blood vessels (such as arteriovenous malformations).

Who Gets It?

Intracerebral hemorrhage occurs at all ages. The average age is lower than for ischemic stroke. Less common than ischemic strokes, hemorrhagic strokes make up about 12 percent of all strokes.

Subarachnoid Hemorrhage

Subarachnoid hemorrhage occurs when a blood vessel just outside the brain ruptures. The area of the skull surrounding the brain (the subarachnoid space) rapidly fills with blood. A patient with subarachnoid hemorrhage may have a sudden, intense headache, neck pain, and nausea or vomiting. Sometimes this is described as the worst headache of one's life. The sudden buildup of pressure outside the brain may also cause rapid loss of consciousness or death.

What Causes It?

Subarachnoid hemorrhage is most often caused by abnormalities of the arteries at the base of the brain, called cerebral aneurysms. These are small areas of rounded or irregular swellings in the arteries. Where the swelling is most severe, the blood vessel wall becomes weak and prone to rupture.

Who Gets It?

The cause of cerebral aneurysms is not known. They may develop from birth or in childhood and grow very slowly. Some people have multiple aneurysms. Subarachnoid hemorrhage can occur at any age, including in teenagers and young adults and is slightly more common in women than men.

Section 11.2

Cerebral Aneurysm

From "Cerebral Aneurysms Information Page,"
by the National Institute of Neurological Disorders and Stroke
(NINDS, www.ninds.nih.gov), September 14, 2011.

What is a cerebral aneurysm?

A cerebral aneurysm (also known as an intracranial or intracerebral aneurysm) is a weak or thin spot on a blood vessel in the brain that balloons out and fills with blood. The bulging aneurysm can put pressure on a nerve or surrounding brain tissue. It may also leak or rupture, spilling blood into the surrounding tissue (called a hemorrhage). Some cerebral aneurysms, particularly those that are very small, do not bleed or cause other problems. Cerebral aneurysms can occur anywhere in the brain, but most are located along a loop of arteries that run between the underside of the brain and the base of the skull.

What causes a cerebral aneurysm?

Cerebral aneurysms can be congenital, resulting from an inborn abnormality in an artery wall. Cerebral aneurysms are also more common in people with certain genetic diseases, such as connective tissue disorders and polycystic kidney disease, and certain circulatory disorders, such as arteriovenous malformations (snarled tangles of arteries and veins in the brain that disrupt blood flow).

Other causes include trauma or injury to the head, high blood pressure, infection, tumors, atherosclerosis (a blood vessel disease in which fats build up on the inside of artery walls) and other diseases of the vascular system, cigarette smoking, and drug abuse. Some investigators have speculated that oral contraceptives may increase the risk of developing aneurysms.

Aneurysms that result from an infection in the arterial wall are called mycotic aneurysms. Cancer-related aneurysms are often associated with primary or metastatic tumors of the head and neck. Drug abuse, particularly the habitual use of cocaine, can inflame blood vessels and lead to the development of brain aneurysms.

96

How are aneurysms classified?

There are three types of cerebral aneurysm. A saccular aneurysm is a rounded or pouch-like sac of blood that is attached by a neck or stem to an artery or a branch of a blood vessel. Also known as a berry aneurysm (because it resembles a berry hanging from a vine), this most common form of cerebral aneurysm is typically found on arteries at the base of the brain. Saccular aneurysms occur most often in adults. A lateral aneurysm appears as a bulge on one wall of the blood vessel, while a fusiform aneurysm is formed by the widening along all walls of the vessel.

Aneurysms are also classified by size. Small aneurysms are less than 11 millimeters in diameter (about the size of a large pencil eraser), larger aneurysms are 11–25 millimeters (about the width of a dime), and giant aneurysms are greater than 25 millimeters in diameter (more than the width of a quarter).

Who is at risk?

Brain aneurysms can occur in anyone, at any age. They are more common in adults than in children and slightly more common in women than in men. People with certain inherited disorders are also at higher risk.

All cerebral aneurysms have the potential to rupture and cause bleeding within the brain. The incidence of reported ruptured aneurysm is about 10 in every 100,000 persons per year (about 27,000 individuals per year in the United States), most commonly in people between ages 30 and 60 years. Possible risk factors for rupture include hypertension, alcohol abuse, drug abuse (particularly cocaine), and smoking. In addition, the condition and size of the aneurysm affects the risk of rupture.

What are the dangers?

Aneurysms may burst and bleed into the brain, causing serious complications, including hemorrhagic stroke, permanent nerve damage, or death. Once it has burst, the aneurysm may burst again and bleed into the brain, and additional aneurysms may also occur. More commonly, rupture may cause a subarachnoid hemorrhage—bleeding into the space between the skull bone and the brain. A delayed but serious complication of subarachnoid hemorrhage is hydrocephalus, in which the excessive buildup of cerebrospinal fluid in the skull dilates fluid pathways called ventricles that can swell and press on the brain tissue. Another delayed postrupture complication is vasospasm, in which other blood vessels in the brain contract and limit blood flow to vital areas of the brain. This reduced blood flow can cause stroke or tissue damage.

What are the symptoms?

Most cerebral aneurysms do not show symptoms until they either become very large or burst. Small, unchanging aneurysms generally will not produce symptoms, whereas a larger aneurysm that is steadily growing may press on tissues and nerves. Symptoms may include pain above and behind the eye; numbness, weakness, or paralysis on one side of the face; dilated pupils; and vision changes. When an aneurysm hemorrhages, an individual may experience a sudden and extremely severe headache, double vision, nausea, vomiting, stiff neck, and/or loss of consciousness. Individuals usually describe the headache as "the worst headache of my life" and it is generally different in severity and intensity from other headaches people may experience. Sentinel or warning headaches may result from an aneurysm that leaks for days to weeks prior to rupture. Only a minority of individuals have a sentinel headache prior to aneurysm rupture.

Other signs that a cerebral aneurysm has burst include nausea and vomiting associated with a severe headache, a drooping eyelid, sensitivity to light, and change in mental status or level of awareness. Some individuals may have seizures. Individuals may lose consciousness briefly or go into prolonged coma. People experiencing this worst headache, especially when it is combined with any other symptoms, should seek immediate medical attention.

How are cerebral aneurysms diagnosed?

Most cerebral aneurysms go unnoticed until they rupture or are detected by brain imaging that may have been obtained for another condition. Several diagnostic methods are available to provide information about the aneurysm and the best form of treatment. The tests are usually obtained after a subarachnoid hemorrhage, to confirm the diagnosis of an aneurysm.

Angiography is a dye test used to analyze the arteries or veins. An intracerebral angiogram can detect the degree of narrowing or obstruction of an artery or blood vessel in the brain, head, or neck, and can identify changes in an artery or vein such as a weak spot like an aneurysm. It is used to diagnose stroke and to precisely determine the location, size, and shape of a brain tumor, aneurysm, or blood vessel that has bled. This test is usually performed in a hospital angiography suite. Following the injection of a local anesthetic, a flexible catheter is inserted into an artery and threaded through the body to the affected artery. A small amount of contrast dye (one that is highlighted on x-rays) is released into the bloodstream and allowed to travel into the head and neck. A series of x-rays is taken and changes, if present, are noted.

Computed tomography (CT) of the head is a fast, painless, noninvasive diagnostic tool that can reveal the presence of a cerebral aneurysm and determine, for those aneurysms that have burst, if blood has leaked into the brain. This is often the first diagnostic procedure ordered by a physician following suspected rupture. X-rays of the head are processed by a computer as two-dimensional cross-sectional images, or "slices," of the brain and skull. Occasionally a contrast dye is injected into the bloodstream prior to scanning. This process, called CT angiography, produces sharper, more detailed images of blood flow in the brain arteries. CT is usually conducted at a testing facility or hospital outpatient setting.

Magnetic resonance imaging (MRI) uses computer-generated radio waves and a powerful magnetic field to produce detailed images of the brain and other body structures. Magnetic resonance angiography (MRA) produces more detailed images of blood vessels. The images may be seen as either three-dimensional pictures or two-dimensional cross-slices of the brain and vessels. These painless, noninvasive procedures can show the size and shape of an unruptured aneurysm and can detect bleeding in the brain.

Cerebrospinal fluid analysis may be ordered if a ruptured aneurysm is suspected. Following application of a local anesthetic, a small amount of this fluid (which protects the brain and spinal cord) is removed from the subarachnoid space—located between the spinal cord and the membranes that surround it—by surgical needle and tested to detect any bleeding or brain hemorrhage. In individuals with suspected subarachnoid hemorrhage, this procedure is usually done in a hospital.

How are cerebral aneurysms treated?

Not all cerebral aneurysms burst. Some people with very small aneurysms may be monitored to detect any growth or onset of symptoms and to ensure aggressive treatment of coexisting medical problems and risk factors. Each case is unique, and considerations for treating an unruptured aneurysm include the type, size, and location of the aneurysm; risk of rupture; the individual's age, health, and personal and family medical history; and risk of treatment.

Two surgical options are available for treating cerebral aneurysms, both of which carry some risk to the individual (such as possible damage to other blood vessels, the potential for aneurysm recurrence and rebleeding, and the risk of post-operative stroke).

Microvascular clipping involves cutting off the flow of blood to the aneurysm. Under anesthesia, a section of the skull is removed and the aneurysm is located. The neurosurgeon uses a microscope to isolate the blood vessel that feeds the aneurysm and places a small, metal, clothespin-like clip on the aneurysm's neck, halting its blood supply. The clip remains in the person and prevents the risk of future bleeding. The piece of the skull is then replaced and the scalp is closed. Clipping has been shown to be highly effective, depending on the location, shape, and size of the aneurysm. In general, aneurysms that are completely clipped surgically do not return.

A related procedure is an occlusion, in which the surgeon clamps off (occludes) the entire artery that leads to the aneurysm. This procedure is often performed when the aneurysm has damaged the artery. An occlusion is sometimes accompanied by a bypass, in which a small blood vessel is surgically grafted to the brain artery, rerouting the flow of blood away from the section of the damaged artery.

Endovascular embolization is an alternative to surgery. Once the individual has been anesthetized, the doctor inserts a hollow plastic tube (a catheter) into an artery (usually in the groin) and threads it, using angiography, through the body to the site of the aneurysm. Using a guide wire, detachable coils (spirals of platinum wire) or small latex balloons are passed through the catheter and released into the aneurysm. The coils or balloons fill the aneurysm, block it from circulation, and cause the blood to clot, which effectively destroys the aneurysm. The procedure may need to be performed more than once during the person's lifetime.

People who receive treatment for aneurysm must remain in bed until the bleeding stops. Underlying conditions, such as high blood pressure, should be treated. Other treatment for cerebral aneurysm is symptomatic and may include anticonvulsants to prevent seizures and analgesics to treat headache. Vasospasm can be treated with calcium channel-blocking drugs and sedatives may be ordered if the person is restless. A shunt may be surgically inserted into a ventricle several months following rupture if the buildup of cerebrospinal fluid is causing harmful pressure on surrounding tissue. Individuals who have suffered a subarachnoid hemorrhage often need rehabilitative, speech, and occupational therapy to regain lost function and learn to cope with any permanent disability.

Can cerebral aneurysms be prevented?

There are no known ways to prevent a cerebral aneurysm from forming. People with a diagnosed brain aneurysm should carefully control high blood pressure, stop smoking, and avoid cocaine use or other stimulant drugs. They should also consult with a doctor about the benefits and risks of taking aspirin or other drugs that thin the blood. Women should check with their doctors about the use of oral contraceptives.

What is the prognosis?

An unruptured aneurysm may go unnoticed throughout a person's lifetime. A burst aneurysm, however, may be fatal or could lead to hemorrhagic stroke, vasospasm (the leading cause of disability or death following a burst aneurysm), hydrocephalus, coma, or short-term and/or permanent brain damage.

The prognosis for persons whose aneurysm has burst is largely dependent on the age and general health of the individual, other preexisting neurological conditions, location of the aneurysm, extent of bleeding (and rebleeding), and time between rupture and medical attention. It is estimated that about 40 percent of individuals whose aneurysm has ruptured do not survive the first 24 hours; up to another 25 percent die from complications within 6 months. People who experience subarachnoid hemorrhage may have permanent neurological damage. Other individuals may recover with little or no neurological deficit. Delayed complications from a burst aneurysm may include hydrocephalus and vasospasm. Early diagnosis and treatment are important.

Individuals who receive treatment for an unruptured aneurysm generally require less rehabilitative therapy and recover more quickly than persons whose aneurysm has burst. Recovery from treatment or rupture may take weeks to months.

Results of the International Subarachnoid Aneurysm Trial (ISAT), sponsored primarily by health ministries in the United Kingdom, France, and Canada and announced in October 2002, found that outcome for individuals who are treated with endovascular coiling may be superior in the short-term (1 year) to outcome for those whose aneurysm is treated with surgical clipping. Long-term results of coiling procedures are unknown and investigators need to conduct more research on this topic, since some aneurysms can recur after coiling. Individuals may want to consult a specialist in both endovascular and surgical repair of aneurysms, to help provide greater understanding of treatment options.

What research is being done?

The National Institute of Neurological Disorders and Stroke (NINDS), a component of the National Institutes of Health (NIH) within the U.S. Department of Health and Human Services, is the nation's primary supporter of research on the brain and nervous system. As part of its mission, the NINDS conducts research on intracranial aneurysms and other vascular lesions of the nervous system and supports studies through grants to medical institutions across the country.

The NINDS sponsored the International Study of Unruptured Intracranial Aneurysms, which included more than 4,000 people at 61 sites in the United States, Canada, and Europe. The findings suggest that the risk of rupture for most very small aneurysms (less than 7 millimeters in size) is small. The results also provide a more comprehensive look at these vascular defects and offer guidance to individuals and physicians facing the difficult decision about whether or not to treat an aneurysm surgically.

NINDS scientists are studying the effects of an experimental drug in treating vasospasm that occurs following rupture of a cerebral aneurysm. The drug, developed at the NIH, delivers nitric oxide to the arteries and has been shown to reverse and prevent brain artery spasms in animals.

Other scientists hope to improve diagnosis and prediction of cerebral vasospasm by developing antibodies to molecules known to cause vasospasm. These molecules can be detected in the cerebrospinal fluid of people with subarachnoid hemorrhage. An additional study will compare standard treatment for subarachnoid hemorrhage to standard treatment plus transluminal balloon angioplasty immediately after severe bleeding. Transluminal balloon angioplasty involves the insertion, via catheter, of a deflated balloon through the affected artery and into the clot. The balloon is inflated to widen the artery and restore blood flow (the deflated balloon and catheter are then withdrawn).

Researchers are building a new, noninvasive, high-resolution x-ray detector system that can be used to guide the placement of stents (small tube-like devices that keep blood vessels open) used to modify blood flow during treatment for brain aneurysms.

Several groups of NINDS-funded researchers are conducting genetic linkage studies to identify risk factors for familial intracranial aneurysm and/or subarachnoid hemorrhage. One study hopes to establish patterns of inheritance in individuals of different ethnic backgrounds. Another project is aimed at targeting and providing prevention and treatment strategies for persons who are genetically at high risk for the development of brain aneurysms. And other investigators will establish a blood and tissue sampling bank for genetic linkage and molecular analyses.

Scientists are investigating the use of intraoperative hypothermia during microclip surgery as a means to improve the rate of recovery of cognitive functions and to reduce early and postoperative complications and neurological damage. Other studies are investigating ways to improve or replace the coils used in endovascular embolization.

Additional research being funded by the NINDS includes the development of a new animal model of human saccular aneurysm, a new method for tissue processing that should allow routine evaluation of the biological response to implantation of occlusion devices, and a computer simulation model to evaluate the outcomes of neurosurgery in individuals with cerebral aneurysms.

Chapter 12

Mini Stroke: Transient Ischemic Attack (TIA)

Chapter Contents

Section 12.1

What Is a TIA?

"Transient Ischemic Attack," © 2013 A.D.A.M., Inc.
Reprinted with permission.

A transient ischemic attack (TIA) is when blood flow to a part of the brain stops for a brief period of time. A person will have stroke-like symptoms for up to 24 hours, but in most cases for one to two hours.

A TIA is felt to be a warning sign that a true stroke may happen in the future if something is not done to prevent it.

Causes

A TIA is different than a stroke. After a TIA, the blockage breaks up quickly and dissolves. Unlike a stroke, a TIA does not cause brain tissue to die.

The loss of blood flow to an area of the brain can be caused by:

- a blood clot in an artery of the brain;
- a blood clot that travels to the brain from somewhere else in the body (for example, from the heart);
- an injury to blood vessels;
- narrowing of a blood vessel in the brain or leading to the brain.

High blood pressure is the number one risk for TIAs and stroke. The other major risk factors are:

- atrial fibrillation;
- diabetes;
- family history of stroke;
- high cholesterol;
- increasing age, especially after age 55;
- race (African Americans are more likely to die from stroke).

People who have heart disease or poor blood flow in their legs caused by narrowed arteries are also more likely to have a TIA or stroke.

Symptoms

Symptoms begin suddenly, last only a short time (from a few minutes to one to two hours), and go away completely. They may occur again at a later time.

The symptoms of TIA are the same as the symptoms of a stroke, and include sudden:

- abnormal feeling of movement (vertigo) or dizziness;
- change in alertness (sleepiness, less responsive, unconscious, or in a coma);
- changes in feeling, including touch, pain, temperature, pressure, hearing, and taste;
- confusion or loss of memory;
- difficulty swallowing;
- difficulty writing or reading;
- drooping of the face;
- inability to recognize objects or people;
- lack of control over the bladder or bowels;
- lack of coordination and balance, clumsiness, or trouble walking;
- loss of vision in one or both eyes;
- numbness or tingling on one side of the body;
- personality, mood, or emotional changes;
- trouble saying or understanding words;
- weakness on one side of the body.

Exams and Tests

Almost always, the symptoms and signs of a TIA will have gone away by the time you get to the hospital. A TIA diagnosis may be made based on your medical history alone.

The health care provider will do a complete physical exam to check for heart and blood vessel problems, as well as for problems with nerves and muscles.

Your blood pressure may be high. The doctor will use a stethoscope to listen to your heart and arteries. An abnormal sound called a bruit may be heard when listening to the carotid artery in the neck or other artery. A bruit is caused by irregular blood flow.

Tests will be done to rule out a stroke or other disorders that may cause the symptoms.

- You will almost always have a head CT [computed tomography] scan or brain MRI [magnetic resonance imaging]. A stroke will show changes on these tests, but TIAs will not.

- You will have an angiogram, CT angiogram, or MR angiogram to see which blood vessel is blocked or bleeding.

- You may have an echocardiogram if your doctor thinks you may have a blood clot from the heart.

- Carotid duplex (ultrasound) can show if the carotid arteries in your neck have narrowed.

- You may have an EKG [electrocardiogram] and heart rhythm monitoring tests to check for an irregular heartbeat.

Your doctor may do other tests to check high blood pressure, heart disease, diabetes, high cholesterol, and other causes of, and risk factors for TIAs or stroke.

Treatment

The goal is to prevent a stroke.

If you have had a TIA within the last 48 hours, you will likely be admitted to the hospital so that doctors can search for the cause and observe you.

High blood pressure, heart disease, diabetes, and blood disorders should be treated as needed.

You may receive blood thinners, such as aspirin, to reduce blood clotting. Other options include dipyridamole, clopidogrel, Aggrenox or heparin, Coumadin, or similar medicines. You may be treated for a long period of time.

Some people who have clogged neck arteries may need surgery (carotid endarterectomy). If you have irregular heartbeats (atrial fibrillation), you will be treated to avoid future complications.

Outlook (Prognosis)

TIAs do not cause lasting damage to the brain.

However, TIAs are a warning sign that you may have a true stroke in the coming days or months. More than 10% of people who have a TIA will have a stroke within three months. Half of these strokes happen during the 48 hours after a TIA. The stroke may occur that same day or at a later time. Some people have only a single episode, and some have more than one episode.

You can reduce your chances of a future stroke by following up with your health care provider to manage your risk factors.

When to Contact a Medical Professional

A TIA is a medical emergency. Call 911 or another local emergency number right away. Do not ignore symptoms just because they go away. They may be a warning of a future stroke.

Section 12.2

Having a TIA Shortens Life Expectancy

"Effects of 'Mini Stroke' Can Shorten Life Expectancy," reprinted with permission from www.heart.org. © 2011 American Heart Association, Inc.

Study Highlights

- Having a transient ischemic attack (TIA), or mini stroke, could lower your life expectancy.

- Survival rates after TIA were 20 percent lower than expected nine years later, compared to the general population.

- The long-term effects of TIA were most serious for patients older than 65 and for patients with previous history of stroke and heart problems.

Having a transient ischemic attack (TIA), or mini stroke, can reduce your life expectancy by 20 percent, according to a [November 2011 online ahead of print] study in *Stroke: Journal of the American Heart Association*.

"People experiencing a TIA won't die from it, but they will have a high risk of early stroke and also an increased risk of future problems that may reduce life expectancy," said Melina Gattellari, PhD, senior lecturer at the School of Public Health and Community Medicine in The University of New South Wales, Sydney and Ingham Institute in Liverpool, Australia.

"Our findings suggest that patients and doctors should be careful to intensely manage lifestyle and medical risk factors for years after a transient ischemic attack."

The statistical analysis is the first to comprehensively quantify the impact of hospital-diagnosed TIA on life expectancy.

Researchers identified 22,157 adults hospitalized with a TIA from July 2000 to June 2007 in New South Wales, Australia, and tracked their medical records for a minimum two years (median 4.1 years). They gathered death registry data for the area through June 2009 and compared death rates in the study population to those in the general population. Median ages were 78 for female patients and 73 for male patients; 23.9 percent were younger than 65 and 19.4 percent were older than 85.

At one year after hospitalization, 91.5 percent of TIA patients were still living, compared to 95 percent expected survival in the general population. At five years, survival of TIA patients was 13.2 percent lower than expected—67.2 percent were still alive, compared to an expected survival of 77.4 percent.

By the end of the study, at the nine-year mark, survival of TIA patients was 20 percent lower than expected.

Increasing age was associated with an increasing risk of death compared to the matched population. TIA had only minimal effect on patients younger than 50, but significantly reduced life expectancy in those older than 65. Compared to patients younger than 50, relative risk of death for patients 75–84 was 7.77 times higher and 11.02 times higher for those 85 and older.

"We thought the reverse may be true—that survival rates in older TIA patients would be more like other older people, who, although not affected by TIA, are affected by other conditions that may influence their survival," Gattellari said. "But even a distant history of TIA is major determinant of prognosis; certainly, the risks faced by TIA patients go well beyond their early stroke risk."

Researchers also examined TIA patients' medical records for other common health risks:

- Congestive heart failure was associated with 3.3 times more risk of dying.

- Atrial fibrillation was associated with twice the risk of dying.

- Prior hospitalization for stroke meant 2.63 times the risk of dying compared to patients without it; further, this effect grew over time, peaking at 5.01 times more risk three years after TIA admission.

In general, adults with a history of TIA can maximize their chances of living a long life by adopting healthy lifestyle habits, such as exercising daily, maintaining a healthy weight, quitting smoking, and eating healthy, Gattellari said.

Co-authors are Chris Goumas, MPH; Frances Garden, MBiost; and John M. Worthington, MBBS. Author disclosures are on the manuscript. The Clinical Excellence Commission and the Commonwealth Department of Health and Ageing partly funded the study.

Chapter 13

Recurrent Stroke

Chapter Contents

Section 13.1

What Is Recurrent Stroke?

After stroke, survivors tend to focus on rehabilitation and recovery. But, preventing another (or recurring) stroke is also a key concern. Of the 750,000 Americans who have a stroke each year, 5 to 14 percent will have a second stroke within one year. Within five years, stroke will recur in 24 percent of women and 42 percent of men. See Table 13.1.

Stroke prevention is also crucial for those who have had transient ischemic attacks (TIAs) or mini strokes. TIAs are brief episodes of stroke-like symptoms that last from a few minutes to 24 hours. TIAs usually don't cause permanent damage or disability.

But, they can be a serious warning sign of an impending stroke. Up to one third of people who have a TIA are expected to have a stroke.

Just like the first strokes, many recurrent strokes and TIAs can be prevented through lifestyle changes, surgery, medicine, or a mix of all three.

Table 13.1. Percentage of Recurrence after First Stroke

3% to 10%	30 Days
5% to 14%	1 Year
25% to 40%	5 Years

Your Lifestyle Choices

Everyone has some stroke risk. But, there are two types of stroke risk factors. One type you can't control. The other you can.

Stroke risk factors you can't change include:

- being over age 55;

- being a man;

- being African American;

- someone in your family has had a stroke;

- having diabetes.

Having one or more of these factors doesn't mean you will have a stroke. By making simple lifestyle changes, you may be able to reduce the risk of a first or recurrent stroke.

These simple lifestyle changes can greatly reduce your chance of having a stroke.

Control Your Blood Pressure

- Find out if you have atrial fibrillation (an irregular heartbeat which allows blood to pool in the heart and cause blood clots).

- Quit smoking.

- Limit alcohol.

- Monitor your cholesterol levels.

- Manage your diabetes.

- Exercise often.

- Eat foods low in sodium (salt) and fat.

- Monitor circulation problems with the help of your doctor.

Monitor Your Blood Pressure

High blood pressure is one of the most important and easily controlled stroke risk factors. So it's important to know your blood pressure range.

Blood pressure is given in two numbers, for example 120/80. The first number, the systolic blood pressure, is a measurement of the force your blood exerts on blood vessel walls as your heart pumps.

The second, diastolic blood pressure, is the measurement of the force your blood exerts on blood vessel walls when your heart is at rest.

For people over age 18, normal blood pressure is lower than 120/80. A blood pressure reading consistently 120/80 to 139/89 is pre-hypertension.

If yours falls in this range, you are more likely to progress to high blood pressure. Also called hypertension, high blood pressure is a reading of 140/90 or higher.

Have your blood pressure checked at least once each year—more often if you have high blood pressure, have had a heart attack or stroke, are diabetic, have kidney disease, have high cholesterol or are overweight. If you are at risk for high blood pressure, ask your doctor how to manage it more aggressively.

Often blood pressure can be controlled through diet and exercise. Even light exercise—a brisk walk, bicycle ride, swim, or yard work—can make a difference. Adults should do some form of moderate physical activity for at least 30 minutes five or more days per week, according to the Centers for Disease Control and Prevention. Regular exercise may reduce your risk of stroke. Before you start an exercise program, check with your doctor.

Your Blood Pressure Is High

What do you do if you still have high blood pressure, even though you have made an effort to eat healthy foods and exercise? Then it's time to talk to your doctor.

A doctor can advise you about better lifestyle choices. Medicine may also be needed.

Many drugs can help treat high blood pressure. The most common are calcium channel blockers or ACE [angiotensin-converting-enzyme] inhibitors. You may have to try several different drugs before you find one that works for you. This is common.

So, try not to be discouraged if it happens. Once you find a drug that works, take it as directed and exactly as prescribed, even when you feel fine.

Medicines

Medicine may help reduce stroke risk. In addition to those that treat high blood pressure, drugs are also available to control high cholesterol and treat heart disease. There are also drugs that can interfere with the blood's tendency to form potential stroke causing blood clots.

Heart Disease

Many forms of heart disease can increase your stroke risk. One form—known as atrial fibrillation or AF—causes blood to form clots that can travel to the brain and cause a stroke. AF is an irregular heartbeat.

Warfarin (Coumadin) and aspirin are often prescribed to treat AF. People taking warfarin should be monitored carefully by a doctor.

Also, people taking this drug should limit foods rich in vitamin K, which in large quantities may offset the drug's effects.

Examples of these foods include green leafy vegetables, alfalfa, egg yolks, soy bean oil, and fish livers.

Two new oral medications, dabigatran (Pradaxa) and rivaroxaban (Xarelto) have been recently approved for strokes associated with atrial fibrillation. They do not require the dietary restrictions or blood testing needed with warfarin. Several additional similar drugs are also nearing approval. However, because all of these drugs are relatively new, it is not yet clear whether they should be preferred over warfarin for clots associated with atrial fibrillation.

High Cholesterol

High levels of cholesterol may also increase stroke risk by not letting blood move freely through the arteries. Cholesterol build-up can break off. This can cause a clot to form or a stroke to occur. A few drugs, such as statins, may help lower cholesterol. Some statins have helped reduce the risk of stroke or TIA in people who have had a heart attack. They have even helped some with average or only slightly high cholesterol.

Blood Clotting

There are also a few drugs that can prevent clots, helping reduce risk of a second stroke.

Aspirin is the least costly and longest lasting of these drugs. A newer, more effective option is a combination of aspirin and extended-release dipyridamole, called Aggrenox. Or, your doctor might choose to treat you with clopidogrel (Plavix). Warfarin is often prescribed to prevent clots from forming in those with atrial fibrillation, and dabigatran (Pradaxa) and rivaroxaban (Xarelto) have also been approved for this purpose.

Surgical Options

For those whose first stroke was caused by a blockage in the carotid arteries (vessels that carry blood from the heart to the brain), surgery known as carotid endarterectomy may help reduce risk of another stroke.

During surgery, blockages and build-up in the arteries are removed to restore the free flow of blood. Your doctor is the best judge to decide if this is a good option for you.

Compliance Is Critical

The key to preventing recurrent stroke is simple: Follow your doctor's suggestions about diet, exercise, and weight loss, and take any modicine as directed. Your doctor will decide what's best for you based on your general health and your medical history. By understanding the basis for these decisions, you'll be better able to follow the suggestions and make informed choices that will help reduce your risk of stroke.

Rehabilitation is a lifetime commitment and an important part of recovering from a stroke.

Through rehabilitation, you relearn basic skills such as talking, eating, dressing, and walking.

Rehabilitation can also improve your strength, flexibility, and endurance. The goal is to regain as much independence as possible.

Remember to ask your doctor, "Where am I on my stroke recovery journey?"

Section 13.2

Patients at Risk of Recurrent Stroke Fare Better with Intense Medical Management

"NIH stroke prevention trial has immediate implications for clinical practice," by the National Institutes of Health (NIH, www.nih.gov), September 7, 2011.

Patients at a high risk for a second stroke who received intensive medical treatment had fewer strokes and deaths than patients who received a brain stent in addition to the medical treatment, a large nationwide clinical trial has shown. The investigators published the results in the online first edition of the *New England Journal of Medicine*. The National Institute of Neurological Disorders and Stroke (NINDS), part of the National Institutes of Health, funded the trial. The medical regimen included daily blood-thinning medications and aggressive control of blood pressure and cholesterol.

New enrollment in the study was stopped in April [2011] because early data showed significantly more strokes and deaths occurred among the stented patients at the 30-day mark compared to the group who received the medical management alone.

In addition to the intensive medical program, half of the patients in the study received an intervention of a self-expanding stent that widens a major artery in the brain and facilitates blood flow. One possible explanation for the higher stroke rate in the stented group is that patients who have had recent stroke symptoms sometimes have unstable plaque in their arteries which the stent could have dislodged, the study authors suggest. The study device, the Gateway-Wingspan intracranial angioplasty and stenting system, is the only system currently approved by the U.S. Food and Drug Administration (FDA) for certain high-risk stroke patients. The authors noted that although similar stenting systems that do not have FDA approval are being used in clinical practice, they did not evaluate those devices in this study.

The authors also emphasize that the study participants were in the highest risk category, with blockage or narrowing of arteries of 70 to 99 percent. Stroke patients with moderate cerebral arterial blockage (50–69 percent) were excluded because their risk of stroke is low with usual medical management, and researchers thought this group would be unlikely to benefit from stenting.

"This study provides an answer to a longstanding question by physicians—what to do to prevent a devastating second stroke in a high risk population. Although technological advances have brought intracranial stenting into practice, we have now learned that, when tested in a large group, this particular device did not lead to a better health outcome," said Walter Koroshetz, MD, deputy director of NINDS.

Stroke is the fourth leading cause of death in the United States. Stenosis, a blockage or narrowing of brain arteries caused by the buildup of plaque, accounts for more than 50,000 of the 795,000 strokes that occur annually nationwide. Stenosis is particularly common in African-Americans, Hispanics, Asian Americans, and people with diabetes.

The NIH Stenting vs. Aggressive Medical Management for Preventing Recurrent Stroke in Intracranial Stenosis (SAMMPRIS) study enrolled 451 patients at 50 sites across the United States. The investigators looked at whether patients had a second stroke or died within 30 days of enrollment, or had a stroke in the same area of the brain from 30 days to the end of follow-up. They had hypothesized that compared to intensive medical therapy alone, the addition of an intracranial stenting system would decrease the risk of a stroke or death by 35 percent over two years.

Instead they found that 14.7 percent of patients (33) in the stenting group experienced a stroke or died within the first 30 days after enrollment, compared with 5.8 percent (13) of patients treated with medical therapy alone. There were five stroke-related deaths within 30 days, all in the stenting group, and one non-stroke-related death in the medical management group. During a follow-up period of just less than one year, 20.5 percent of patients in the stenting group and 11.5 percent of patients in the medical group had a stroke or death, or a stroke in the same area of the brain beyond 30 days, a highly significant difference in favor of the patients in the study's medical group. Based on these data, the Data and Safety Monitoring Board recommended that the NINDS stop new enrollment, and the NIH issued a clinical alert. All patients will continue to be followed for two years to determine the long-term effects of both interventions.

SAMMPRIS is the first stroke prevention trial to compare intracranial stenting with medical therapy and to incorporate intensive medical management into the study design. This includes a daily dosage of 325 milligrams of aspirin; 75 milligrams a day of clopidogrel, a medication used to prevent blood clots, for 90 days after enrollment; and aggressive management of key stroke risk factors—high blood pressure and high levels of low density lipoprotein (LDL), the unhealthy form of cholesterol. All patients also participated in a lifestyle modification program which focused on quitting smoking, increasing exercise, and controlling diabetes and cholesterol.

In a previous NIH trial, stroke patients with criteria similar to those enrolled in SAMMPRIS were treated with less intensive medical management. Their comparable 30-day and one year rates were 10.7 percent and 25 percent, respectively. The investigators note that comparisons with historical controls have limitations, but the much lower event rates in the medical group in SAMMPRIS suggest that the intensive medical management was effective in lowering the stroke risk.

"The SAMMPRIS study results have immediate implications for clinical practice. Stroke patients with recent symptoms and intracranial arterial blockage of 70 percent or greater should be treated with aggressive medical therapy alone that follows the regimen used in this trial as closely as possible," said Marc Chimowitz, MBChB, of the department of neurosciences at the Medical University of South Carolina in Charleston, and first author of the *NEJM* article.

Patients in the study were between 30 and 80 years old and had experienced a recent transient ischemic attack, a type of stroke that resolves within 24 hours, or another type of non-disabling stroke, which was caused by a large degree of stenosis in a cerebral artery.

Part Three

Stroke Risk Factors and Prevention

Chapter 14

Atherosclerosis and Carotid Artery Disease

Atherosclerosis

Atherosclerosis is a disease in which plaque builds up inside your arteries. Arteries are blood vessels that carry oxygen-rich blood to your heart and other parts of your body.

Plaque is made up of fat, cholesterol, calcium, and other substances found in the blood. Over time, plaque hardens and narrows your arteries. This limits the flow of oxygen-rich blood to your organs and other parts of your body.

Atherosclerosis can lead to serious problems, including heart attack, stroke, or even death.

Atherosclerosis-Related Diseases

Atherosclerosis can affect any artery in the body, including arteries in the heart, brain, arms, legs, pelvis, and kidneys. As a result, different diseases may develop based on which arteries are affected.

Coronary Heart Disease

Coronary heart disease (CHD), also called coronary artery disease, is the #1 killer of both men and women in the United States. CHD

This chapter contains text from "Atherosclerosis," by the National Heart, Lung, and Blood Institute (NHLBI, www.nhlbi.nih.gov), part of the National Institutes of Health, July 1, 2011, and text excerpted from "Carotid Artery Disease," by the NHLBI, November 1, 2010.

occurs if plaque builds up in the coronary arteries. These arteries supply oxygen-rich blood to your heart.

Plaque narrows the coronary arteries and reduces blood flow to your heart muscle. Plaque buildup also makes it more likely that blood clots will form in your arteries. Blood clots can partially or completely block blood flow.

If blood flow to your heart muscle is reduced or blocked, you may have angina (chest pain or discomfort) or a heart attack.

Plaque also can form in the heart's smallest arteries. This disease is called coronary microvascular disease (MVD). In coronary MVD, plaque doesn't cause blockages in the arteries as it does in CHD.

Carotid Artery Disease

Carotid artery disease occurs if plaque builds up in the arteries on each side of your neck (the carotid arteries). These arteries supply oxygen-rich blood to your brain. If blood flow to your brain is reduced or blocked, you may have a stroke.

Peripheral Arterial Disease

Peripheral arterial disease (PAD) occurs if plaque builds up in the major arteries that supply oxygen-rich blood to your legs, arms, and pelvis.

If blood flow to these parts of your body is reduced or blocked, you may have numbness, pain, and, sometimes, dangerous infections.

Chronic Kidney Disease

Chronic kidney disease can occur if plaque builds up in the renal arteries. These arteries supply oxygen-rich blood to your kidneys.

Over time, chronic kidney disease causes a slow loss of kidney function. The main function of the kidneys is to remove waste and extra water from the body.

Outlook

Improved treatments have reduced the number of deaths from atherosclerosis-related diseases. These treatments also have improved the quality of life for people who have these diseases. However, atherosclerosis remains a common health problem.

You may be able to prevent or delay atherosclerosis and the diseases it can cause. Making lifestyle changes and getting ongoing care can help you avoid the problems of atherosclerosis and live a long, healthy life.

Other Names for Atherosclerosis

- Arteriosclerosis

- Hardening of the arteries

Causes of Atherosclerosis

The exact cause of atherosclerosis isn't known. However, studies show that atherosclerosis is a slow, complex disease that may start in childhood. It develops faster as you age.

Atherosclerosis may start when certain factors damage the inner layers of the arteries. These factors include the following:

- Smoking

- High amounts of certain fats and cholesterol in the blood

- High blood pressure

- High amounts of sugar in the blood due to insulin resistance or diabetes

Plaque may begin to build up where the arteries are damaged. Over time, plaque hardens and narrows the arteries. Eventually, an area of plaque can rupture (break open).

When this happens, blood cell fragments called platelets stick to the site of the injury. They may clump together to form blood clots. Clots narrow the arteries even more, limiting the flow of oxygen-rich blood to your body.

Depending on which arteries are affected, blood clots can worsen angina (chest pain) or cause a heart attack or stroke.

Researchers continue to look for the causes of atherosclerosis. They hope to find answers to questions such as the following:

- Why and how do the arteries become damaged?

- How does plaque develop and change over time?

- Why does plaque rupture and lead to blood clots?

Risk Factors for Atherosclerosis

Coronary heart disease (atherosclerosis of the coronary arteries) is the number-one killer of both men and women in the United States.

The exact cause of atherosclerosis isn't known. However, certain traits, conditions, or habits may raise your risk for the disease. These conditions are known as risk factors. The more risk factors you have, the more likely it is that you'll develop atherosclerosis.

You can control most risk factors and help prevent or delay atherosclerosis. Other risk factors can't be controlled.

Major Risk Factors

- Unhealthy blood cholesterol levels: This includes high LDL [low-density lipoprotein] cholesterol (sometimes called bad cholesterol) and low HDL [high-density lipoprotein] cholesterol (sometimes called good cholesterol).

- High blood pressure: Blood pressure is considered high if it stays at or above 140/90 mmHg over time. If you have diabetes or chronic kidney disease, high blood pressure is defined as 130/80 mmHg or higher. (The mmHg is millimeters of mercury—the units used to measure blood pressure.)

- Smoking: Smoking can damage and tighten blood vessels, raise cholesterol levels, and raise blood pressure. Smoking also doesn't allow enough oxygen to reach the body's tissues.

- Insulin resistance: This condition occurs if the body can't use its insulin properly. Insulin is a hormone that helps move blood sugar into cells where it's used as an energy source. Insulin resistance may lead to diabetes.

- Diabetes: With this disease, the body's blood sugar level is too high because the body doesn't make enough insulin or doesn't use its insulin properly.

- Overweight or obesity: The terms overweight and obesity refer to body weight that's greater than what is considered healthy for a certain height.

- Lack of physical activity: A lack of physical activity can worsen other risk factors for atherosclerosis, such as unhealthy blood cholesterol levels, high blood pressure, diabetes, and overweight and obesity.

- Unhealthy diet: An unhealthy diet can raise your risk for atherosclerosis. Foods that are high in saturated and trans fats, cholesterol, sodium (salt), and sugar can worsen other atherosclerosis risk factors.

- Older age: As you get older, your risk for atherosclerosis increases. Genetic or lifestyle factors cause plaque to build up in your arteries as you age. By the time you're middle-aged or older, enough plaque has built up to cause signs or symptoms. In men, the risk increases after age 45. In women, the risk increases after age 55.

- Family history of early heart disease: Your risk for atherosclerosis increases if your father or a brother was diagnosed with heart disease before 55 years of age, or if your mother or a sister was diagnosed with heart disease before 65 years of age.

Although age and a family history of early heart disease are risk factors, it doesn't mean that you'll develop atherosclerosis if you have one or both. Controlling other risk factors often can lessen genetic influences and prevent atherosclerosis, even in older adults.

Studies show that an increasing number of children and youth are at risk for atherosclerosis. This is due to a number of causes, including rising childhood obesity rates.

Emerging Risk Factors

Scientists continue to study other possible risk factors for atherosclerosis.

High levels of a protein called C-reactive protein (CRP) in the blood may raise the risk for atherosclerosis and heart attack. High levels of CRP are a sign of inflammation in the body.

Inflammation is the body's response to injury or infection. Damage to the arteries' inner walls seems to trigger inflammation and help plaque grow.

People who have low CRP levels may develop atherosclerosis at a slower rate than people who have high CRP levels. Research is under way to find out whether reducing inflammation and lowering CRP levels also can reduce the risk for atherosclerosis.

High levels of triglycerides in the blood also may raise the risk for atherosclerosis, especially in women. Triglycerides are a type of fat.

Studies are under way to find out whether genetics may play a role in atherosclerosis risk.

Other Factors That Affect Atherosclerosis

Other factors also may raise your risk for atherosclerosis, such as the following:

- Sleep apnea: Sleep apnea is a disorder that causes one or more pauses in breathing or shallow breaths while you sleep. Untreated sleep apnea can raise your risk for high blood pressure, diabetes, and even a heart attack or stroke.

- Stress: Research shows that the most commonly reported trigger for a heart attack is an emotionally upsetting event, especially one involving anger.

- Alcohol: Heavy drinking can damage the heart muscle and worsen other risk factors for atherosclerosis. Men should have no more than two drinks containing alcohol a day. Women should have no more than one drink containing alcohol a day.

Signs and Symptoms of Atherosclerosis

Atherosclerosis usually doesn't cause signs and symptoms until it severely narrows or totally blocks an artery. Many people don't know they have the disease until they have a medical emergency, such as a heart attack or stroke.

Some people may have signs and symptoms of the disease. Signs and symptoms will depend on which arteries are affected.

Coronary Arteries

The coronary arteries supply oxygen-rich blood to your heart. If plaque narrows or blocks these arteries (a disease called coronary heart disease, or CHD), a common symptom is angina. Angina is chest pain or discomfort that occurs when your heart muscle doesn't get enough oxygen-rich blood.

Angina may feel like pressure or squeezing in your chest. You also may feel it in your shoulders, arms, neck, jaw, or back. Angina pain may even feel like indigestion. The pain tends to get worse with activity and go away with rest. Emotional stress also can trigger the pain.

Other symptoms of CHD are shortness of breath and arrhythmias. Arrhythmias are problems with the rate or rhythm of the heartbeat.

Plaque also can form in the heart's smallest arteries. This disease is called coronary microvascular disease (MVD). Symptoms of coronary MVD include angina, shortness of breath, sleep problems, fatigue (tiredness), and lack of energy.

Carotid Arteries

The carotid arteries supply oxygen-rich blood to your brain. If plaque narrows or blocks these arteries (a disease called carotid artery disease), you may have symptoms of a stroke. These symptoms may include the following:

- Sudden weakness

- Paralysis (an inability to move) or numbness of the face, arms, or legs, especially on one side of the body

- Confusion

- Trouble speaking or understanding speech

- Trouble seeing in one or both eyes

- Problems breathing

- Dizziness, trouble walking, loss of balance or coordination, and unexplained falls

- Loss of consciousness

- Sudden and severe headache

Peripheral Arteries

Plaque also can build up in the major arteries that supply oxygen-rich blood to the legs, arms, and pelvis (a disease called peripheral arterial disease).

If these major arteries are narrowed or blocked, you may have numbness, pain, and, sometimes, dangerous infections.

Renal Arteries

The renal arteries supply oxygen-rich blood to your kidneys. If plaque builds up in these arteries, you may develop chronic kidney disease. Over time, chronic kidney disease causes a slow loss of kidney function.

Early kidney disease often has no signs or symptoms. As the disease gets worse it can cause tiredness, changes in how you urinate (more often or less often), loss of appetite, nausea (feeling sick to the stomach), swelling in the hands or feet, itchiness or numbness, and trouble concentrating.

Atherosclerosis Diagnosis

Your doctor will diagnose atherosclerosis based on your medical and family histories, a physical exam, and test results.

Specialists Involved

If you have atherosclerosis, a primary care doctor, such as an internist or family practitioner, may handle your care. Your doctor may recommend other health care specialists if you need expert care, such as the following:

- A cardiologist: This is a doctor who specializes in diagnosing and treating heart diseases and conditions. You may go to a cardiologist if you have coronary heart disease (CHD) or coronary microvascular disease (MVD).

- A vascular specialist: This is a doctor who specializes in diagnosing and treating blood vessel problems. You may go to a vascular specialist if you have peripheral arterial disease (PAD).

- A neurologist: This is a doctor who specializes in diagnosing and treating nervous system disorders. You may see a neurologist if you've had a stroke due to carotid artery disease.

- A nephrologist: This is a doctor who specializes in diagnosing and treating kidney diseases and conditions. You may go to a nephrologist if you have chronic kidney disease.

Physical Exam

During the physical exam, your doctor may listen to your arteries for an abnormal whooshing sound called a bruit. Your doctor can hear a bruit when placing a stethoscope over an affected artery. A bruit may indicate poor blood flow due to plaque buildup.

Your doctor also may check to see whether any of your pulses (for example, in the leg or foot) are weak or absent. A weak or absent pulse can be a sign of a blocked artery.

Diagnostic Tests

Your doctor may recommend one or more tests to diagnose atherosclerosis. These tests also can help your doctor learn the extent of your disease and plan the best treatment.

Blood Tests

Blood tests check the levels of certain fats, cholesterol, sugar, and proteins in your blood. Abnormal levels may be a sign that you're at risk for atherosclerosis.

EKG (Electrocardiogram)

An EKG is a simple, painless test that detects and records the heart's electrical activity. The test shows how fast the heart is beating and its rhythm (steady or irregular). An EKG also records the strength and timing of electrical signals as they pass through the heart.

An EKG can show signs of heart damage caused by CHD. The test also can show signs of a previous or current heart attack.

Chest X-Ray

A chest X-ray takes pictures of the organs and structures inside your chest, such as your heart, lungs, and blood vessels. A chest X-ray can reveal signs of heart failure.

Ankle / Brachial Index

This test compares the blood pressure in your ankle with the blood pressure in your arm to see how well your blood is flowing. This test can help diagnose PAD.

Echocardiography

Echocardiography (echo) uses sound waves to create a moving picture of your heart. The test provides information about the size and shape of your heart and how well your heart chambers and valves are working.

Echo also can identify areas of poor blood flow to the heart, areas of heart muscle that aren't contracting normally, and previous injury to the heart muscle caused by poor blood flow.

Computed Tomography Scan

A computed tomography (CT) scan creates computer-generated pictures of the heart, brain, or other areas of the body. The test can show hardening and narrowing of large arteries.

A cardiac CT scan also can show whether calcium has built up in the walls of the coronary (heart) arteries. This may be an early sign of CHD.

Stress Testing

During stress testing, you exercise to make your heart work hard and beat fast while heart tests are done. If you can't exercise, you may be given medicine to make your heart work hard and beat fast.

When your heart is working hard, it needs more blood and oxygen. Plaque-narrowed arteries can't supply enough oxygen-rich blood to meet your heart's needs.

A stress test can show possible signs and symptoms of CHD, such as the following:

- Abnormal changes in your heart rate or blood pressure

- Shortness of breath or chest pain

- Abnormal changes in your heart rhythm or your heart's electrical activity

As part of some stress tests, pictures are taken of your heart while you exercise and while you rest. These imaging stress tests can show how well blood is flowing in various parts of your heart. They also can show how well your heart pumps blood when it beats.

Angiography

Angiography is a test that uses dye and special X-rays to show the inside of your arteries. This test can show whether plaque is blocking your arteries and how severe the blockage is.

A thin, flexible tube called a catheter is put into a blood vessel in your arm, groin (upper thigh), or neck. Dye that can be seen on an X-ray picture is injected through the catheter into the arteries. By looking at the X-ray picture, your doctor can see the flow of blood through your arteries.

Other Tests

Other tests are being studied to see whether they can give a better view of plaque buildup in the arteries. Examples of these tests include magnetic resonance imaging (MRI) and positron emission tomography (PET).

Atherosclerosis Treatment

Treatments for atherosclerosis may include lifestyle changes, medicines, and medical procedures or surgery.

The goals of treatment include the following:

- Relieving symptoms

- Reducing risk factors in an effort to slow or stop the buildup of plaque

- Lowering the risk of blood clots forming

- Widening or bypassing plaque-clogged arteries

- Preventing atherosclerosis-related diseases

Lifestyle Changes

Making lifestyle changes often can help prevent or treat atherosclerosis. For some people, these changes may be the only treatment needed.

A healthy diet is an important part of a healthy lifestyle. Following a healthy diet can prevent or reduce high blood pressure and high blood cholesterol and help you maintain a healthy weight.

Your doctor may recommend TLC [Therapeutic Lifestyle Changes] if you have high blood cholesterol. TLC is a three-part program that includes a healthy diet, physical activity, and weight management.

With the TLC diet, less than 7 percent of your daily calories should come from saturated fat. This kind of fat is found in some meats, dairy products, chocolate, baked goods, and deep-fried and processed foods.

No more than 25 to 35 percent of your daily calories should come from all fats, including saturated, trans, monounsaturated, and polyunsaturated fats.

You also should have less than 200 mg a day of cholesterol. The amounts of cholesterol and the types of fat in prepared foods can be found on the foods' Nutrition Facts labels.

Foods high in soluble fiber also are part of a healthy diet. They help prevent the digestive tract from absorbing cholesterol. These foods include the following:

- Whole-grain cereals such as oatmeal and oat bran

- Fruits such as apples, bananas, oranges, pears, and prunes

- Legumes such as kidney beans, lentils, chick peas, black-eyed peas, and lima beans

A diet rich in fruits and vegetables can increase important cholesterol-lowering compounds in your diet. These compounds, called plant stanols or sterols, work like soluble fiber.

A healthy diet also includes some types of fish, such as salmon, tuna (canned or fresh), and mackerel. These fish are a good source of omega-3 fatty acids. These acids may help protect the heart from blood clots and inflammation and reduce the risk for heart attack. Try to have about two fish meals every week.

You should try to limit the amount of sodium (salt) that you eat. This means choosing low-salt and "no added salt" foods and seasonings at the table or while cooking. The Nutrition Facts label on food packaging shows the amount of sodium in the item.

Try to limit drinks with alcohol. Too much alcohol will raise your blood pressure and triglyceride level. (Triglycerides are a type of fat found in the blood.) Alcohol also adds extra calories, which will cause weight gain.

Men should have no more than two drinks containing alcohol a day. Women should have no more than one drink containing alcohol a day. One drink is a glass of wine, beer, or a small amount of hard liquor.

Your doctor may recommend the Dietary Approaches to Stop Hypertension (DASH) eating plan if you have high blood pressure. The DASH eating plan focuses on fruits, vegetables, whole grains, and other foods that are heart healthy and low in fat, cholesterol, and salt.

DASH also focuses on fat-free or low-fat milk and dairy products, fish, poultry, and nuts. The DASH eating plan is reduced in red meats (including lean red meats), sweets, added sugars, and sugar-containing beverages. The plan is rich in nutrients, protein, and fiber.

The DASH eating plan is a good heart healthy eating plan, even for those who don't have high blood pressure.

Be Physically Active

Regular physical activity can lower many atherosclerosis risk factors, including LDL (bad) cholesterol, high blood pressure, and excess weight.

Physical activity also can lower your risk for diabetes and raise your HDL cholesterol level. HDL is the good cholesterol that helps prevent atherosclerosis.

Talk with your doctor before you start a new exercise plan. Ask him or her how much and what kinds of physical activity are safe for you.

People gain health benefits from as little as 60 minutes of moderate-intensity aerobic activity per week. For major health benefits, do at least 150 minutes (2 hours and 30 minutes) of moderate-intensity aerobic activity or 75 minutes (1 hour and 15 minutes) of vigorous-intensity aerobic activity each week. The more active you are, the more you will benefit.

Maintain a Healthy Weight

Maintaining a healthy weight can lower your risk for atherosclerosis. A general goal to aim for is a body mass index (BMI) of less than 25.

BMI measures your weight in relation to your height and gives an estimate of your total body fat.

A BMI between 25 and 29.9 is considered overweight. A BMI of 30 or more is considered obese. A BMI of less than 25 is the goal for preventing and treating atherosclerosis. Your doctor or health care provider can help you set an appropriate BMI goal.

Quit Smoking

If you smoke or use tobacco, quit. Smoking can damage and tighten blood vessels and raise your risk for atherosclerosis. Talk with your doctor about programs and products that can help you quit. Also, try to avoid secondhand smoke.

If you have trouble quitting smoking on your own, consider joining a support group. Many hospitals, workplaces, and community groups offer classes to help people quit smoking.

Manage Stress

Research shows that the most commonly reported trigger for a heart attack is an emotionally upsetting event—particularly one involving anger. Also, some of the ways people cope with stress—such as drinking, smoking, or overeating—aren't healthy.

Learning how to manage stress, relax, and cope with problems can improve your emotional and physical health. Having supportive people in your life with whom you can share your feelings or concerns can help relieve stress.

Physical activity, medicine, and relaxation therapy also can help relieve stress. You may want to consider taking part in a stress management program.

Medicines

To slow the progress of plaque buildup, your doctor may prescribe medicines to help lower your cholesterol level or blood pressure. He or she also may prescribe medicines to prevent blood clots from forming.

For successful treatment, take all medicines as your doctor prescribes.

Medical Procedures and Surgery

If you have severe atherosclerosis, your doctor may recommend a medical procedure or surgery.

Angioplasty is a procedure that's used to open blocked or narrowed coronary (heart) arteries. Angioplasty can improve blood flow to the heart and relieve chest pain. Sometimes a small mesh tube called a stent is placed in the artery to keep it open after the procedure.

Coronary artery bypass grafting (CABG) is a type of surgery. In CABG, arteries or veins from other areas in your body are used to bypass (that is, go around) your narrowed coronary arteries. CABG can improve blood flow to your heart, relieve chest pain, and possibly prevent a heart attack.

Bypass grafting also can be used for leg arteries. For this surgery, a healthy blood vessel is used to bypass a narrowed or blocked artery in one of the legs. The healthy blood vessel redirects blood around the blocked artery, improving blood flow to the leg.

Carotid endarterectomy is surgery to remove plaque buildup from the carotid arteries in the neck. This procedure restores blood flow to the brain, which can help prevent a stroke.

Atherosclerosis Prevention

Taking action to control your risk factors can help prevent or delay atherosclerosis and its related diseases. Your risk for atherosclerosis increases with the number of risk factors you have.

One step you can take is to adopt a healthy lifestyle. Following a healthy diet is an important part of a healthy lifestyle.

A healthy diet includes a variety of fruits and vegetables (including beans and peas). It also includes whole grains, lean meats, poultry without skin, seafood, and fat-free or low-fat milk and dairy products. A healthy diet is low in sodium (salt), added sugar, solid fats, and refined grains.

The National Heart, Lung, and Blood Institute's (NHLBI's) Therapeutic Lifestyle Changes (TLC) and Dietary Approaches to Stop Hypertension (DASH) are two programs that promote healthy eating.

If you're overweight or obese, work with your doctor to create a reasonable weight-loss plan. Controlling your weight helps you control atherosclerosis risk factors.

Be as physically active as you can. Physical activity can improve your fitness level and your health. Ask your doctor what types and amounts of activity are safe for you.

If you smoke, quit. Smoking can damage and tighten blood vessels and raise your risk for atherosclerosis. Talk with your doctor about programs and products that can help you quit. Also, try to avoid secondhand smoke.

Know your family history of atherosclerosis. If you or someone in your family has an atherosclerosis-related disease, be sure to tell your doctor.

If lifestyle changes aren't enough, your doctor may prescribe medicines to control your atherosclerosis risk factors. Take all of your medicines as your doctor advises.

Living with Atherosclerosis

Improved treatments have reduced the number of deaths from atherosclerosis-related diseases. These treatments also have improved the quality of life for people who have these diseases.

Adopting a healthy lifestyle may help you prevent or delay atherosclerosis and the problems it can cause. This, along with ongoing medical care, can help you avoid the problems of atherosclerosis and live a long, healthy life.

Researchers continue to look for ways to improve the health of people who have atherosclerosis or may develop it.

Ongoing Care

If you have atherosclerosis, work closely with your doctor and other health care providers to avoid serious problems, such as heart attack and stroke.

Follow your treatment plan and take all of your medicines as your doctor prescribes. Your doctor will let you know how often you should schedule office visits or blood tests. Be sure to let your doctor know if you have new or worsening symptoms.

Having an atherosclerosis-related disease may cause fear, anxiety, depression, and stress. Talk about how you feel with your doctor. Talking to a professional counselor also can help. If you're very depressed, your doctor may recommend medicines or other treatments that can improve your quality of life.

Community resources are available to help you learn more about atherosclerosis. Contact your local public health departments, hospitals, and local chapters of national health organizations to learn more about available resources in your area.

Talk about your lifestyle changes with your family and friends—whoever can provide support or needs to understand why you're changing your habits.

Family and friends may be able to help you make lifestyle changes. For example, they can help you plan healthier meals. Because atherosclerosis tends to run in families, your lifestyle changes may help many of your family members, too.

Carotid Artery Disease

Carotid artery disease is a disease in which a waxy substance called plaque builds up inside the carotid arteries. You have two common carotid arteries, one on each side of your neck. They each divide into internal and external carotid arteries.

The internal carotid arteries supply oxygen-rich blood to your brain. The external carotid arteries supply oxygen-rich blood to your face, scalp, and neck.

Carotid artery disease is serious because it can cause a stroke, also called a brain attack. A stroke occurs if blood flow to your brain is cut off.

If blood flow is cut off for more than a few minutes, the cells in your brain start to die. This impairs the parts of the body that the brain cells control. A stroke can cause lasting brain damage; long-term disability, such as vision or speech problems or paralysis (an inability to move); or death.

Outlook

Carotid artery disease causes more than half of the strokes that occur in the United States. Other conditions, such as certain heart problems and bleeding in the brain, also can cause strokes.

Lifestyle changes, medicines, and medical procedures can help prevent or treat carotid artery disease and may reduce the risk of stroke.

If you think you're having a stroke, you need urgent treatment. Call 911 right away if you have symptoms of a stroke. Do not drive yourself to the hospital.

You have the best chance for full recovery if treatment to open a blocked artery is given within four hours of symptom onset. The sooner treatment occurs, the better your chances of recovery.

What Causes Carotid Artery Disease?

Carotid artery disease seems to start when damage occurs to the inner layers of the carotid arteries. Major factors that contribute to damage include the following:

- Smoking

- High levels of certain fats and cholesterol in the blood

- High blood pressure

- High levels of sugar in the blood due to insulin resistance or diabetes

When damage occurs, your body starts a healing process. The healing may cause plaque to build up where the arteries are damaged.

The plaque in an artery can crack or rupture. If this happens, blood cell fragments called platelets will stick to the site of the injury and may clump together to form blood clots.

The buildup of plaque or blood clots can severely narrow or block the carotid arteries. This limits the flow of oxygen-rich blood to your brain, which can cause a stroke.

Who Is at Risk for Carotid Artery Disease?

Certain traits, conditions, or habits may raise your risk for carotid artery disease. These conditions are known as risk factors. The more risk factors you have, the more likely you are to get the disease. Some risk factors you can control, but others you can't.

The major risk factors for carotid artery disease also are the major risk factors for coronary heart disease (also called coronary artery disease) and peripheral arterial disease.

- **Unhealthy blood cholesterol levels:** This includes high LDL cholesterol (low-density lipoprotein cholesterol, sometimes called bad cholesterol) and low HDL cholesterol (high-density lipoprotein cholesterol, sometimes called good cholesterol).

- **High blood pressure:** Blood pressure is considered high if it stays at or above 140/90 mmHg over time. If you have diabetes or chronic kidney disease, high blood pressure is defined as 130/80 mmHg or higher. (The mmHg is millimeters of mercury—the units used to measure blood pressure.)

- **Smoking:** Smoking can damage and tighten blood vessels, lead to unhealthy cholesterol levels, and raise blood pressure. Smoking also can limit how much oxygen reaches the body's tissues.

- **Insulin resistance:** This condition occurs if the body can't use its own insulin properly. Insulin is a hormone that helps move blood sugar into cells where it's used as an energy source. Insulin resistance may lead to diabetes.

- **Diabetes:** With this disease, the body's blood sugar level is too high because the body doesn't make enough insulin or doesn't use its insulin properly. People who have diabetes are four times more likely to have carotid artery disease than people who don't have diabetes.

- **Overweight or obesity:** The terms overweight and obesity refer to body weight that's greater than what is considered healthy for a certain height.

- **Metabolic syndrome:** Metabolic syndrome is the name for a group of risk factors that raise your risk for stroke and other health problems, such as diabetes and heart disease. The five metabolic risk factors are a large waistline (abdominal obesity), a high triglyceride level (a type of fat found in the blood), a low HDL cholesterol level, high blood pressure, and high blood sugar.

139

Metabolic syndrome is diagnosed if you have at least three of these metabolic risk factors.

- **Lack of physical activity:** Lack of physical activity can worsen some other risk factors for carotid artery disease, such as unhealthy blood cholesterol levels, high blood pressure, diabetes, and overweight or obesity.

- **Unhealthy diet:** An unhealthy diet can raise your risk for carotid artery disease. Foods that are high in saturated and trans fats, cholesterol, sodium (salt), and sugar can worsen other carotid artery disease risk factors.

- **Older age:** As you get older, your risk for carotid artery disease increases. Genetic or lifestyle factors cause plaque to build up in your arteries as you age. Before age 75, the risk is greater in men than women. However, after age 75, the risk is greater in women.

- **Family history of atherosclerosis:** This increases your risk.

Having any of these risk factors doesn't guarantee that you'll develop carotid artery disease. However, if you know that you have one or more risk factors, you can take steps to help prevent or delay the disease.

Steps include following a healthy lifestyle and taking medicines as your doctor prescribes.

If you have plaque buildup in your carotid arteries, you also may have plaque buildup in other arteries. People who have carotid artery disease also are at increased risk for coronary heart disease.

Signs and Symptoms of Carotid Artery Disease

Carotid artery disease may not cause signs or symptoms until it severely narrows or blocks a carotid artery. Signs and symptoms may include a bruit, a transient ischemic attack (TIA), or a stroke.

Bruit

During a physical exam, your doctor may listen to your carotid arteries with a stethoscope. He or she may hear a whooshing sound called a bruit. This sound may suggest changed or reduced blood flow due to plaque buildup. To find out more, your doctor may recommend tests.

Not all people who have carotid artery disease have bruits.

Transient Ischemic Attack (Mini-Stroke)

For some people, having a TIA, or mini-stroke, is the first sign of carotid artery disease. During a mini-stroke, you may have some or all of the symptoms of a stroke. However, the symptoms usually go away on their own within 24 hours.

The symptoms may include the following:

- Sudden weakness or numbness in the face or limbs, often on just one side of the body

- The inability to move one or more of your limbs

- Trouble speaking or understanding speech

- Sudden trouble seeing in one or both eyes

- Dizziness or loss of balance

- A sudden, severe headache with no known cause

Even if the symptoms stop quickly, you should see a doctor right away. Call 911 for help. Do not drive yourself to the hospital. It's important to get checked and to get treatment started as soon as possible.

A mini-stroke is a warning sign that you're at high risk of having a stroke. You shouldn't ignore these symptoms. About one-third of people who have mini-strokes will later have strokes. Getting medical care can help find possible causes of a mini-stroke and help you manage risk factors. These actions might prevent a future stroke.

Although a mini-stroke may warn of a stroke, it doesn't predict when a stroke will happen. A stroke may occur days, weeks, or even months after a mini-stroke. In about half of the cases of strokes that follow TIAs, the strokes occur within one year.

Stroke

The symptoms of a stroke are the same as those of a mini-stroke, but the results are not. A stroke can cause lasting brain damage; long-term disability, such as vision or speech problems or paralysis (an inability to move); or death. Most people who have strokes have not previously had warning mini-strokes.

Getting treatment for a stroke right away is very important. You have the best chance for full recovery if treatment to open a blocked artery is given within four hours of symptom onset. The sooner treatment occurs, the better your chances of recovery.

Call 911 for help as soon as symptoms occur. Do not drive yourself to the hospital. It's very important to get checked and to get treatment started as soon as possible.

Make those close to you aware of stroke symptoms and the need for urgent action. Learning the signs and symptoms of a stroke will allow you to help yourself or someone close to you lower the risk of brain damage or death due to a stroke.

How Is Carotid Artery Disease Treated?

Treatments for carotid artery disease may include lifestyle changes, medicines, and medical procedures. The goals of treatment are to stop the disease from getting worse and to prevent a stroke.

Your treatment will depend on your symptoms, how severe the disease is, and your age and overall health.

Lifestyle Changes

Making lifestyle changes can help prevent carotid artery disease or keep it from getting worse. For some people, these changes may be the only treatment needed:

- Follow a healthy diet to prevent or lower high blood pressure and high blood cholesterol and to maintain a healthy weight.

- Be physically active. Check with your doctor first to find out how much and what kinds of activity are safe for you.

- If you're overweight or obese, lose weight.

- If you smoke, quit. Also, try to avoid secondhand smoke.

Follow a Healthy Diet

A healthy diet is an important part of a healthy lifestyle. Following a healthy diet can prevent or reduce high blood pressure and high blood cholesterol and help you maintain a healthy weight.

Your doctor may recommend a three-part program called Therapeutic Lifestyle Changes (TLC) if you have high blood cholesterol. TLC includes a healthy diet, physical activity, and weight management.

With the TLC diet, less than 7 percent of your daily calories should come from saturated fat. This kind of fat is found mainly in meat, poultry, and dairy products. No more than 25 to 35 percent of your daily calories should come from all fats, including saturated, trans, monounsaturated, and polyunsaturated fats.

You also should have less than 200 mg a day of cholesterol. The amounts of cholesterol and the different kinds of fat in prepared foods can be found on the foods' Nutrition Facts labels.

Foods high in soluble fiber also are part of a healthy diet. They help block the digestive tract from absorbing cholesterol. These foods include the following:

- Whole-grain cereals such as oatmeal and oat bran

- Fruits such as apples, bananas, oranges, pears, and prunes

- Legumes such as kidney beans, lentils, chick peas, black-eyed peas, and lima beans

A diet rich in fruits and vegetables can increase important cholesterol-lowering compounds in your diet. These compounds, called plant stanols or sterols, work like soluble fiber.

Fish are an important part of a healthy diet. They're a good source of omega-3 fatty acids, which help lower blood cholesterol levels. Try to have about two fish meals every week. Fish high in omega-3 fatty acids are salmon, tuna (canned or fresh), and mackerel.

You also should try to limit the amount of sodium (salt) that you eat. Too much sodium can raise your risk of high blood pressure. Choose low-sodium and no added salt foods and seasonings at the table or when cooking. The Nutrition Facts label on food packaging shows the amount of sodium in an item.

Try to limit drinks with alcohol. Too much alcohol will raise your blood pressure and triglyceride level. (Triglycerides are a type of fat found in the blood.) Alcohol also adds extra calories, which will cause weight gain.

Men should have no more than two drinks containing alcohol a day. Women should have no more than one drink containing alcohol a day. One drink is a glass of wine, beer, or a small amount of hard liquor.

Your doctor may recommend the Dietary Approaches to Stop Hypertension (DASH) eating plan if you have high blood pressure. The DASH eating plan focuses on fruits, vegetables, whole grains, and other foods that are heart healthy and low in fat, cholesterol, and sodium.

DASH also focuses on fat-free or low-fat milk and dairy products, fish, poultry, and nuts. The DASH eating plan is reduced in red meats (including lean red meats), sweets, added sugars, and sugar-containing beverages. It's rich in nutrients, protein, and fiber.

The DASH eating plan is a good healthy eating plan, even for those who don't have high blood pressure.

Be Physically Active

Regular physical activity can lower many carotid artery disease risk factors, including LDL (bad) cholesterol, high blood pressure, and excess weight.

Physical activity also can lower your risk for diabetes and raise your HDL cholesterol level. HDL cholesterol is the good cholesterol that helps prevent plaque buildup.

Talk with your doctor before you start a new exercise plan. Ask him or her how much and what kinds of physical activity are safe for you.

People gain health benefits from as little as 60 minutes of moderate-intensity aerobic activity per week. The more active you are, the more you will benefit.

Maintain a Healthy Weight

Maintaining a healthy weight can lower your risk for carotid artery disease and stroke. Even a modest weight gain can increase your risk of having a stroke.

If you're overweight, aim to reduce your weight by 7 to 10 percent during your first year of treatment. This amount of weight loss can lower your risk for carotid artery disease and other health problems.

After the first year, you may have to continue to lose weight so you can lower your body mass index (BMI) to less than 25.

BMI measures your weight in relation to your height. A BMI between 25 and 29.9 is considered overweight for adults. A BMI of 30 or more is considered obese for adults. A BMI of less than 25 is the goal for preventing and treating carotid artery disease.

Quit Smoking

If you smoke or use tobacco, quit. Smoking can damage your arteries and raise your risk for stroke and other health problems. Also, try to avoid secondhand smoke.

Talk with your doctor about programs and products that can help you quit.

Medicines

You may need medicines to treat diseases and conditions that damage the carotid arteries. High blood pressure, high blood cholesterol, and diabetes can worsen carotid artery disease.

Some people can control these risk factors with lifestyle changes. Others also need medicines to achieve and maintain control.

You may need anticlotting medicines to prevent blood clots from forming in your carotid arteries and causing a stroke. Damage and plaque buildup make blood clots more likely.

Aspirin and clopidogrel are two common anticlotting medicines. They stop platelets from clumping together to form clots. These medicines are a mainstay of treatment for people who have known carotid artery disease.

Your health care team will help find a treatment plan that's right for you. Sticking to this plan will help avoid further harm to your carotid arteries.

If you have a stroke due to a blood clot, you may be given a clot-dissolving, or clot-busting, medicine. This type of medicine must be given within 4 hours of symptom onset.

The sooner treatment occurs, the better your chances of recovery. Thus, it's important to know the signs and symptoms of a stroke and call 911 right away for emergency care.

Medical Procedures

You may need a medical procedure to treat carotid artery disease. Doctors use one of two methods to open narrowed or blocked carotid arteries: carotid endarterectomy and carotid artery angioplasty and stenting.

Chapter 15

C-Reactive Protein and Stroke Risk

What is CRP?

C-reactive protein (CRP) is a substance that is released into the blood in response to inflammation, the process by which the body responds to injury. Elevated levels of CRP in the blood mean that there is inflammation somewhere in the body, but other tests are needed to determine the cause and location of the inflammation.

Physicians now believe that atherosclerosis, hardening of the arteries that can lead to a stroke or heart attack, is an inflammatory process. Atherosclerosis causes only a small amount of CRP to be released into the blood. Therefore, a very sensitive test called a high-sensitivity CRP test (hs-CRP) is used to measure CRP levels. A CRP test may be performed to help determine your risk of heart disease or stroke, or if you are hospitalized for heart attack or unstable chest pain.

What are CRP levels?

CRP is measured in milligrams per liter of blood (mg/L). The risk categories in Table 15.1 were established by the American Heart Association (AHA) and the Centers for Disease Control and Prevention (CDC) in 2003 using information drawn from largely white populations. In people whose CRP is tested for heart attack or unstable chest pain, a higher cutoff is used—a level above 10 mg/L is considered high

"CRP and Stroke Risk," Office on Women's Health, U.S. Department of Health and Human Services (www.womenshealth.gov), 2010.

in these cases. CRP is affected by some drugs—for example, hormone therapy increases CRP levels.

Table 15.1. CRP Risk Levels

Risk Category	CRP (mg/L)
Low	Less than 1.0
Average	1.0 to 3.0
High	Above 3.0

Are CRP levels higher in women?

When the AHA and CDC set cutoffs for high and low CRP, it was assumed that levels were similar in men and women. Research now shows that women have higher levels of CRP than men. A Dallas study of nearly 2750 people aged 30 to 65 years (more than half were women) found that on average CRP levels were almost twice as high in women as in men (3.3 vs. 1.8 mg/L). Even after accounting for traditional heart disease risk factors and the use of hormone therapy or the cholesterol-lowering statin drugs (both are closely tied to CRP levels), white women were 60% and African-American women were 70% more likely to have high CRP than white men. Being overweight or obese is also very strongly associated with high CRP, and excess weight appears to raise women's CRP levels more than men's.

Aside from being naturally higher in women, many other medical conditions can raise CRP levels, including arthritis, diabetes, high blood pressure, bacterial and viral infections, sleep disturbance, too much or too little physical activity, drinking too much alcohol, and depression.

Are CRP levels higher in certain races/ethnicities?

An analysis of the Women's Health Study that included more than 25,000 female health professionals older than 45 years showed that CRP levels vary by race. African-American women had higher CRP levels (2.96 mg/L) than Hispanic (2.06 mg/L), white (2.02 mg/L), or Asian (1.12 mg/L) women. Among Asians, South Asians (2.59 mg/L) appear to have higher levels compared with Chinese men and women (1.18 mg/L).

CRP testing of more than 3200 Native Americans aged 45 to 74 years (64% were women) found that levels were much higher than those reported for other populations. The AHA and CDC cutoffs were not useful for predicting the risk of heart attack or dying from heart disease in this population. The authors suggested an alternative upper cutoff (above 4.0 mg/L) for Native Americans.

Does high CRP increase the risk of stroke in women?

Several studies have shown that even a small elevation of CRP in the blood of apparently healthy individuals is a strong predictor of future cardiovascular events, including stroke. In one study of 1400 people (60% women) with an average age of 70 years, having high CRP levels tripled the risk of stroke in women and doubled it in men, even after other stroke risk factors were taken into account.

Another study involving nearly 28,000 women showed that CRP is a stronger predictor than LDL cholesterol of cardiovascular events including stroke, and high CRP levels increase postmenopausal women's risk of stroke even in cases where their LDL (bad) cholesterol levels are normal (below 130 mg/dL). Women with the highest CRP levels (greater than 2.09 mg/L) had double the risk of a first cardiovascular event compared with women with the lowest CRP levels, even after accounting for other risk factors such as age, smoking, diabetes and high blood pressure. Even in women with low LDL cholesterol, those with high CRP levels were 50% more likely to have a first cardiovascular event than women with low CRP.

High CRP levels have also been strongly linked with 30-day outcome following a procedure in which a stent is implanted in the carotid artery (the main artery leading to the brain) to open a blockage, restoring blood flow to the brain and preventing strokes. Slightly more than 22% of patients with CRP greater than 5 mg/L had another stroke or died within 30 days of the procedure, compared with only 3% of patients with lower CRP. You may want to speak with your doctor about your CRP levels if you are considering carotid stenting.

How does CRP influence stroke risk?

CRP is produced in response to inflammation somewhere in the body. This inflammation can be caused by many things—for example, CRP levels temporarily increase when you are fighting an infection. It is thought that high long-term levels of CRP are caused by the same inflammation and damage to your blood vessels as atherosclerosis, and that the presence of plaque in your arteries stimulates more production of CRP. In this way, CRP acts like a barometer of the damage occurring to your blood vessels—the higher your CRP level, the more damage is occurring, and the higher your risk of cardiovascular events such as stroke.

In addition to being a marker of inflammation, CRP may itself contribute to vessel injury. Researchers say that CRP may stimulate the formation of plaque on the interior walls of blood vessels, and reduce the vessel's ability to heal itself. CRP does this by causing the proliferation of immune cells that help to create a blockage on the inside of a blood vessel, at the same time reducing the vessel's ability to create new healthy cells to counteract the injury.

Is high CRP a stronger risk factor for stroke for women?

High levels of CRP are a strong predictor of stroke in both men and women. A large study showed that CRP levels were higher in women of all ethnic groups compared with men, even after accounting for higher body mass index and other variables. However, it is not clear if women are consistently at higher risk of stroke than men because of their comparatively high levels of CRP.

Should I have a CRP test?

According to the AHA, if a person's cardiovascular risk score is low (the possibility of developing cardiovascular disease is less than 10% in 10 years), then no test is needed. If the risk score is in the intermediate range (10% to 20% in 10 years), the test can help predict a cardiovascular or stroke event and help the patient take immediate, preventive action. However, a person with a high risk score (greater than 20% in 10 years) or established heart disease or stroke should be treated intensively regardless of CRP levels and does not need CRP testing.

There is an ongoing debate about how useful CRP really is. A review of the scientific literature prompted some researchers to conclude there is not sufficient evidence to recommend measurement of CRP in people who have never had a stroke, because it is not known whether early detection, or intervention based on detection, improves health outcomes. However, since CRP levels also serve as an indicator of risk of cardiovascular disease, testing is probably valuable. For prevention of additional strokes in those who have had one already, elevated CRP adds to existing information, but there are currently no specific treatments based on CRP levels alone that are known to prevent recurrent stroke.

Chapter 16

Atrial Fibrillation and Stroke

What is atrial fibrillation?

The heartbeat is controlled by an electrical conduction system that sends impulses to the heart muscle causing it to rhythmically expand and contract. Sometimes the heart's electrical conduction system loses its regular pattern, which can cause many different heart rhythm problems. One of these is atrial fibrillation (AF or Afib).

In AF, the electrical impulses are no longer coming from the heart's natural pacemaker (the sinus node), but from the heart's top chambers (atria). Compared to the typical impulses, which occur 60 to 70 times per minute, in AF the charges are very rapid, more than 300 times per minute. The rapid, uncoordinated muscle contractions that result prevent the heart from pumping effectively. The abnormal impulses in the atria also spill over to the heart's main pumping chambers (the ventricles), causing them to beat rapidly and irregularly as well.

AF can be continuous (persistent AF), or episodes may alternate with periods of normal heart rhythm, a condition known as paroxysmal AF. When the rhythm disturbance has lasted for more than a week, it is considered persistent AF.

"Atrial Fibrillation," Office on Women's Health, U.S. Department of Health and Human Services (www.womenshealth.gov), 2010.

What are the symptoms of atrial fibrillation?

Symptoms of AF typically include a racing, irregular, or uncomfortable heartbeat, or a sensation of a flopping in the chest. Some people also experience dizziness, chest pain, and sweating. Not all people with AF experience symptoms.

How common is atrial fibrillation?

AF is the most common heart rhythm disorder, affecting an estimated 2.2 million Americans, or about 1 in 100 people. According to the U.S. Census Bureau, the number of people affected by AF is projected to be more than 12 million by the year 2050.

Although men are 1.5 times more likely than women to develop AF, the actual numbers of women and men with AF are roughly the same because AF is more common in older people and women tend to live longer than men. As with many heart problems, women who develop AF tend to do so later in life than men, at an average age of 75 (compared to 67 in men).

AF itself is not usually deadly, but it can lead to other problems such as chronic fatigue, heart failure, and, most importantly, stroke. There is no difference in the mortality rate between men and women with AF.

What does atrial fibrillation have to do with stroke?

In people with AF, the atria's rapid, irregular beat moves blood inefficiently, and the blood inside the chambers tends to form clots. These clots can break loose and travel through the bloodstream to the brain, where they become lodged in an artery, causing a blocked-vessel (ischemic) stroke.

What impact does atrial fibrillation have on my stroke risk?

AF is responsible for 15% to 20% of all strokes. It increases the risk of a first stroke three- to four-fold, and doubles the risk of a recurrent stroke. The stroke risk is the same whether the AF is persistent or paroxysmal (comes and goes).

Several studies have found that AF is a more important stroke risk factor in women than in men. In one observational study of 1,581 patients (half were women) who had experienced a first stroke, women were almost twice as likely to have had AF that preceded the stroke (31% versus 19% of men).

If you have AF, your personal stroke risk varies widely based on other conditions you may have: Doctors use a formula called the CHADS$_2$ [Congestive heart failure; hypertension; age equal to or greater than 75 years; diabetes mellitus; prior stroke or transient ischemic attack/TIA or thromboembolism] score to determine your approximate risk. To find out your stroke risk, add up all your CHADS$_2$ points in Table 16.1, and then look up your corresponding yearly stroke risk in Table 16.2.

In addition to increasing your chances of stroke, AF also tends to make strokes more severe: One study found that people with AF who had a stroke were more than twice as likely to be bedridden than those who had strokes from other causes.

Table 16.1. CHADS$_2$ Score for Predicting Stroke Risk in Patients with AF

Risk Factor	Points
Heart Failure	+1
Systolic blood pressure higher than 160 mm Hg	+1
Being 75 years or older	+1
Diabetes	+1
Previous Stroke or TIA	+2

Table 16.2. Your Stroke Risk

CHADS$_2$ Score	Risk Level	Yearly Stroke Risk
0	Low	1.0%
1	Low to Moderate	1.5%
2*	Moderate	2.5%
3	High	5.0%
4, 5, or 6	Very High	More than 7%

*Note: If you have had a stroke or TIA you are considered to be at high risk, even if you have no other risk factors.

Chapter 17

Blood Clotting Disorders and Stroke

What is a hypercoagulable state?

When a person has an abnormally strong tendency for the blood to thicken and clot, it is called a hypercoagulable state. It can be the result of environmental factors (such as the effects of hormones, surgery, or cancer), or it can be caused by an inherited defect in one of the molecules involved in blood clotting. Blood clotting problems like these are more likely to increase your risk of developing harmful blood clots in the deep veins of the legs (deep vein thrombosis or DVT) than blood clots in the arteries that can result in a heart attack or stroke. A blood clot or thrombus in the veins of the legs can break off and travel through the bloodstream to block an artery in the lungs, causing the life-threatening condition pulmonary embolism.

What causes blood clotting problems?

There are several causes for blood clotting problems. You are more prone to developing blood clots after surgery (especially hip or knee), or when you are immobilized for more than four days, or as a result of injuries from a severe accident. Cancer can also lead to a hypercoagulable state: 1% to 15% of cancer patients develop blood clots in their veins.

Some people have a higher risk of blood clotting problems because they inherit mutations (variations) in the genes for blood clotting proteins.

"Blood Clotting Problems and Stroke Risk," Office on Women's Health, U.S. Department of Health and Human Services (www.womenshealth.gov), 2010.

Hormones, including estrogen found in hormone therapy and birth control pills, can increase your risk of developing blood clots, especially if you have an inherited blood clotting disorder or have a history of unexplained blood clots.

Can inherited blood clotting problems increase my risk of having a stroke?

Blood clotting disorders may be to blame for 5% to 10% of blocked-vessel (ischemic) strokes—possibly more in younger, otherwise healthy people. Typical clotting disorders result in a greater likelihood of clots forming inside of blood vessels, which can cause a blocked-vessel stroke. Clotting disorders that predispose to the formation of blood clots are not risk factors for bleeding (hemorrhagic) stroke. There are some rare inherited disorders that make the blood unable to clot, which does increase the chances of a bleeding stroke.

What is Factor V Leiden?

The most commonly inherited blood clotting problem is called Factor V Leiden (FVL), so-called because it affects the Factor V (5) clotting protein. FVL occurs in about 5% of white women and men; rates are lower for Hispanics and it is rare in people of Asian or African descent.

Does FVL increase my risk of stroke?

Inheriting the FVL mutation may increase your risk of stroke in the presence of other risk factors, such as birth control pills. The mutation by itself accounts for an increase in stroke risk less than that associated with the birth control pill alone. However, women with a single defective FVL gene have a 30-fold higher risk of developing blood clots while using birth control pills, a 15-fold higher risk with postmenopausal hormone therapy, and a 7-fold higher risk during pregnancy compared with women without this mutation. Women who carry two abnormal FVL genes have an even greater risk of developing blood clots. It is likely that these women will experience at least one blood clotting event during their lifetime. Whether the FVL mutation increases stroke risk in younger people without other risk factors is controversial. A recent European study of 240 stroke patients found that FVL together with another genetic clotting condition (prothrombin) accounted for an overall four-fold increased risk of stroke compared with patients with similar risk factors but no genetic clotting condition. Compared with men, women in this study had a greater stroke risk (five-fold) associated with these disorders.

What other inherited blood clotting problems may be linked to stroke?

A common genetic risk factor for blood clots is a mutation in the gene encoding the clotting factor prothrombin. The mutation is found in about 1 in 50 persons in the United States. It raises the risk of blood clots for both women and men of all ages, but appears to increase stroke risk only if you have other risk factors such as a congenital heart defect (especially patent foramen ovale), other clotting problems, or are taking birth control pills. If you know you have an inherited blood clotting disorder, or have had a blood clot before, it is very important you address your other risk factors for stroke such as quitting smoking, managing high blood pressure, and talking to your doctor about birth control pills.

Results from the Framingham Heart Study showed that one particular blood marker was an independent risk factor for blocked-vessel stroke and transient ischemic attack (TIA) in women but not in men. The blood marker in question is called an anticardiolipin antibody (aCL). aCL is a protein found in the blood that, if present in excessive amounts, is associated with clotting abnormalities as well as multiple pregnancy miscarriages. The study in question found that women with a high level of aCL in their blood were almost three times as likely to suffer a blocked-vessel stroke as women with normal aCL levels. No association between stroke and aCL was found for men.

Should I be tested for blood clotting problems?

Currently, the American Stroke Association maintains that there is not sufficient evidence to make recommendations for the prevention of stroke based on inherited blood clotting conditions such as FVL and prothrombin. Unless you are young (under 50) and have had a blood clot or unexplained stroke, or if you have other stroke risk factors including family history, testing is usually not necessary.

Tests that measure blood clotting proteins do not help predict whether you will develop cardiovascular disease any better than the well-established risk factors (such as high blood pressure and high cholesterol).

Although tests for inherited blood clotting problems are not usually done, you may be sent for one if you meet any of the following criteria:

- Blood clotting problem before age 50
- Blood clots in unusual parts of the body (not the legs)
- Repeated blood clots in the veins

- Family history of blood clot problems before age 50
- Blood clot and a strong family history
- Blood clot during pregnancy or while using birth control pills
- You had a stroke before age 50 and you smoke

How can I prevent stroke if I have a blood clotting problem?

If you had a blood clot and were diagnosed with an inherited blood clotting problem, you may have to take blood thinning medications for the rest of your life. Some people only need to take medications in situations that put them at high risk for developing blood clots, such as during pregnancy or surgery.

Some of the risk factors that increase your likelihood of blood clotting problems include smoking, physical inactivity, higher body mass index (BMI), and diabetes or early signs of diabetes (insulin resistance). Quitting smoking and getting more exercise helps lower levels of blood clotting proteins and has also been proven to lower your risk of stroke.

Chapter 18

Peripheral Artery Disease

What is it?

Peripheral artery disease (PAD) is a disease of the arteries outside the heart and brain. PAD affects about 8 million Americans, including 12% to 20% of women and men aged 65 or older.

Common early symptoms of PAD are cramping, heaviness, fatigue, pain, or discomfort in the legs or buttocks during activity, called intermittent claudication. However, not all people with PAD have symptoms: In one study of 933 disabled women older than 65, 63% of those with PAD had no leg pain with activity.

The standard test for diagnosing PAD is a simple comparison of blood pressure measurements in the arm and leg called the Ankle Brachial Index, or ABI. If your ABI number is low (less than 0.9), other imaging tests may be needed.

How is it related to stroke?

Like CAD [coronary artery disease], PAD is related to stroke because they are both a result of the same disease process: Atherosclerosis. In PAD, the fatty buildup blocks circulation in arteries leading to the kidneys, stomach, legs, arms, or feet. PAD is often the first sign of atherosclerosis that is affecting the arteries of your heart and brain as well, and could eventually lead to a heart attack or stroke.

"Peripheral Artery Disease," Office on Women's Health, U.S. Department of Health and Human Services (www.womenshealth.gov), 2010.

How does it affect my stroke risk?

Compared to those without PAD, people with PAD have four to five times the risk of dying of cardiovascular disease. Overall, studies indicate that PAD increases your chances of suffering a stroke by about 40%.

PAD is generally accepted to be a risk factor for stroke in both women and men, although so far evidence from clinical trials linking PAD to stroke risk in women is lacking. The ARIC [Atherosclerosis Risk in Communities] study of more than 15,000 people (55% were women) found that men with PAD in the legs were four to five times as likely to have a stroke or transient ischemic attack (TIA), but there was no significant difference in stroke risk between women with and without PAD after adjustment for other factors. These results suggest that, at least in women, PAD may not increase stroke risk on its own; rather, PAD and stroke share enough risk factors that a woman with one disease is likely to be at high risk for the other.

What can I do to prevent stroke?

Despite being a very common disease, only one out of every four people with PAD are undergoing treatment. PAD often goes undiagnosed, so it is important to go to your doctor with any symptoms that could signal PAD—pain in your legs or buttocks with activity that goes away with rest is not a normal part of aging. Since PAD can be the first sign of widespread artery disease, you should consider it an opportunity to get your risk factors under control before they lead to a potentially fatal heart attack or stroke.

Like CAD, PAD shares many risk factors for stroke, and the treatments that are recommended for relieving your PAD symptoms and preventing the disease from getting any worse will also help lower your stroke risk. The most important things are to quit smoking (80% of people with PAD are smokers), control your diabetes, cholesterol, and blood pressure, and make lifestyle changes such as eating a diet low in saturated fat and starting an exercise regimen. You may also start taking blood-thinning medication to prevent the formation of clots that can lead to a stroke. Medication is also available to relieve some of the leg pain caused by PAD.

Chapter 19

Diabetes and Stroke Risk

Having diabetes or prediabetes puts you at increased risk for heart disease and stroke. You can lower your risk by keeping your blood glucose (also called blood sugar), blood pressure, and blood cholesterol close to the recommended target numbers-the levels suggested by diabetes experts for good health.

If you have already had a heart attack or a stroke, taking care of yourself can help prevent future health problems.

What is diabetes?

Diabetes is a disorder of metabolism—the way our bodies use digested food for energy. Most of the food we eat is broken down into glucose, the form of sugar in the blood. Glucose is the body's main source of fuel.

After digestion, glucose enters the bloodstream. Then glucose goes to cells throughout the body where it is used for energy. However, a hormone called insulin must be present to allow glucose to enter the cells. Insulin is a hormone produced by the pancreas, a large gland behind the stomach.

In people who do not have diabetes, the pancreas automatically produces the right amount of insulin to move glucose from blood into

Excerpted from "Diabetes, Heart Disease, and Stroke," by the National Institute for Diabetes and Digestive and Kidney Diseases (NIDDK, www.niddk .nih.gov), part of the National Institutes of Health, December 6, 2011.

the cells. However, diabetes develops when the pancreas does not make enough insulin, or the cells in the muscles, liver, and fat do not use insulin properly, or both. As a result, the amount of glucose in the blood increases while the cells are starved of energy.

Over time, high blood glucose levels damage nerves and blood vessels, leading to complications such as heart disease and stroke, the leading causes of death among people with diabetes. Uncontrolled diabetes can eventually lead to other health problems as well, such as vision loss, kidney failure, and amputations.

What is the connection between diabetes, heart disease, and stroke?

If you have diabetes, you are at least twice as likely as someone who does not have diabetes to have heart disease or a stroke. People with diabetes also tend to develop heart disease or have strokes at an earlier age than other people. If you are middle-aged and have type 2 diabetes, some studies suggest that your chance of having a heart attack is as high as someone without diabetes who has already had one heart attack. Women who have not gone through menopause usually have less risk of heart disease than men of the same age. But women of all ages with diabetes have an increased risk of heart disease because diabetes cancels out the protective effects of being a woman in her child-bearing years.

People with diabetes who have already had one heart attack run an even greater risk of having a second one. In addition, heart attacks in people with diabetes are more serious and more likely to result in death. High blood glucose levels over time can lead to increased deposits of fatty materials on the insides of the blood vessel walls. These deposits may affect blood flow, increasing the chance of clogging and hardening of blood vessels (atherosclerosis).

What are the risk factors for heart disease and stroke in people with diabetes?

Diabetes itself is a risk factor for heart disease and stroke. Also, many people with diabetes have other conditions that increase their chance of developing heart disease and stroke. These conditions are called risk factors. One risk factor for heart disease and stroke is having a family history of heart disease. If one or more members of your family had a heart attack at an early age (before age 55 for men or 65 for women), you may be at increased risk.

You can't change whether heart disease runs in your family, but you can take steps to control the other risk factors for heart disease listed here:

- **Having central obesity:** Central obesity means carrying extra weight around the waist, as opposed to the hips. A waist measurement of more than 40 inches for men and more than 35 inches for women means you have central obesity. Your risk of heart disease is higher because abdominal fat can increase the production of LDL (low-density lipoprotein, or bad) cholesterol, the type of blood fat that can be deposited on the inside of blood vessel walls.

- **Having abnormal blood fat (cholesterol) levels:** LDL cholesterol can build up inside your blood vessels, leading to narrowing and hardening of your arteries—the blood vessels that carry blood from the heart to the rest of the body. Arteries can then become blocked. Therefore, high levels of LDL cholesterol raise your risk of getting heart disease. Triglycerides are another type of blood fat that can raise your risk of heart disease when the levels are high. HDL (good) cholesterol removes deposits from inside your blood vessels and takes them to the liver for removal. Low levels of HDL cholesterol increase your risk for heart disease.

- **Having high blood pressure:** If you have high blood pressure, also called hypertension, your heart must work harder to pump blood. High blood pressure can strain the heart, damage blood vessels, and increase your risk of heart attack, stroke, eye problems, and kidney problems.

- **Smoking:** Smoking doubles your risk of getting heart disease. Stopping smoking is especially important for people with diabetes because both smoking and diabetes narrow blood vessels. Smoking also increases the risk of other long-term complications, such as eye problems. In addition, smoking can damage the blood vessels in your legs and increase the risk of amputation.

Chapter 20

High Blood Pressure and High Cholesterol

Chapter Contents

Section 20.1

High Blood Pressure

Excerpted from "High Blood Pressure," National Heart, Lung,
and Blood Institute (NHLBI, www.nhlbi.nih.gov), part of the
National Institutes of Health, August 2, 2012.

High blood pressure (HBP) is a serious condition that can lead to
coronary heart disease, heart failure, stroke, kidney failure, and other
health problems.

Blood pressure is the force of blood pushing against the walls of
the arteries as the heart pumps blood. If this pressure rises and stays
high over time, it can damage the body in many ways.

Overview

About one in three adults in the United States has HBP. The condition itself usually has no signs or symptoms. You can have it for years
without knowing it. During this time, though, HBP can damage your
heart, blood vessels, kidneys, and other parts of your body.

Knowing your blood pressure numbers is important, even when
you're feeling fine. If your blood pressure is normal, you can work with
your health care team to keep it that way. If your blood pressure is
too high, treatment may help prevent damage to your body's organs.

Blood Pressure Numbers

Blood pressure is measured as systolic and diastolic pressures.
Systolic refers to blood pressure when the heart beats while pumping blood. Diastolic refers to blood pressure when the heart is at rest
between beats.

You most often will see blood pressure numbers written with the
systolic number above or before the diastolic number, such as 120/80
mmHg. (The mmHg is millimeters of mercury—the units used to measure blood pressure.)

Table 20.1 shows normal blood pressure numbers for adults. It also
shows which numbers put you at greater risk for health problems.

Table 20.1. Categories for Blood Pressure Levels in Adults (measured in millimeters of mercury, or mmHg)

Category	Systolic (top number)		Diastolic (bottom number)
Normal	Less than 120	And	Less than 80
Prehypertension	120–139	Or	80–89
High blood pressure			
Stage 1	140–159	Or	90–99
Stage 2	160 or higher	Or	100 or higher

The ranges in Table 20.1 apply to most adults (aged 18 and older) who don't have short-term serious illnesses.

Blood pressure doesn't stay the same all the time. It lowers as you sleep and rises when you wake up. Blood pressure also rises when you're excited, nervous, or active. If your numbers stay above normal most of the time, you're at risk for health problems. The risk grows as blood pressure numbers rise. Prehypertension means you may end up with HBP, unless you take steps to prevent it.

If you're being treated for HBP and have repeat readings in the normal range, your blood pressure is under control. However, you still have the condition. You should see your doctor and follow your treatment plan to keep your blood pressure under control.

Your systolic and diastolic numbers may not be in the same blood pressure category. In this case, the more severe category is the one you're in. For example, if your systolic number is 160 and your diastolic number is 80, you have stage 2 HBP. If your systolic number is 120 and your diastolic number is 95, you have stage 1 HBP.

If you have diabetes or chronic kidney disease, HBP is defined as 130/80 mmHg or higher. HBP numbers also differ for children and teens.

Outlook

Blood pressure tends to rise with age. Following a healthy lifestyle helps some people delay or prevent this rise in blood pressure.

People who have HBP can take steps to control it and reduce their risk for related health problems. Key steps include following a healthy lifestyle, having ongoing medical care, and following your treatment plan.

Other Names for High Blood Pressure

High blood pressure (HBP) also is called hypertension.

- When HBP has no known cause, it might be called essential hypertension, primary hypertension, or idiopathic hypertension.

- When another condition causes HBP, it's sometimes called secondary hypertension.

Some people only have high systolic blood pressure. This condition is called isolated systolic hypertension (ISH). Many older adults have this condition. ISH can cause as much harm as HBP in which both numbers are too high.

What Causes High Blood Pressure?

Blood pressure tends to rise with age, unless you take steps to prevent or control it.

Some medical problems—such as chronic kidney disease, thyroid disease, and sleep apnea—may cause blood pressure to rise. Some medicines also may raise your blood pressure. Examples include asthma medicines (for example, corticosteroids) and cold-relief products.

Other medicines also can cause high blood pressure (HBP). If you have HBP, let your doctor know about all of the medicines you take, including over-the-counter products.

In some women, birth control pills, pregnancy, or hormone therapy (HT) may cause blood pressure to rise.

Women taking birth control pills usually have a small rise in both systolic and diastolic blood pressures. If you already have HBP and want to use birth control pills, make sure your doctor knows about your HBP. Talk with him or her about how often you should have your blood pressure checked and how to control it while taking the pill.

Taking HT to reduce the symptoms of menopause can cause a small rise in systolic blood pressure. If you already have HBP and want to start using HT, talk with your doctor about the risks and benefits. If you decide to take hormones, find out how to control your blood pressure and how often you should have it checked.

Children younger than 10 years old who have HBP often have another condition that's causing it (such as kidney disease). Treating the underlying condition may resolve the HBP.

The older a child is when HBP is diagnosed, the more likely he or she is to have essential hypertension. This means that doctors don't know what's causing the HBP.

Who Is at Risk for High Blood Pressure?

High blood pressure (HBP) is a common condition. In the United States, about one in three adults has HBP.

Certain traits, conditions, and habits can raise your risk for HBP. The major risk factors for HBP are described in the following.

Older Age

Blood pressure tends to rise with age. About 65 percent of Americans aged 60 or older have HBP.

Isolated systolic hypertension (ISH) is the most common form of HBP in older adults. ISH occurs when only systolic blood pressure (the top number) is high. About two out of three people over age 60 with HBP have ISH.

HBP doesn't have to be a routine part of aging. You can take steps to keep your blood pressure at a normal level.

Race/Ethnicity

HBP can affect anyone. However, it's more common in African-American adults than in Caucasian or Hispanic-American adults. In relation to these groups, African Americans:

- tend to get HBP earlier in life;

- often have more severe HBP;

- are more likely to be aware that they have HBP and to get treatment;

- are less likely than Caucasians to achieve target control levels with HBP treatment;

- have higher rates than Caucasians of early death from HBP-related problems, such as coronary heart disease, stroke, and kidney failure.

HBP risks vary among different groups of Hispanic-American adults. For instance, Puerto Rican-American adults have higher rates of HBP-related death than all other Hispanic groups and Caucasians. However, Cuban Americans have lower rates of HBP-related death than Caucasians.

Overweight or Obesity

You're more likely to develop prehypertension or HBP if you're overweight or obese. The terms overweight and obesity refer to body weight that's greater than what is considered healthy for a certain height.

Gender

Men and women are equally likely to develop HBP during their lifetimes. However, before age 45, men are more likely to have HBP than women. After age 65, the condition is more likely to affect women than men.

Also, men younger than 55 are more likely to have uncontrolled HBP than women. However, after age 65, women are more likely to have uncontrolled HBP.

Unhealthy Lifestyle Habits

Many unhealthy lifestyle habits can raise your risk for HBP, including:

- eating too much sodium (salt);
- drinking too much alcohol;
- not getting enough potassium in your diet;
- lack of physical activity;
- smoking.

Other Risk Factors

A family history of HBP raises your risk for the condition. Long-lasting stress also can put you at risk for HBP.

You're also more likely to develop HBP if you have prehypertension. Prehypertension means that your blood pressure is in the 120–139/80–89 mmHg range.

Risk Factors for Children and Teens

Prehypertension and HBP are becoming more common in children and teens. This is due in part to a rise in overweight and obesity among children and teens.

African-American and Mexican-American youth are more likely to have HBP and prehypertension than Caucasian youth. Also, boys are at higher risk for HBP than girls.

Like adults, children and teens need to have routine blood pressure checks, especially if they're overweight.

What Are the Signs and Symptoms of High Blood Pressure?

High blood pressure (HBP) itself usually has no signs or symptoms. Rarely, headaches may occur.

You can have HBP for years without knowing it. During this time, the condition can damage your heart, blood vessels, kidneys, and other parts of your body.

Some people only learn that they have HBP after the damage has caused problems, such as coronary heart disease, stroke, or kidney failure.

Knowing your blood pressure numbers is important, even when you're feeling fine. If your blood pressure is normal, you can work with your health care team to keep it that way. If your blood pressure is too high, you can take steps to lower it. Lowering your blood pressure will help reduce your risk for related health problems.

Complications of High Blood Pressure

When blood pressure stays high over time, it can damage the body. HBP can cause the following:

- It can cause the heart to get larger or weaker, which may lead to heart failure. Heart failure is a condition in which the heart can't pump enough blood to meet the body's needs.

- It can cause aneurysms to form in blood vessels. An aneurysm is an abnormal bulge in the wall of an artery. Common spots for aneurysms are the main artery that carries blood from the heart to the body; the arteries in the brain, legs, and intestines; and the artery leading to the spleen.

- It can cause blood vessels in the kidneys to narrow. This may cause kidney failure.

- It can cause arteries throughout the body to narrow in some places, which limits blood flow (especially to the heart, brain, kidneys, and legs). This can cause a heart attack, stroke, kidney failure, or amputation of part of the leg.

- It can cause blood vessels in the eyes to burst or bleed. This may lead to vision changes or blindness.

How Is High Blood Pressure Diagnosed?

High blood pressure (HBP) is diagnosed using a blood pressure test. This test will be done several times to make sure the results are correct. If your numbers are high, your doctor may have you return for repeat tests to check your blood pressure over time.

If your blood pressure is 140/90 mmHg or higher over time, your doctor will likely diagnose you with HBP. If you have diabetes or chronic kidney disease, a blood pressure of 130/80 mmHg or higher is considered HBP.

The ranges for HBP in children are different, as discussed in the following text.

How Is Blood Pressure Tested?

A blood pressure test is easy and painless. This test is done at a doctor's office or clinic.

To prepare for the test:

- Don't drink coffee or smoke cigarettes for 30 minutes prior to the test. These actions may cause a short-term rise in your blood pressure.

- Go to the bathroom before the test. Having a full bladder can change your blood pressure reading.

- Sit for five minutes before the test. Movement can cause short-term rises in blood pressure.

- To measure your blood pressure, your doctor or nurse will use some type of a gauge, a stethoscope (or electronic sensor), and a blood pressure cuff.

Most often, you will sit or lie down with the cuff around your arm as your doctor or nurse checks your blood pressure. If he or she doesn't tell you what your blood pressure numbers are, you should ask.

Diagnosing High Blood Pressure in Children and Teens

Doctors measure blood pressure in children and teens the same way they do in adults. Your child should have routine blood pressure checks starting at three years of age.

Blood pressure normally rises with age and body size. Newborn babies often have very low blood pressure numbers, while older teens have numbers similar to adults.

The ranges for normal blood pressure and HBP generally are lower for youth than for adults. To find out whether a child has HBP, a doctor will compare the child's blood pressure numbers to average numbers for his or her age, gender, and height.

172

What Does a Diagnosis of High Blood Pressure Mean?

If you're diagnosed with HBP, your doctor will prescribe treatment. Your blood pressure will be tested again to see how the treatment affects it.

Once your blood pressure is under control, you'll still need treatment. "Under control" means that your blood pressure numbers are in the normal range. Your doctor will likely recommend routine blood pressure tests. He or she can tell you how often you should be tested.

The sooner you find out about HBP and treat it, the better. Early treatment may help you avoid problems such as heart attack, stroke, and kidney failure.

How Is High Blood Pressure Treated?

High blood pressure (HBP) is treated with lifestyle changes and medicines.

Most people who have HBP will need lifelong treatment. Sticking to your treatment plan is important. It can help prevent or delay problems related to HBP and help you live and stay active longer.

Goals of Treatment

The treatment goal for most adults is to get and keep blood pressure below 140/90 mmHg. For adults who have diabetes or chronic kidney disease, the goal is to get and keep blood pressure below 130/80 mmHg.

Lifestyle Changes

Healthy lifestyle habits can help you control HBP. These habits include the following:

- Following a healthy diet

- Being physically active

- Maintaining a healthy weight

- Quitting smoking

- Managing your stress and learning to cope with stress

If you combine healthy lifestyle habits, you can achieve even better results than taking single steps.

You may find it hard to make lifestyle changes. Start by making one healthy lifestyle change and then adopt others.

173

Some people can control their blood pressure with lifestyle changes alone, but many people can't. Keep in mind that the main goal is blood pressure control.

If your doctor prescribes medicines as a part of your treatment plan, keep up your healthy lifestyle habits. They will help you better control your blood pressure.

Following a Healthy Diet

Your doctor may recommend the DASH (Dietary Approaches to Stop Hypertension) eating plan if you have HBP. The DASH eating plan focuses on fruits, vegetables, whole grains, and other foods that are heart healthy and low in fat, cholesterol, and sodium (salt).

DASH also focuses on fat-free or low-fat dairy products, fish, poultry, and nuts. The DASH eating plan is reduced in red meats (including lean red meats), sweets, added sugars, and sugar-containing beverages. It's rich in nutrients, protein, and fiber.

To help control HBP, you should limit the amount of salt that you eat. This means choosing low-sodium and no added salt foods and seasonings at the table and while cooking. The Nutrition Facts label on food packaging shows the amount of sodium in an item. You should eat no more than about 1 teaspoon of salt a day.

Also, try to limit alcoholic drinks. Too much alcohol will raise your blood pressure. Men should have no more than two alcoholic drinks a day. Women should have no more than one alcoholic drink a day. One drink is a glass of wine, beer, or a small amount of hard liquor.

Being Physically Active

Routine physical activity can lower HBP and reduce your risk for other health problems. Talk with your doctor before you start a new exercise plan. Ask him or her how much and what kinds of physical activity are safe for you.

People gain health benefits from as little as 60 minutes of moderate-intensity aerobic activity per week. The more active you are, the more you will benefit.

Maintaining a Healthy Weight

Maintaining a healthy weight can help you control HBP and reduce your risk for other health problems.

If you're overweight or obese, aim to reduce your weight by 5 to 10 percent during your first year of treatment. This amount of weight loss can lower your risk for health problems related to HBP.

To lose weight, cut back your calorie intake and do more physical activity. Eat smaller portions and choose lower calorie foods. Don't feel that you have to finish the entrees served at restaurants. Many restaurant portions are oversized and have too many calories for the average person.

After your first year of treatment, you may have to continue to lose weight so you can lower your body mass index (BMI) to less than 25. BMI measures your weight in relation to your height and gives an estimate of your total body fat.

A BMI between 25 and 29.9 is considered overweight. A BMI of 30 or more is considered obese. A BMI of less than 25 is the goal for controlling blood pressure.

You can use the NHLBI's online BMI calculator to figure out your BMI, or your doctor can help you.

Quit Smoking

If you smoke or use tobacco, quit. Smoking can damage your blood vessels and raise your risk for HBP. Smoking also can worsen health problems related to HBP.

Talk with your doctor about programs and products that can help you quit smoking. Also, try to avoid secondhand smoke.

If you have trouble quitting smoking on your own, consider joining a support group. Many hospitals, workplaces, and community groups offer classes to help people quit smoking.

Managing Stress

Learning how to manage stress, relax, and cope with problems can improve your emotional and physical health.

Physical activity helps some people cope with stress. Other people listen to music or focus on something calm or peaceful to reduce stress. Some people learn yoga, tai chi, or how to meditate.

Medicines

Today's blood pressure medicines can safely help most people control their blood pressure. These medicines are easy to take. The side effects, if any, tend to be minor.

If you have side effects from your medicines, talk with your doctor. He or she might adjust the doses or prescribe other medicines. You shouldn't decide on your own to stop taking your medicines.

Blood pressure medicines work in different ways to lower blood pressure. Some remove extra fluid and salt from the body to lower blood pressure. Others slow down the heartbeat or relax and widen blood vessels. Often, two or more medicines work better than one.

Diuretics

Diuretics sometimes are called water pills. They help your kidneys flush excess water and salt from your body. This reduces the amount of fluid in your blood, and your blood pressure goes down.

Diuretics often are used with other HBP medicines and sometimes combined into one pill.

Beta Blockers

Beta blockers help your heart beat slower and with less force. As a result, your heart pumps less blood through your blood vessels. This causes your blood pressure to go down.

ACE Inhibitors

ACE [angiotensin-converting enzyme] inhibitors keep your body from making a hormone called angiotensin II. This hormone normally causes blood vessels to narrow. ACE inhibitors prevent this, so your blood pressure goes down.

Angiotensin II Receptor Blockers

Angiotensin II receptor blockers are newer blood pressure medicines that protect your blood vessels from the angiotensin II hormone. As a result, blood vessels relax and widen, and your blood pressure goes down.

Calcium Channel Blockers

Calcium channel blockers keep calcium from entering the muscle cells of your heart and blood vessels. This allows blood vessels to relax, and your blood pressure goes down.

Alpha Blockers

Alpha blockers reduce nerve impulses that tighten blood vessels. This allows blood to flow more freely, causing blood pressure to go down.

Alpha-Beta Blockers

Alpha-beta blockers reduce nerve impulses the same way alpha blockers do. However, they also slow the heartbeat like beta blockers. As a result, blood pressure goes down.

Nervous System Inhibitors

Nervous system inhibitors increase nerve impulses from the brain to relax and widen blood vessels. This causes blood pressure to go down.

Vasodilators

Vasodilators relax the muscles in blood vessel walls. This causes blood pressure to go down.

Treatment for Children and Teens

If another condition is causing your child's HBP, treating it often resolves the HBP. When the cause of a child or teen's HBP isn't known, the first line of treatment is lifestyle changes (as it is for adults).

If lifestyle changes don't control blood pressure, children and teens also may need to take medicines. Most of the medicines listed above for adults have special doses for children.

How Can High Blood Pressure Be Prevented?

If You Have Normal Blood Pressure

If you don't have high blood pressure (HBP), you can take steps to prevent it. Healthy lifestyle habits can help you maintain normal blood pressure.

- Follow a healthy diet. Limit the amount of sodium (salt) and alcohol that you consume. The National Heart, Lung, and Blood Institute's DASH (Dietary Approaches to Stop Hypertension) eating plan promotes healthy eating.

- Be physically active. Routine physical activity can lower HBP and reduce your risk for other health problems.

- Maintain a healthy weight. Staying at a healthy weight can help you control HBP and reduce your risk for other health problems.

- Quit smoking. Smoking can damage your blood vessels and raise your risk for HBP. Smoking also can worsen health problems related to HBP.

- Learn to manage and cope with stress. Learning how to manage stress, relax, and cope with problems can improve your emotional and physical health.

• Many people who adopt these healthy lifestyle habits are able to prevent or delay HBP. The more lifestyle changes you make, the more likely you are to lower your blood pressure and avoid related health problems.

If You Have High Blood Pressure

If you have HBP, you can still take steps to prevent the long-term problems it can cause. Healthy lifestyle habits (listed above) and medicines can help you live a longer, more active life.

Follow the treatment plan your doctor prescribes to control your blood pressure. Treatment can help you prevent or delay coronary heart disease, stroke, kidney disease, and other health problems.

Children and Teens

A healthy lifestyle also can help prevent HBP in children and teens. Key steps include having a child:

• Follow a healthy diet that focuses on plenty of fruits, vegetables, and, for children older than four years old, low-fat dairy products. A healthy diet also is low in saturated and trans fats and salt.

• Be active for at least one to two hours per day. Limit screen time in front of the TV or computer to two hours per day at most.

• Maintain a healthy weight. If your child is overweight, ask his or her doctor about how your child can safely lose weight.

• Make these healthy habits part of a family health plan to help your child adopt and maintain a healthy lifestyle.

Living with High Blood Pressure

If you have high blood pressure (HBP), you'll need to treat and control it for life. This means making lifestyle changes, taking prescribed medicines, and getting ongoing medical care.

Treatment can help control blood pressure, but it will not cure HBP. If you stop treatment, your blood pressure and risk for related health problems will rise.

For a healthy future, follow your treatment plan closely. Work with your health care team for lifelong blood pressure control.

Lifestyle Changes

Making healthy lifestyle changes can help control HBP. A healthy lifestyle includes following a healthy diet, being physically active, maintaining a healthy weight, and not smoking.

Medicines

Take all blood pressure medicines that your doctor prescribes. Know the names and doses of your medicines and how to take them. If you have questions about your medicines, talk with your doctor or pharmacist.

Make sure you refill your medicines before they run out. Take your medicines exactly as your doctor directs—don't skip days or cut pills in half.

If you're having side effects from your medicines, talk with your doctor. He or she may need to adjust the doses or prescribe other medicines. You shouldn't decide on your own to stop taking your medicines.

Ongoing Care

If you have HBP, have medical checkups or tests as your doctor advises. Your doctor may need to change or add medicines to your treatment plan over time. Routine checkups allow your doctor to change your treatment right away if your blood pressure goes up again.

Keeping track of your blood pressure is important. Have your blood pressure checked on the schedule your doctor advises.

You may want to learn how to check your blood pressure at home. Your doctor can help you learn how to do this. Each time you check your own blood pressure, you should write down your numbers and the date.

The National Heart, Lung, and Blood Institute's (NHLBI's) "My Blood Pressure Wallet Card" can help you track your blood pressure. You also can write down the names and doses of your medicines and keep track of your lifestyle changes with this handy card.

During checkups, you can ask your doctor or health care team any questions you have about your treatments.

High Blood Pressure and Pregnancy

Many pregnant women who have HBP have healthy babies. However, HBP can cause problems for both the mother and the fetus. HBP can harm the mother's kidneys and other organs. It also can cause the baby to be born early and with a low birth weight.

If you're thinking about having a baby and you have HBP, talk with your health care team. You can take steps to control your blood pressure before and while you're pregnant.

Some women get HBP for the first time while they're pregnant. In the most serious cases, the mother has a condition called pre-eclampsia.

This condition can threaten the lives of both the mother and the unborn child. You'll need special care to reduce your risk. With such care, most women and babies have good outcomes.

Section 20.2

High Cholesterol

Excerpted from "High Blood Cholesterol," by the National Heart, Lung, and Blood Institute (NHLBI, www.nhlbi.nih.gov), part of the National Institutes of Health, September 19, 2012.

To understand high blood cholesterol, it helps to learn about cholesterol. Cholesterol is a waxy, fat-like substance that's found in all cells of the body.

Your body needs some cholesterol to make hormones, vitamin D, and substances that help you digest foods. Your body makes all the cholesterol it needs. However, cholesterol also is found in some of the foods you eat.

Cholesterol travels through your bloodstream in small packages called lipoproteins. These packages are made of fat (lipid) on the inside and proteins on the outside.

Two kinds of lipoproteins carry cholesterol throughout your body: low-density lipoproteins (LDL) and high-density lipoproteins (HDL). Having healthy levels of both types of lipoproteins is important.

LDL cholesterol sometimes is called bad cholesterol. A high LDL level leads to a buildup of cholesterol in your arteries. (Arteries are blood vessels that carry blood from your heart to your body.)

HDL cholesterol sometimes is called good cholesterol. This is because it carries cholesterol from other parts of your body back to your liver. Your liver removes the cholesterol from your body.

What Is High Blood Cholesterol?

High blood cholesterol is a condition in which you have too much cholesterol in your blood. By itself, the condition usually has no signs or symptoms. Thus, many people don't know that their cholesterol levels are too high.

People who have high blood cholesterol have a greater chance of getting coronary heart disease, also called coronary artery disease.

The higher the level of LDL cholesterol in your blood, the GREATER your chance is of getting heart disease. The higher the level of HDL cholesterol in your blood, the LOWER your chance is of getting heart disease.

Coronary heart disease is a condition in which plaque builds up inside the coronary (heart) arteries. Plaque is made up of cholesterol, fat, calcium, and other substances found in the blood. When plaque builds up in the arteries, the condition is called atherosclerosis.

Over time, plaque hardens and narrows your coronary arteries. This limits the flow of oxygen-rich blood to the heart.

Eventually, an area of plaque can rupture (break open). This causes a blood clot to form on the surface of the plaque. If the clot becomes large enough, it can mostly or completely block blood flow through a coronary artery.

If the flow of oxygen-rich blood to your heart muscle is reduced or blocked, angina or a heart attack may occur.

Angina is chest pain or discomfort. It may feel like pressure or squeezing in your chest. The pain also may occur in your shoulders, arms, neck, jaw, or back. Angina pain may even feel like indigestion.

A heart attack occurs if the flow of oxygen-rich blood to a section of heart muscle is cut off. If blood flow isn't restored quickly, the section of heart muscle begins to die. Without quick treatment, a heart attack can lead to serious problems or death.

Plaque also can build up in other arteries in your body, such as the arteries that bring oxygen-rich blood to your brain and limbs. This can lead to problems such as carotid artery disease, stroke, and peripheral arterial disease (PAD).

Outlook

Lowering your cholesterol may slow, reduce, or even stop the build-up of plaque in your arteries. It also may reduce the risk of plaque rupturing and causing dangerous blood clots.

What Causes High Blood Cholesterol?

Many factors can affect the cholesterol levels in your blood. You can control some factors, but not others.

Factors You Can Control

Diet

Cholesterol is found in foods that come from animal sources, such as egg yolks, meat, and cheese. Some foods have fats that raise your cholesterol level.

For example, saturated fat raises your low-density lipoprotein (LDL) cholesterol level more than anything else in your diet. Saturated fat is found in some meats, dairy products, chocolate, baked goods, and deep-fried and processed foods.

Trans fatty acids (trans fats) raise your LDL cholesterol and lower your high-density lipoprotein (HDL) cholesterol. Trans fats are made when hydrogen is added to vegetable oil to harden it. Trans fats are found in some fried and processed foods.

Limiting foods with cholesterol, saturated fat, and trans fats can help you control your cholesterol levels.

Physical Activity and Weight

Lack of physical activity can lead to weight gain. Being overweight tends to raise your LDL level, lower your HDL level, and increase your total cholesterol level. (Total cholesterol is a measure of the total amount of cholesterol in your blood, including LDL and HDL.)

Routine physical activity can help you lose weight and lower your LDL cholesterol. Being physically active also can help you raise your HDL cholesterol level.

Factors You Can't Control

Heredity

High blood cholesterol can run in families. An inherited condition called familial hypercholesterolemia causes very high LDL cholesterol. (Inherited means the condition is passed from parents to children through genes.) This condition begins at birth, and it may cause a heart attack at an early age.

Age and Sex

Starting at puberty, men often have lower levels of HDL cholesterol than women. As women and men age, their LDL cholesterol levels often rise. Before age 55, women usually have lower LDL cholesterol levels than men. However, after age 55, women can have higher LDL levels than men.

What Are the Signs and Symptoms of High Blood Cholesterol?

High blood cholesterol usually has no signs or symptoms. Thus, many people don't know that their cholesterol levels are too high.

If you're 20 years old or older, have your cholesterol levels checked at least once every 5 years. Talk with your doctor about how often you should be tested.

How Is High Blood Cholesterol Diagnosed?

Your doctor will diagnose high blood cholesterol by checking the cholesterol levels in your blood. A blood test called a lipoprotein panel can measure your cholesterol levels. Before the test, you'll need to fast (not eat or drink anything but water) for 9 to 12 hours.

The lipoprotein panel will give your doctor information about the following:

- Total cholesterol: Total cholesterol is a measure of the total amount of cholesterol in your blood, including low-density lipo-protein (LDL) cholesterol and high-density lipoprotein (HDL) cholesterol.

- LDL cholesterol: LDL, or bad, cholesterol is the main source of cholesterol buildup and blockages in the arteries.

- HDL cholesterol: HDL, or good, cholesterol helps remove cholesterol from your arteries.

- Triglycerides: Triglycerides are a type of fat found in your blood. Some studies suggest that a high level of triglycerides in the blood may raise the risk of coronary heart disease, especially in women.

If it's not possible to have a lipoprotein panel, knowing your total cholesterol and HDL cholesterol can give you a general idea about your cholesterol levels.

Testing for total and HDL cholesterol does not require fasting. If your total cholesterol is 200 mg/dL or more, or if your HDL cholesterol is less than 40 mg/dL, your doctor will likely recommend that you have a lipoprotein panel. (Cholesterol is measured as milligrams (mg) of cholesterol per deciliter (dL) of blood.)

Triglycerides also can raise your risk for heart disease. If your triglyceride level is borderline high (150–199 mg/dL) or high (200 mg/dL or higher), you may need treatment.

Factors that can raise your triglyceride level include the following:

- Overweight and obesity

- Lack of physical activity

- Cigarette smoking

- Excessive alcohol use

- A very high carbohydrate diet

- Certain diseases and medicines

- Some genetic disorders

How Is High Blood Cholesterol Treated?

High blood cholesterol is treated with lifestyle changes and medicines. The main goal of treatment is to lower your low-density lipoprotein (LDL) cholesterol level enough to reduce your risk for coronary heart disease, heart attack, and other related health problems.

Your risk for heart disease and heart attack goes up as your LDL cholesterol level rises and your number of heart disease risk factors increases.

Some people are at high risk for heart attacks because they already have heart disease. Other people are at high risk for heart disease because they have diabetes or more than one heart disease risk factor.

Talk with your doctor about lowering your cholesterol and your risk for heart disease.

The two main ways to lower your cholesterol (and, thus, your heart disease risk) include the following:

- Therapeutic Lifestyle Changes (TLC): TLC is a three-part program that includes a healthy diet, weight management, and physical activity. TLC is for anyone whose LDL cholesterol level is above goal.

- Medicines: If cholesterol-lowering medicines are needed, they're used with the TLC program to help lower your LDL cholesterol level.

Your doctor will set your LDL goal. The higher your risk for heart disease, the lower he or she will set your LDL goal.

Lowering Cholesterol Using Therapeutic Lifestyle Changes

TLC is a set of lifestyle changes that can help you lower your LDL cholesterol. The main parts of the TLC program are a healthy diet, weight management, and physical activity.

With the TLC diet, less than 7 percent of your daily calories should come from saturated fat. This kind of fat is found in some meats, dairy products, chocolate, baked goods, and deep-fried and processed foods.

No more than 25 to 35 percent of your daily calories should come from all fats, including saturated, trans, monounsaturated, and polyunsaturated fats.

You also should have less than 200 mg a day of cholesterol. The amounts of cholesterol and the types of fat in prepared foods can be found on the foods' Nutrition Facts labels.

Foods high in soluble fiber also are part of the TLC diet. They help prevent the digestive tract from absorbing cholesterol. These foods include the following:

- Whole-grain cereals such as oatmeal and oat bran

- Fruits such as apples, bananas, oranges, pears, and prunes

- Legumes such as kidney beans, lentils, chick peas, black-eyed peas, and lima beans

A diet rich in fruits and vegetables can increase important cholesterol-lowering compounds in your diet. These compounds, called plant stanols or sterols, work like soluble fiber.

A healthy diet also includes some types of fish, such as salmon, tuna (canned or fresh), and mackerel. These fish are a good source of omega-3 fatty acids. These acids may help protect the heart from blood clots and inflammation and reduce the risk of heart attack. Try to have about two fish meals every week.

You also should try to limit the amount of sodium (salt) that you eat. This means choosing low-salt and "no added salt" foods and seasonings at the table or while cooking. The Nutrition Facts label on food packaging shows the amount of sodium in the item.

Try to limit drinks with alcohol. Too much alcohol will raise your blood pressure and triglyceride level. (Triglycerides are a type of fat found in the blood.) Alcohol also adds extra calories, which will cause weight gain.

Men should have no more than two drinks containing alcohol a day. Women should have no more than one drink containing alcohol a day. One drink is a glass of wine, beer, or a small amount of hard liquor.

Weight Management

If you're overweight or obese, losing weight can help lower LDL cholesterol. Maintaining a healthy weight is especially important if you have a condition called metabolic syndrome.

Metabolic syndrome is the name for a group of risk factors that raise your risk for heart disease and other health problems, such as diabetes and stroke.

The five metabolic risk factors are a large waistline (abdominal obesity), a high triglyceride level, a low HDL cholesterol level, high blood pressure, and high blood sugar. Metabolic syndrome is diagnosed if you have at least three of these metabolic risk factors.

Physical Activity

Routine physical activity can lower LDL cholesterol and triglycerides and raise your HDL cholesterol level.

People gain health benefits from as little as 60 minutes of moderate-intensity aerobic activity per week. The more active you are, the more you will benefit.

Cholesterol-Lowering Medicines

In addition to lifestyle changes, your doctor may prescribe medicines to help lower your cholesterol. Even with medicines, you should continue the TLC program.

Medicines can help control high blood cholesterol, but they don't cure it. Thus, you must continue taking your medicine to keep your cholesterol level in the recommended range.

The five major types of cholesterol-lowering medicines are statins, bile acid sequestrants, nicotinic acid, fibrates, and ezetimibe.

Statins work well at lowering LDL cholesterol. These medicines are safe for most people. Rare side effects include muscle and liver problems.

Bile acid sequestrants also help lower LDL cholesterol. These medicines usually aren't prescribed as the only medicine to lower cholesterol. Sometimes they're prescribed with statins.

Nicotinic acid lowers LDL cholesterol and triglycerides and raises HDL cholesterol. You should only use this type of medicine with a doctor's supervision.

Fibrates lower triglycerides, and they may raise HDL cholesterol. When used with statins, fibrates may increase the risk of muscle problems.

Ezetimibe lowers LDL cholesterol. This medicine works by blocking the intestine from absorbing cholesterol.

While you're being treated for high blood cholesterol, you'll need ongoing care. Your doctor will want to make sure your cholesterol levels are controlled. He or she also will want to check for other health problems.

If needed, your doctor may prescribe medicines for other health problems. Take all medicines exactly as your doctor prescribes. The combination of medicines may lower your risk for heart disease and heart attack.

While trying to manage your cholesterol, take steps to manage other heart disease risk factors too. For example, if you have high blood pressure, work with your doctor to lower it.

If you smoke, quit. Talk with your doctor about programs and products that can help you quit smoking. Also, try to avoid secondhand smoke. If you're overweight or obese, try to lose weight. Your doctor can help you create a reasonable weight-loss plan.

Chapter 21

Overweight, Obesity, and Stroke Risk

The terms "overweight" and "obesity" refer to body weight that's greater than what is considered healthy for a certain height.

The most useful measure of overweight and obesity is body mass index (BMI). BMI is calculated from your height and weight.

Overview

Millions of Americans and people worldwide are overweight or obese. Being overweight or obese puts you at risk for many health problems. The more body fat that you have and the more you weigh, the more likely you are to develop the following:

- Coronary heart disease

- High blood pressure

- Type 2 diabetes

- Gallstones

- Breathing problems

- Certain cancers

From "What Are Overweight and Obesity?" by the National Heart, Lung, and Blood Institute (NHLBI, www.nhlbi.nih.gov), part of the National Institutes of Health, July 13, 2012.

Your weight is the result of many factors. These factors include environment, family history and genetics, metabolism (the way your body changes food and oxygen into energy), behavior or habits, and more.

You can't change some factors, such as family history. However, you can change other factors, such as your lifestyle habits.

For example, follow a healthy eating plan and keep your calorie needs in mind. Be physically active and try to limit the amount of time that you're inactive.

Weight-loss medicines and surgery also are options for some people if lifestyle changes aren't enough.

Outlook

Reaching and staying at a healthy weight is a long-term challenge for people who are overweight or obese. But it also is a chance to lower your risk for other serious health problems. With the right treatment and motivation, it's possible to lose weight and lower your long-term disease risk.

What Causes Overweight and Obesity?

Lack of Energy Balance

A lack of energy balance most often causes overweight and obesity. Energy balance means that your energy IN equals your energy OUT.

Energy IN is the amount of energy or calories you get from food and drinks. Energy OUT is the amount of energy your body uses for things like breathing, digesting, and being physically active.

To maintain a healthy weight, your energy IN and OUT don't have to balance exactly every day. It's the balance over time that helps you maintain a healthy weight.

The same amount of energy IN and energy OUT over time = weight stays the same

- More energy IN than energy OUT over time = weight gain
- More energy OUT than energy IN over time = weight loss

Overweight and obesity happen over time when you take in more calories than you use.

Other Causes

An inactive lifestyle: Many Americans aren't very physically active. One reason for this is that many people spend hours in front of TVs and computers doing work, schoolwork, and leisure activities. In fact, more than two hours a day of regular TV viewing time has been linked to overweight and obesity.

Other reasons for not being active include: relying on cars instead of walking, fewer physical demands at work or at home because of modern technology and conveniences, and lack of physical education classes in schools.

People who are inactive are more likely to gain weight because they don't burn the calories that they take in from food and drinks. An inactive lifestyle also raises your risk for coronary heart disease, high blood pressure, diabetes, colon cancer, and other health problems.

Environment: Our environment doesn't support healthy lifestyle habits; in fact, it encourages obesity. Some reasons include:

- Lack of neighborhood sidewalks and safe places for recreation: Not having area parks, trails, sidewalks, and affordable gyms makes it hard for people to be physically active.

- Work schedules: People often say that they don't have time to be physically active because of long work hours and time spent commuting.

- Oversized food portions: Americans are exposed to huge food portions in restaurants, fast food places, gas stations, movie theaters, supermarkets, and even at home. Some of these meals and snacks can feed two or more people. Eating large portions means too much energy IN. Over time, this will cause weight gain if it isn't balanced with physical activity.

- Lack of access to healthy foods: Some people don't live in neighborhoods that have supermarkets that sell healthy foods, such as fresh fruits and vegetables. Or, for some people, these healthy foods are too costly.

- Food advertising: Americans are surrounded by ads from food companies. Often children are the targets of advertising for high-calorie, high-fat snacks and sugary drinks. The goal of these ads is to sway people to buy these high-calorie foods, and often they do.

Genes and Family History

Studies of identical twins who have been raised apart show that genes have a strong influence on a person's weight. Overweight and obesity tend to run in families. Your chances of being overweight are greater if one or both of your parents are overweight or obese.

Your genes also may affect the amount of fat you store in your body and where on your body you carry the extra fat. Because families also share food and physical activity habits, a link exists between genes and the environment.

Children adopt the habits of their parents. A child who has overweight parents who eat high-calorie foods and are inactive will likely become overweight too. However, if the family adopts healthy food and physical activity habits, the child's chance of being overweight or obese is reduced.

Health Conditions

Some hormone problems may cause overweight and obesity, such as underactive thyroid (hypothyroidism), Cushing syndrome, and polycystic ovarian syndrome (PCOS).

Underactive thyroid is a condition in which the thyroid gland doesn't make enough thyroid hormone. Lack of thyroid hormone will slow down your metabolism and cause weight gain. You'll also feel tired and weak.

Cushing syndrome is a condition in which the body's adrenal glands make too much of the hormone cortisol. Cushing syndrome also can develop if a person takes high doses of certain medicines, such as prednisone, for long periods.

People who have Cushing syndrome gain weight, have upper-body obesity, a rounded face, fat around the neck, and thin arms and legs.

PCOS is a condition that affects about 5–10 percent of women of childbearing age. Women who have PCOS often are obese, have excess hair growth, and have reproductive problems and other health issues. These problems are caused by high levels of hormones called androgens.

Medicines

Certain medicines may cause you to gain weight. These medicines include some corticosteroids, antidepressants, and seizure medicines.

These medicines can slow the rate at which your body burns calories, increase your appetite, or cause your body to hold on to extra water. All of these factors can lead to weight gain.

Emotional Factors

Some people eat more than usual when they're bored, angry, or stressed. Over time, overeating will lead to weight gain and may cause overweight or obesity.

Smoking

Some people gain weight when they stop smoking. One reason is that food often tastes and smells better after quitting smoking.

Another reason is because nicotine raises the rate at which your body burns calories, so you burn fewer calories when you stop smoking. However, smoking is a serious health risk, and quitting is more important than possible weight gain.

Age

As you get older, you tend to lose muscle, especially if you're less active. Muscle loss can slow down the rate at which your body burns calories. If you don't reduce your calorie intake as you get older, you may gain weight.

Midlife weight gain in women is mainly due to aging and lifestyle, but menopause also plays a role. Many women gain about five pounds during menopause and have more fat around the waist than they did before.

Pregnancy

During pregnancy, women gain weight to support their babies' growth and development. After giving birth, some women find it hard to lose the weight. This may lead to overweight or obesity, especially after a few pregnancies.

Lack of Sleep

Research shows that lack of sleep increases the risk of obesity. For example, one study of teenagers showed that with each hour of sleep lost, the odds of becoming obese went up. Lack of sleep increases the risk of obesity in other age groups as well.

People who sleep fewer hours also seem to prefer eating foods that are higher in calories and carbohydrates, which can lead to overeating, weight gain, and obesity.

Sleep helps maintain a healthy balance of the hormones that make you feel hungry (ghrelin) or full (leptin). When you don't get enough sleep, your level of ghrelin goes up and your level of leptin goes down. This makes you feel hungrier than when you're well-rested.

Sleep also affects how your body reacts to insulin, the hormone that controls your blood glucose (sugar) level. Lack of sleep results in a higher than normal blood sugar level, which may increase your risk for diabetes.

What Are the Health Risks of Overweight and Obesity?

Being overweight or obese isn't a cosmetic problem. These conditions greatly raise your risk for other health problems.

Coronary Heart Disease

As your body mass index rises, so does your risk for coronary heart disease (CHD). CHD is a condition in which a waxy substance called plaque builds up inside the coronary arteries. These arteries supply oxygen-rich blood to your heart.

Plaque can narrow or block the coronary arteries and reduce blood flow to the heart muscle. This can cause angina or a heart attack. (Angina is chest pain or discomfort.)

Obesity also can lead to heart failure. This is a serious condition in which your heart can't pump enough blood to meet your body's needs.

High Blood Pressure

Blood pressure is the force of blood pushing against the walls of the arteries as the heart pumps blood. If this pressure rises and stays high over time, it can damage the body in many ways.

Your chances of having high blood pressure are greater if you're overweight or obese.

Stroke

Being overweight or obese can lead to a buildup of plaque in your arteries. Eventually, an area of plaque can rupture, causing a blood clot to form.

If the clot is close to your brain, it can block the flow of blood and oxygen to your brain and cause a stroke. The risk of having a stroke rises as BMI increases.

Type 2 Diabetes

Diabetes is a disease in which the body's blood glucose, or blood sugar, level is too high. Normally, the body breaks down food into glucose and then carries it to cells throughout the body. The cells use a hormone called insulin to turn the glucose into energy.

In type 2 diabetes, the body's cells don't use insulin properly. At first, the body reacts by making more insulin. Over time, however, the body can't make enough insulin to control its blood sugar level.

Diabetes is a leading cause of early death, CHD, stroke, kidney disease, and blindness. Most people who have type 2 diabetes are overweight.

Abnormal Blood Fats

If you're overweight or obese, you're at increased risk of having abnormal levels of blood fats. These include high levels of triglycerides and LDL (bad) cholesterol and low levels of HDL (good) cholesterol.

Abnormal levels of these blood fats are a risk factor for CHD.

Metabolic Syndrome

Metabolic syndrome is the name for a group of risk factors that raises your risk for heart disease and other health problems, such as diabetes and stroke.

You can develop any one of these risk factors by itself, but they tend to occur together. A diagnosis of metabolic syndrome is made if you have at least three of the following risk factors:

- A large waistline: This is called abdominal obesity or "having an apple shape." Having extra fat in the waist area is a greater risk factor for CHD than having extra fat in other parts of the body, such as on the hips.

- A higher than normal triglyceride level (or you're on medicine to treat high triglycerides)

- A lower than normal HDL cholesterol level (or you're on medicine to treat low HDL cholesterol)

- Higher than normal blood pressure (or you're on medicine to treat high blood pressure)

- Higher than normal fasting blood sugar (or you're on medicine to treat diabetes)

Cancer

Being overweight or obese raises your risk for colon, breast, endometrial, and gallbladder cancers.

Osteoarthritis

Osteoarthritis is a common joint problem of the knees, hips, and lower back. The condition occurs if the tissue that protects the joints wears away. Extra weight can put more pressure and wear on joints, causing pain.

Sleep Apnea

Sleep apnea is a common disorder in which you have one or more pauses in breathing or shallow breaths while you sleep.

A person who has sleep apnea may have more fat stored around the neck. This can narrow the airway, making it hard to breathe.

Obesity Hypoventilation Syndrome

Obesity hypoventilation syndrome (OHS) is a breathing disorder that affects some obese people. In OHS, poor breathing results in too much carbon dioxide (hypoventilation) and too little oxygen in the blood (hypoxemia).

OHS can lead to serious health problems and may even cause death.

Reproductive Problems

Obesity can cause menstrual issues and infertility in women.

Gallstones

Gallstones are hard pieces of stone-like material that form in the gallbladder. They're mostly made of cholesterol. Gallstones can cause stomach or back pain.

People who are overweight or obese are at increased risk of having gallstones. Also, being overweight may result in an enlarged gallbladder that doesn't work well.

Overweight and Obesity-Related Health Problems in Children and Teens

Overweight and obesity also increase the health risks for children and teens. Type 2 diabetes once was rare in American children, but an increasing number of children are developing the disease.

Also, overweight children are more likely to become overweight or obese as adults, with the same disease risks.

Who Is at Risk for Overweight and Obesity?

Overweight and obesity affect Americans of all ages, sexes, and racial/ethnic groups. This serious health problem has been growing over the last 30 years.

Adults

According to the National Health and Nutrition Examination Survey (NHANES) 2009–2010, almost 70 percent of Americans are overweight or obese. The survey also shows differences in overweight and obesity among racial/ethnic groups.

In women, overweight and obesity are highest among non-Hispanic Black women (about 82 percent), compared with about 76 percent for Hispanic women and 64 percent for non-Hispanic White women.

In men, overweight and obesity are highest among Hispanic men (about 82 percent), compared with about 74 percent for non-Hispanic White men and about 70 percent for non-Hispanic Black men.

Children and Teens

Children also have become heavier. In the past 30 years, obesity has tripled among school-aged children and teens.

According to NHANES 2009–2010, about 1 in 6 American children ages 2–19 are obese. The survey also suggests that overweight and obesity are having a greater effect on minority groups, including Blacks and Hispanics.

What Are the Signs and Symptoms of Overweight and Obesity?

Weight gain usually happens over time. Most people know when they've gained weight. Some of the signs of overweight and obesity include the following:

- Clothes feeling tight and needing a larger size

- The scale showing that you've gained weight

- Having extra fat around the waist

- A higher than normal body mass index and waist circumference

How Are Overweight and Obesity Diagnosed?

The most common way to find out whether you're overweight or obese is to figure out your body mass index (BMI). BMI is an estimate of body fat, and it's a good gauge of your risk for diseases that occur with more body fat.

BMI is calculated from your height and weight.

Waist Circumference

Health care professionals also may take your waist measurement. This helps screen for the possible health risks related to overweight and obesity in adults.

If you have abdominal obesity and most of your fat is around your waist rather than at your hips, you're at increased risk for coronary heart disease and type 2 diabetes. The risk goes up with a waist size that's greater than 35 inches for women or greater than 40 inches for men.

You also can measure your waist size. To do so correctly, stand and place a tape measure around your middle, just above your hipbones. Measure your waist just after you breathe out.

Specialists Involved

A primary care doctor (or pediatrician for children and teens) will assess your BMI, waist measurement, and overall health risk. If you're overweight or obese, or if you have a large waist size, your doctor should explain the health risks and find out whether you're interested and willing to lose weight.

If you are, you and your doctor can work together to create a treatment plan. The plan may include weight-loss goals and treatment options that are realistic for you.

Your doctor may send you to other health care specialists if you need expert care. These specialists may include the following:

- An endocrinologist if you need to be treated for type 2 diabetes or a hormone problem, such as an underactive thyroid

- A registered dietitian or nutritionist to work with you on ways to change your eating habits

- An exercise physiologist or trainer to figure out your level of fitness and show you how to do physical activities suitable for you

- A bariatric surgeon if weight-loss surgery is an option for you

- A psychiatrist, psychologist, or clinical social worker to help treat depression or stress

How Are Overweight and Obesity Treated?

Successful weight-loss treatments include setting goals and making lifestyle changes, such as eating fewer calories and being physically active. Medicines and weight-loss surgery also are options for some people if lifestyle changes aren't enough.

Setting realistic weight-loss goals is an important first step to losing weight.

For Adults

Try to lose 5 to 10 percent of your current weight over 6 months. This will lower your risk for coronary heart disease (CHD) and other conditions.

The best way to lose weight is slowly. A weight loss of one to two pounds a week is do-able, safe, and will help you keep off the weight. It also will give you the time to make new, healthy lifestyle changes.

If you've lost 10 percent of your body weight, have kept it off for 6 months, and are still overweight or obese, you may want to consider further weight loss.

For Children and Teens

If your child is overweight or at risk for overweight or obesity, the goal is to maintain his or her current weight and to focus on eating healthy and being physically active. This should be part of a family effort to make lifestyle changes.

If your child is overweight or obese and has a health condition related to overweight or obesity, your doctor may refer you to a pediatric obesity treatment center.

Lifestyle Changes

Lifestyle changes can help you and your family achieve long-term weight-loss success. Example of lifestyle changes include:

- Focusing on balancing energy IN (calories from food and drinks) with energy OUT (physical activity)

- Following a healthy eating plan

- Learning how to adopt healthy lifestyle habits

Over time, these changes will become part of your everyday life.

Calories

Cutting back on calories (energy IN) will help you lose weight. To lose 1 to 2 pounds a week, adults should cut back their calorie intake by 500 to 1,000 calories a day.

In general, having 1,000 to 1,200 calories a day will help most women lose weight safely.

In general, having 1,200 to 1,600 calories a day will help most men lose weight safely. This calorie range also is suitable for women who weigh 165 pounds or more or who exercise routinely.

These calorie levels are a guide and may need to be adjusted. If you eat 1,600 calories a day but don't lose weight, then you may want to cut back to 1,200 calories. If you're hungry on either diet, then you may want to add 100 to 200 calories a day.

Very low-calorie diets with fewer than 800 calories a day shouldn't be used unless your doctor is monitoring you.

For overweight children and teens, it's important to slow the rate of weight gain. However, reduced-calorie diets aren't advised unless you talk with a health care provider.

Healthy Eating Plan

A healthy eating plan gives your body the nutrients it needs every day. It has enough calories for good health, but not so many that you gain weight.

A healthy eating plan is low in saturated fat, trans fat, cholesterol, sodium (salt), and added sugar. Following a healthy eating plan will lower your risk for heart disease and other conditions.

Healthy foods include the following:

- Fat-free and low-fat dairy products, such as low-fat yogurt, cheese, and milk

- Protein foods, such as lean meat, fish, poultry without skin, beans, and peas

- Whole-grain foods, such as whole-wheat bread, oatmeal, and brown rice

- Other grain foods include pasta, cereal, bagels, bread, tortillas, couscous, and crackers

- Fruits, which can be fresh, canned, frozen, or dried

- Vegetables, which can be fresh, canned (without salt), frozen, or dried

Canola and olive oils, and soft margarines made from these oils, are heart healthy. However, you should use them in small amounts because they're high in calories.

You also can include unsalted nuts, like walnuts and almonds, in your diet as long as you limit the amount you eat (nuts also are high in calories).

The National Heart, Lung, and Blood Institute's "Aim for a Healthy Weight" patient booklet provides more information about following a healthy eating plan.

Foods to limit: Foods that are high in saturated and trans fats and cholesterol raise blood cholesterol levels and also might be high in calories. Fats and cholesterol raise your risk for heart disease, so they should be limited.

Saturated fat is found mainly in the following:

- Fatty cuts of meat, such as ground beef, sausage, and processed meats (for example, bologna, hot dogs, and deli meats)

- Poultry with the skin

- High-fat dairy products like whole-milk cheeses, whole milk, cream, butter, and ice cream

- Lard, coconut, and palm oils, which are found in many processed foods

Trans fat is found mainly in the following:

- Foods with partially hydrogenated oils, such as many hard margarines and shortening

- Baked products and snack foods, such as crackers, cookies, doughnuts, and breads

- Foods fried in hydrogenated shortening, such as french fries and chicken

Cholesterol mainly is found in the following:

- Egg yolks

- Organ meats, such as liver

- Shrimp

- Whole milk or whole-milk products, such as butter, cream, and cheese

Limiting foods and drinks with added sugars, like high-fructose corn syrup, is important. Added sugars will give you extra calories without nutrients like vitamins and minerals. Added sugars are found in many desserts, canned fruit packed in syrup, fruit drinks, and nondiet drinks.

Check the list of ingredients on food packages for added sugars like high-fructose corn syrup. Drinks that contain alcohol also will add calories, so it's a good idea to limit your alcohol intake.

Portion size: A portion is the amount of food that you choose to eat for a meal or snack. It's different from a serving, which is a measured amount of food and is noted on the Nutrition Facts label on food packages.

Anyone who has eaten out lately is likely to notice how big the portions are. In fact, over the past 40 years, portion sizes have grown significantly. These growing portion sizes have changed what we think of as a normal portion.

Cutting back on portion size is a good way to eat fewer calories and balance your energy IN.

Food weight: Studies have shown that we all tend to eat a constant "weight" of food. Ounce for ounce, our food intake is fairly consistent. Knowing this, you can lose weight if you eat foods that are lower in calories and fat for a given amount of food.

For example, replacing a full-fat food product that weighs two ounces with a low-fat product that weighs the same helps you cut back on calories. Another helpful practice is to eat foods that contain a lot of water, such as vegetables, fruits, and soups.

Physical Activity

Being physically active and eating fewer calories will help you lose weight and keep weight off over time. Physical activity also will benefit you in other ways. It will do the following:

- Lower your risk for heart disease, heart attack, diabetes, and cancers (such as breast, uterine, and colon cancers)
- Strengthen your heart and help your lungs work better
- Strengthen your muscles and keep your joints in good condition
- Slow bone loss
- Give you more energy
- Help you relax and better cope with stress
- Allow you to fall asleep more quickly and sleep more soundly
- Give you an enjoyable way to share time with friends and family

The four main types of physical activity are aerobic, muscle-strengthening, bone strengthening, and stretching. You can do physical activity with light, moderate, or vigorous intensity. The level of intensity depends on how hard you have to work to do the activity.

People vary in the amount of physical activity they need to control their weight. Many people can maintain their weight by doing 150 to 300 minutes (2 hours and 30 minutes to 5 hours) of moderate-intensity activity per week, such as brisk walking.

People who want to lose a large amount of weight (more than 5 percent of their body weight) may need to do more than 300 minutes of moderate-intensity activity per week. This also may be true for people who want to keep off weight that they've lost.

You don't have to do the activity all at once. You can break it up into short periods of at least 10 minutes each.

If you have a heart problem or chronic disease, such as heart disease, diabetes, or high blood pressure, talk with your doctor about what types of physical activity are safe for you. You also should talk with your doctor about safe physical activities if you have symptoms such as chest pain or dizziness.

Children should get at least 60 minutes or more of physical activity every day. Most physical activity should be moderate-intensity aerobic activity. Activity should vary and be a good fit for the child's age and physical development.

Many people lead inactive lives and might not be motivated to do more physical activity. When starting a physical activity program, some people may need help and supervision to avoid injury.

If you're obese, or if you haven't been active in the past, start physical activity slowly and build up the intensity a little at a time.

When starting out, one way to be active is to do more everyday activities, such as taking the stairs instead of the elevator and doing household chores and yard work. The next step is to start walking, biking, or swimming at a slow pace, and then build up the amount of time you exercise or the intensity level of the activity.

To lose weight and gain better health, it's important to get moderate-intensity physical activity. Choose activities that you enjoy and that fit into your daily life.

A daily, brisk walk is an easy way to be more active and improve your health. Use a pedometer to count your daily steps and keep track of how much you're walking. Try to increase the number of steps you take each day. Other examples of moderate-intensity physical activity include dancing, gardening, and water aerobics.

For greater health benefits, try to step up your level of activity or the length of time you're active. For example, start walking for 10 to 15 minutes three times a week, and then build up to brisk walking for 60 minutes, 5 days a week.

Behavioral Changes

Changing your behaviors or habits related to food and physical activity is important for losing weight. The first step is to understand which habits lead you to overeat, or have an inactive lifestyle. The next step is to change these habits.

Below are some simple tips to help you adopt healthier habits.

- Change your surroundings. You might be more likely to overeat when watching TV, when treats are available at work, or when you're with a certain friend. You also might find it hard to motivate yourself to be physically active. However, you can change these habits.

- Instead of watching TV, dance to music in your living room or go for a walk.

- Leave the office break room right after you get a cup of coffee.

- Bring a change of clothes to work. Head straight to an exercise class on the way home from work.

- Put a note on your calendar to remind yourself to take a walk or go to your exercise class.

- Keep a record. A record of your food intake and the amount of physical activity that you do each day will help inspire you. You also can keep track of your weight. For example, when the record shows that you've been meeting your physical activity goals, you'll want to keep it up. A record also is an easy way to track how you're doing, especially if you're working with a registered dietitian or nutritionist.

- Seek support. Ask for help or encouragement from your friends, family, and health care provider. You can get support in person, through e-mail, or by talking on the phone. You also can join a support group.

- Reward success. Reward your success for meeting your weight-loss goals or other achievements with something you would like to do, not with food. Choose rewards that you'll enjoy, such as a movie, music CD, an afternoon off from work, a massage, or personal time.

Weight-Loss Medicines

Weight-loss medicines approved by the Food and Drug Administration (FDA) might be an option for some people.

If you're not successful at losing one pound a week after six months of using lifestyle changes, medicines may help. You should only use medicines as part of a program that includes diet, physical activity, and behavioral changes.

Weight-loss medicines might be suitable for adults who are obese (a BMI of 30 or greater). People who have BMIs of 27 or greater, and who are at risk for heart disease and other health conditions, also may benefit from weight-loss medicines.

Sibutramine (Meridia)

As of October 2010, the weight-loss medicine sibutramine (Meridia) was taken off the market in the United States. Research showed that the medicine may raise the risk of heart attack and stroke.

Orlistat (Xenical and Alli)

Orlistat (Xenical) causes a weight loss between 5 and 10 pounds, although some people lose more weight. Most of the weight loss occurs within the first 6 months of taking the medicine.

People taking Xenical need regular checkups with their doctors, especially during the first year of taking the medicine. During checkups, your doctor will check your weight, blood pressure, and pulse and may recommend other tests. He or she also will talk with you about any medicine side effects and answer your questions.

The FDA also has approved Alli, an over-the-counter (OTC) weight-loss aid for adults. Alli is the lower dose form of orlistat. Alli is meant to be used along with a reduced-calorie, low-fat diet and physical activity. In studies, most people taking Alli lost 5 to 10 pounds over 6 months.

Both Xenical and Alli reduce the absorption of fats, fat calories, and vitamins A, D, E, and K to promote weight loss. Both medicines also can cause mild side effects, such as oily and loose stools.

Although rare, some reports of liver disease have occurred with the use of orlistat. More research is needed to find out whether the medicine plays a role in causing liver disease. Talk with your doctor if you're considering using Xenical or Alli to lose weight. He or she can discuss the risks and benefits with you.

You also should talk with your doctor before starting orlistat if you're taking blood-thinning medicines or being treated for diabetes or thyroid disease. Also, ask your doctor whether you should take a multivitamin due to the possible loss of some vitamins.

Lorcaserin Hydrochloride (Belviq) and Qsymia

In July 2012, the FDA approved two new medicines for chronic (ongoing) weight management. Lorcaserin hydrochloride (Belviq) and Qsymia are approved for adults who have a BMI of 30 or greater.

(Qsymia is a combination of two FDA-approved medicines: phentermine and topiramate.)

These medicines also are approved for adults with a BMI of 27 or greater who have at least one weight-related condition, such as high blood pressure, type 2 diabetes, or high blood cholesterol.

Both medicines are meant to be used along with a reduced-calorie diet and physical activity.

Other Medicines

Some prescription medicines are used for weight loss, but aren't FDA-approved for treating obesity. They include:

- Medicines to treat depression: Some medicines for depression cause an initial weight loss and then a regain of weight while taking the medicine.

- Medicines to treat seizures: Two medicines used for seizures, topiramate and zonisamide, have been shown to cause weight loss. These medicines are being studied to see whether they will be useful in treating obesity.

- Medicines to treat diabetes: Metformin may cause small amounts of weight loss in people who have obesity and diabetes. It's not known how this medicine causes weight loss, but it has been shown to reduce hunger and food intake.

Over-the-Counter Products

Some OTC products claim to promote weight loss. The FDA doesn't regulate these products because they're considered dietary supplements, not medicines.

However, many of these products have serious side effects and generally aren't recommended. Some of these OTC products include the following:

Ephedra (also called ma huang): Ephedra comes from plants and has been sold as a dietary supplement. The active ingredient in the plant is called ephedrine. Ephedra can cause short-term weight loss, but it also has serious side effects. It causes high blood pressure and stresses the heart. In 2004, the FDA banned the sale of dietary supplements containing ephedra in the United States.

Chromium: This is a mineral that's sold as a dietary supplement to reduce body fat. While studies haven't found any weight-loss benefit from chromium, there are few serious side effects from taking it.

Diuretics and herbal laxatives: These products cause you to lose water weight, not fat. They also can lower your body's potassium levels, which may cause heart and muscle problems.

Hoodia: Hoodia is a cactus that's native to Africa. It's sold in pill form as an appetite suppressant. However, no firm evidence shows that hoodia works. No large-scale research has been done on humans to show whether hoodia is effective or safe.

Weight-Loss Surgery

Weight-loss surgery might be an option for people who have extreme obesity (BMI of 40 or more) when other treatments have failed.

Weight-loss surgery also is an option for people who have a BMI of 35 or more and life-threatening conditions, such as the following:

- Severe sleep apnea (a condition in which you have one or more pauses in breathing or shallow breaths while you sleep)

- Obesity-related cardiomyopathy

- Severe type 2 diabetes

Types of Weight-Loss Surgery

Two common weight-loss surgeries include banded gastroplasty and Roux-en-Y gastric bypass. For gastroplasty, a band or staples are used to create a small pouch at the top of your stomach. This surgery limits the amount of food and liquids the stomach can hold.

For gastric bypass, a small stomach pouch is created with a bypass around part of the small intestine where most of the calories you eat are absorbed. This surgery limits food intake and reduces the calories your body absorbs.

Weight-loss surgery can improve your health and weight. However, the surgery can be risky, depending on your overall health. Gastroplasty has few long-term side effects, but you must limit your food intake dramatically.

Gastric bypass has more side effects. They include nausea (feeling sick to your stomach), bloating, diarrhea, and faintness. These side effects are all part of a condition called dumping syndrome. After gastric bypass, you may need multivitamins and minerals to prevent nutrient deficiencies.

Lifelong medical followup is needed after both surgeries. Your doctor also may recommend a program both before and after surgery to help you with diet, physical activity, and coping skills.

If you think you would benefit from weight-loss surgery, talk with your doctor. Ask whether you're a candidate for the surgery and discuss the risks, benefits, and what to expect.

Weight-Loss Maintenance

Maintaining your weight loss over time can be a challenge. For adults, weight loss is a success if you lose at least 10 percent of your initial weight and you don't regain more than six or seven pounds in two years. You also must keep a lower waist circumference (at least two inches lower than your waist circumference before you lost weight).

After six months of keeping off the weight, you can think about losing more if the following are true:

- You've already lost 5 to 10 percent of your body weight.

- You're still overweight or obese.

The key to losing more weight or maintaining your weight loss is to continue with lifestyle changes. Adopt these changes as a new way of life.

If you want to lose more weight, you may need to eat fewer calories and increase your activity level. For example, if you eat 1,600 calories a day but don't lose weight, you may want to cut back to 1,200 calories. It's also important to make physical activity part of your normal daily routine.

How Can Overweight and Obesity Be Prevented?

Following a healthy lifestyle can help you prevent overweight and obesity. Many lifestyle habits begin during childhood. Thus, parents and families should encourage their children to make healthy choices, such as following a healthy diet and being physically active.

Make following a healthy lifestyle a family goal. For example:

- Follow a healthy eating plan. Make healthy food choices, keep your calorie needs and your family's calorie needs in mind, and focus on the balance of energy IN and energy OUT.

- Focus on portion size. Watch the portion sizes in fast food and other restaurants. The portions served often are enough for two or three people. Children's portion sizes should be smaller than those for adults. Cutting back on portion size will help you balance energy IN and energy OUT.

- Be active. Make personal and family time active. Find activities that everyone will enjoy. For example, go for a brisk walk, bike or rollerblade, or train together for a walk or run.

- Reduce screen time. Limit the use of TVs, computers, DVDs, and videogames because they limit time for physical activity. Health experts recommend 2 hours or less a day of screen time that's not work- or homework-related.

- Keep track of your weight, body mass index, and waist circumference. Also, keep track of your children's growth.

- Being overweight or obese isn't a cosmetic problem. These conditions greatly raise your risk for other health problems.

Overweight and Obesity-Related Health Problems in Children and Teens

Overweight and obesity also increase the health risks for children and teens. Type 2 diabetes once was rare in American children, but an increasing number of children are developing the disease.

Also, overweight children are more likely to become overweight or obese as adults, with the same disease risks.

Chapter 22

Other Stroke Risk Factors

Chapter Contents

Section 22.1

Inactivity, Exercise, and Stroke

"Exercise & Stroke Risk," Office on Women's Health, U.S. Department of Health and Human Services (www.womenshealth.gov), 2010.

Does exercise lower my risk of stroke?

Yes, especially for the type of stroke caused by a blocked vessel (ischemic stroke). Exercise reduces your stroke risk by the same amount that it reduces your risk of heart disease. This is not surprising since stroke and heart disease share many risk factors that exercise helps to control. Findings from the Nurses' Health Study of over 72,000 women aged 40 to 65 show that regular exercise can cut your risk of blocked-vessel stroke in half. Even moderate or brisk walking—done on a regular basis—reduces the risk of stroke by 30% to 50%.

It has been known for a while that lifelong regular exercise—beginning at around age 15—is associated with up to a 70% reduced risk of blocked-vessel stroke later in life, but there is accumulating evidence that starting exercise in mid-life also helps. Increasing your level of activity by 3.5 hours per week can reduce your stroke risk by almost 40%, regardless of the age at which the increase is made.

How does exercise protect against stroke?

Regular physical activity helps reduce risk factors for stroke (and heart disease) including high blood pressure, high cholesterol and triglycerides, diabetes, and obesity. If you already have these risk factors, being active can stop them from getting worse. Exercise also keeps your arteries flexible (stiff arteries are prone to clogging) and can reverse or stall the buildup of fatty plaque in blood vessels, which can lead to clots and stroke. If you are not used to regular exercise, talk to your doctor before starting an exercise program because the risk of heart attack and stroke may increase during and immediately after strenuous exercise.

A study involving nearly 30,000 women (ages 45 to 90) from the Women's Health Study finds that almost 60% of the effects of exercise on cardiovascular risk reduction are due to changes in known risk factors, mostly inflammatory blood markers and high blood pressure.

Lowering inflammatory blood markers through exercise reduced risk of heart disease and stroke by 33%, and lowering blood pressure reduced risk by 27%.

Another major risk factor for stroke is obesity. Adopting a healthy lifestyle, including exercise, to get to a healthy weight is the best way to modify this risk. Women with a BMI (body mass index) greater than 30 have a 72% increased risk of blocked-vessel stroke in comparison to women with a BMI less than 25.

Exercise also reduces the likelihood of developing type 2 diabetes—a major risk factor for stroke—by increasing the body's sensitivity to insulin. This in turn makes it easier for your body to maintain suitably low blood sugar levels.

How much exercise do I need?

The amount of exercise that you need for optimal control of your stroke risk factors generally depends on how intense the exercise is. The good news is that studies show that any exercise at all appears to reduce stroke risk, and the more you exercise the more your risk decreases.

A large study of about 1,000 people (57% women) looked at the effects of both light and moderate-to-heavy exercise on stroke risk. The average age of participants was 69, and the average amount of exercise they got was 4 to 5 hours/week. Researchers found that any form of exercise reduced stroke risk in all groups, but both higher intensity exercise and longer periods of any exercise translated to a lower stroke risk. Light activity reduced risk by 61%, and moderate-to-heavy exercise reduced risk by 77%. Less than 2 hours of exercise per week was associated with a 58% risk reduction, while exercising for more than 5 hours per week was associated with a 69% risk reduction. Light-moderate exercise included walking, calisthenics, dancing, golf, bowling, horseback riding, and gardening. Heavy exercise included hiking, tennis, swimming, bicycle riding, jogging, aerobic dancing, handball, racquetball, and squash.

Will I benefit from exercise if I already had a stroke?

Exercise may help to prevent recurrent stroke, and it can aid stroke recovery. After a stroke, many patients, especially the elderly, have a decreased tolerance for physical activity that could be due to limited range of movement, depression, or fatigue from lack of exercise during the recovery period. Research studies show that aggressive rehabilitation beyond the usual 6-week period increases aerobic capacity and motor function in stroke patients, and an aerobic exercise program can improve multiple cardiovascular risk factors. Compared with usual stroke care and recovery, an exercise-intensive program can lead to better outcomes in patients' endurance, balance, and mobility.

The key to preventing further strokes is the control of your risk factors by lifestyle modification and medication. Current data suggest that less than half of stroke patients have their risk factors adequately controlled for preventing another stroke. One of the most prevalent risk factors that persist after stroke is high blood sugar. Many people who suffer stroke in the first place have diabetes, a major risk factor for stroke. In addition, a paralyzing stroke makes it harder for subsequently weaker muscles to metabolize sugar (glucose), which contributes to insulin insensitivity and high blood sugar, thereby increasing the risk of recurrent stroke. Improving sugar metabolism is therefore crucial to staving off further strokes.

Preliminary studies suggest that exercise may be one way of improving sugar metabolism. A small study of 12 stroke patients with abnormal sugar metabolism found that 6-month exercise therapy improved two measures of abnormal blood sugar—glucose intolerance and insulin response—in 7 (58%) patients, compared with only 1 of the non-exercising patients. Fasting insulin levels decreased by 23% in 6 months in the exercising group, compared with an increase of 9% for the non-exercisers. Larger studies are needed to confirm these results.

Do I need to talk to my health care provider before I start exercising?

You should talk to your health care provider before beginning an exercise program if you:

- have heart disease, have had a stroke, or are at high risk for either;
- are middle-aged (45 to 50) or older and currently inactive;
- have diabetes or are at high risk for it;
- take blood pressure medication;
- are obese (body mass index [BMI] of 30 or more);
- are pregnant;
- have a medical condition or disability that may affect your ability to exercise (for example, knee problems, arthritis).

Section 22.2

Migraine and Stroke Risk

"Migraine and Stroke," Office on Women's Health, U.S. Department of Health and Human Services (www.womenshealth.gov), 2010.

What is a migraine?

A migraine is an intense headache that may be accompanied by nausea, vomiting, fatigue, sensitivity to light and sound, and mild to severe throbbing pain, usually worse on one side of the head. Women are more likely than men to have migraines, especially between the ages of 20 and 44. There are an estimated 28 million migraine sufferers in the United States, and 70% of them are women.

The two most common types of migraine are defined by their warning symptoms:

- **Migraine with aura:** Known as the classical migraine, it affects about 20% of migraine sufferers. This type of migraine has warning symptoms, called auras, that usually affect vision—such as bright flashing lights or spots—and occur 10 to 30 minutes before the migraine. There are other types of auras that affect other senses, such as a ringing in the ear or changes in smell or taste. Migraines with aura may also include other symptoms such as difficulty speaking, weakness of an arm or leg, confusion, pain, nausea, and sensitivity to light.

- **Migraine without aura:** Known as the common migraine because it occurs in 80% of migraine sufferers in the United States, this type of migraine has no visual warning symptoms. However, symptoms such as fatigue, depression, or anxiety may appear hours before the migraine.

Does having migraines increase my risk of stroke?

Women who have migraines with aura have twice the risk of blocked-vessel (ischemic) stroke and heart disease, and are more than twice as likely to die from cardiovascular disease. It is not clear if women who have migraines with aura have an increased risk of stroke because of the migraine alone, or if it is related to other risk factors that also contribute to stroke, such as high blood pressure and smoking. Migraines without aura do not seem to increase your risk of stroke.

The longer you have migraines, the more the blood vessels in your brain are affected by the changes that occur during a migraine. One study of 300 women found that the risk of stroke increased in those who had migraines with aura more than 12 times a year or for more than 12 years. The risk may be even higher in women who smoke, use birth control pills, or have high blood pressure.

What causes migraines?

The exact cause of migraines is not fully understood. The theory is that migraines are related to abnormal activity deep in the brain brought on by internal and external cues, called triggers. This abnormal brain activity causes changes in the size of the blood vessels, which swell up. The nerves in the brain respond to these swollen blood vessels by sending pain signals—a migraine. Migraines are associated with blocked-vessel stroke because of this change in blood vessel size and blood flow in the brain, especially during migraines with aura.

Most migraines are triggered by external factors. Some common external triggers include the following:

- Bright lights
- Alcohol
- Smoking or exposure to smoke
- Lack of sleep or too much sleep
- Stress
- Chocolates, dairy products, nuts, fermented or pickled foods
- Weather changes

Internal factors can also trigger migraines, such as fluctuating hormones in women. Seven out of 10 women report that they have more migraines around their menstrual cycle, usually a couple of days before menstruation begins. This may be due to lower estrogen levels during this time.

Migraines tend to be hereditary; between 70% to 80% of migraine sufferers have a family history of migraines. This leads some to believe that the heightened sensitivity of the nerves in the brain to certain triggers may be genetic.

Section 22.3

Sleep Apnea Increases Risk of Stroke

"Sleep Apnea Tied to Increased Risk of Stroke," by the
National Institutes of Health (NIH, www.nih.gov), April 8, 2010.

Obstructive sleep apnea is associated with an increased risk of stroke in middle-aged and older adults, especially men, according to new results from a landmark study supported by the National Heart, Lung, and Blood Institute (NHLBI) of the National Institutes of Health. Overall, sleep apnea more than doubles the risk of stroke in men. Obstructive sleep apnea is a common disorder in which the upper airway is intermittently narrowed or blocked, disrupting sleep and breathing during sleep.

Researchers from the Sleep Heart Health Study (SHHS) report that the risk of stroke appears in men with mild sleep apnea and rises with the severity of sleep apnea. Men with moderate to severe sleep apnea were nearly three times more likely to have a stroke than men without sleep apnea or with mild sleep apnea. The risk from sleep apnea is independent of other risk factors such as weight, high blood pressure, race, smoking, and diabetes.

They also report for the first time a link between sleep apnea and increased risk of stroke in women. Obstructive Sleep Apnea Hypopnea and Incident Stroke: The Sleep Heart Health Study, was published online March 25 [2010] ahead of print in the *American Journal of Respiratory and Critical Care Medicine*.

Stroke is the second leading cause of death worldwide. "Although scientists have uncovered several risk factors for stroke—such as age, high blood pressure and atrial fibrillation, and diabetes—there are still many cases in which the cause or contributing factors are unknown," noted NHLBI Acting Director Susan B. Shurin, MD. "This is the largest study to date to link sleep apnea with an increased risk of stroke. The time is right for researchers to study whether treating sleep apnea could prevent or delay stroke in some individuals."

Conducted in nine medical centers across the United States, the SHHS is the largest and most comprehensive prospective, multi-center study on the risk of cardiovascular disease and other conditions related to sleep apnea. In the latest report, researchers studied stroke risk in 5,422 participants aged 40 years and older without a history of stroke. At the start of the study, participants performed a standard at-home sleep test, which determined whether they had sleep apnea and, if so, the severity of the sleep apnea.

Researchers followed the participants for an average of about nine years. They report that during the study, 193 participants had a stroke—85 men (of 2,462 men enrolled) and 108 women (out of 2,960 enrolled).

After adjusting for several cardiovascular risk factors, the researchers found that the effect of sleep apnea on stroke risk was stronger in men than in women. In men, a progressive increase in stroke risk was observed as sleep apnea severity increased from mild levels to moderate to severe levels. In women, however, the increased risk of stroke was significant only with severe levels of sleep apnea.

The researchers suggest that the differences between men and women might be because men are more likely to develop sleep apnea at younger ages. Therefore, they tend to have untreated sleep apnea for longer periods of time than women. "It's possible that the stroke risk is related to cumulative effects of sleep apnea adversely influencing health over many years," said Susan Redline, MD, MPH, professor of medicine, pediatrics, and epidemiology and biostatistics, at Case Western Reserve University in Cleveland and lead author of the paper.

"Our findings provide compelling evidence that obstructive sleep apnea is a risk factor for stroke, especially in men," noted Redline. "Overall, the increased risk of stroke in men with sleep apnea is comparable to adding 10 years to a man's age. Importantly, we found that increased stroke risk in men occurs even with relatively mild levels of sleep apnea."

"Research on the effects of sleep apnea not only increases our understanding of how lapses of breathing during sleep affects our health and well-being, but it can also provide important insight into how cardiovascular problems such as stroke and high blood pressure develop," noted Michael J. Twery, PhD, director of the NIH National Center on Sleep Disorders Research, an office administered by the NHLBI.

The new results support earlier findings that have linked sleep apnea to stroke risk. SHHS researchers have also reported that untreated sleep apnea is associated with an increased risk of high blood pressure, heart attack, irregular heartbeats, heart failure, and death from any cause. Other studies have also linked untreated sleep apnea with overweight and obesity and diabetes. It is also linked to excessive daytime sleepiness, which lowers performance in the workplace and at school, and increases the risk of injuries and death from drowsy driving and other accidents.

More than 12 million American adults are believed to have sleep apnea, and most are not diagnosed or treated. Treatments to restore regular breathing during sleep include mouthpieces, surgery, and breathing devices, such as continuous positive airway pressure, or CPAP. In people who are overweight or obese, weight loss can also help.

These treatments can help improve breathing and reduce the severity of symptoms such as loud snoring and excessive daytime sleepiness, thereby improving sleep-related quality of life and performance at work or in school. Randomized clinical trials to test whether treating sleep apnea lowers the risk of stroke, other cardiovascular diseases, or death are needed.

"We now have abundant evidence that sleep apnea is associated with cardiovascular risk factors and diseases. The next logical step is to determine if treating sleep apnea can lower a person's risk of these leading killers," said Redline. "With stimulus funds, our research group is now developing the additional research and resources to begin answering this important question."

Section 22.4

Stress and Stroke Risk

"Stress and Stroke Risk," Office on Women's Health, U.S. Department of Health and Human Services (www.womenshealth.gov), 2010.

What is stress?

Stress is your body's response to outside pressures or demands, called stressors. Your body responds to stressors by releasing chemicals and hormones into your blood, causing your heart to beat faster, your blood pressure to rise, and your muscles to tense. This physical response gives you more energy and strength to deal with the stressor. Once the stressor disappears or you have adapted to it, the body usually goes back to normal. However, extreme stress or stress over long periods of time (called chronic stress) can damage your emotional and physical health. Common symptoms of chronic stress include trouble sleeping, tiredness, headaches, backaches, upset stomach, irritability, and depression.

How does stress affect my stroke risk?

Stress is associated with high blood pressure and atherosclerosis, both strong risk factors for stroke. People who experience more stress and are less able to cope with it emotionally and physically are more at risk for stroke. One recent study of more than 20,000 people (57% were women) who had never had a stroke or heart disease found that stress was associated with an increased stroke risk, even after taking into account other stroke risk factors.

Researchers are divided as to exactly how stress affects stroke risk, but there is evidence that stress can affect your stroke risk in two ways.

First, stress can affect your stroke risk by how you behave in response to stressful situations. Some people under stress tend to engage in unhealthy coping behavior that only makes the stress worse and can make them more sensitive to further stress. If you smoke or eat or drink too much in response to stress, you increase your risk of high blood pressure, heart disease, and stroke.

Second, stress can affect your risk of stroke by how your body responds to stress. When your blood pressure rises in response to stress, your blood vessels expand to accommodate the increase in blood flow. Usually, once the stressful condition disappears or you have adapted to it, your blood pressure and blood vessels go back to normal. However, if the stress doesn't disappear (it's long-term or chronic) or happens repeatedly, the sudden spikes in blood pressure can damage your blood vessels, the same way as if you had persistent high blood pressure.

Repeated or long-lasting blood pressure spikes may result in blood vessel wall damage and atherosclerosis, which can cause a blocked-vessel (ischemic) stroke. A study of 254 postmenopausal women aged 50 to 60 found that strong elevations in blood pressure in response to stress may eventually impair the blood vessel wall's ability to expand. A 4-year study of 726 adults (59% were women) aged 59 to 71 found that high levels of anxiety for a long period of time may increase the hardening (atherosclerosis) of the carotid arteries in your neck.

How someone's blood pressure reacts to stress varies from person to person. Studies have found that people who have above-average blood pressure spikes in response to stress may be at higher risk for stroke than those with less reactive blood pressures.

Section 22.5

Alcohol and Stroke

How is alcohol use linked to stroke?

Scientists are still figuring out how alcohol use can be linked to stroke. The most important thing to remember is that a doctor is the best resource for determining how alcohol use will affect stroke risk. In some studies, drinking lots of alcohol has been negatively linked to stroke. For example, more than two drinks per day may increase stroke risk by 50%. Other studies have indicated that one alcoholic drink a day may lower a person's risk for stroke, provided that there is no other medical reason for avoiding alcohol. Although recommendations for moderate alcohol consumption range from one to two drinks per day, the vast majority of healthcare professionals agree that drinking more than one to two drinks each day can increase stroke risk and lead to other medical problems, including heart and liver disease, and possibly brain damage.

What counts as one drink?

- 12 ounces of beer
- One glass (5 ounces) of wine
- 1 1/4 to 1 1/2 ounces of liquor

Alcohol is also reported in some studies to have a protective effect against stroke because it raises levels of high-density lipoproteins (HDL) cholesterol, often called good cholesterol. HDLs carry cholesterol to the liver where it is filtered out of blood and eliminated. Too much cholesterol in the blood causes plaque to accumulate in blood vessels and arteries, slowing blood flow and possibly leading to stroke. Alcohol is also considered to be a mild blood thinner, which may prevent clots from forming in blood vessels and causing a stroke.

Because conflicting reports exist about alcohol use and its effects on stroke risk, talk to your doctor before consuming alcoholic drinks on a regular basis. Remember that alcohol is a drug and can interact with other drugs you may be taking. If you do not drink, don't start. Many professionals in the healthcare community believe more studies are necessary to determine if the benefits of alcohol outweigh the risks.

Section 22.6

Smoking and Stroke

"Smoking and Stroke Risk," Office on Women's Health, U.S. Department of Health and Human Services (www.womenshealth.gov), 2010.

How does smoking affect my stroke risk?

Smoking affects your metabolism and the chemistry of your blood vessels in several ways, all of which put you at increased risk for stroke:

- The chemicals in cigarettes damage the walls of the arteries, resulting in a buildup of fatty plaque that can harden and narrow the arteries, restricting blood flow to your brain.

- Smoking irritates the lungs and blood vessels, causing irritation inside the body (an inflammatory response) that increases the number of white blood cells and other predictors of increased risk for heart attack, stroke, and sudden death.

- Smoking makes the blood more likely to clot. These clots can travel in your bloodstream until they finally become stuck in one of the blood vessels in your brain, cutting off blood flow and triggering a stroke.

- Smokers tend to have high levels of LDL (low density lipoprotein, or bad) cholesterol and triglycerides—two types of blood fat that increase your risk of heart disease and stroke. Smoking also lowers HDL (high density lipoprotein, or good) cholesterol. HDL cholesterol helps remove LDL (bad) cholesterol from the artery walls.

Is smoking more harmful to women than men?

While smoking appears to have a greater effect on heart disease risk in women compared to men, most studies find that the increased stroke risk due to smoking is similar in women and men.

Of special concern to women is the combined effect of smoking and birth control pills on stroke. In one study conducted by the World Health Organization, women who smoked but did not take birth control pills had only 1.3 times the risk of stroke compared with nonsmoking women who did not take birth control pills. Women who smoked while using birth control pills had a risk seven times higher.

Is light smoking harmful?

The more cigarettes you smoke the higher your stroke risk, but even light smoking is harmful. As few as one to four cigarettes a day doubles the risk of having a heart attack or dying from heart disease. No studies have examined what effect smoking just a few cigarettes a day may have on stroke risk in the long term.

Will quitting smoking help prevent stroke?

Yes. The risk of stroke decreases steadily after quitting smoking. Within 1 year of quitting, the elevated risk associated with smoking is reduced by 50%; former smokers have the same stroke risk as non-smokers 5 years after quitting.

Will cutting back lower my stroke risk?

Your level of stroke risk depends on how many cigarettes you smoke each day and how long you have been smoking. If you are unable to quit, smoking fewer cigarettes each day is preferable to continuing to smoke more. Keep in mind, though, that smoking even a few cigarettes a day is enough to change the chemistry of your blood vessels. Some of the damage that smoking causes occurs the minute you light up—the blood thickens and the arteries stiffen. The most effective way to lower your stroke risk and eliminate your smoking-related stroke risk completely over time is to quit smoking.

The Surgeon General's Report on the Health Consequences of Smoking notes that cigarettes with lower yields of tar and nicotine have not been shown to lower your risk of heart disease or stroke and should not be considered lower-risk alternatives to regular cigarettes.

What are the other health risks of smoking?

In addition to increasing your risk of stroke and heart disease, smoking also increases your risk of cancer, particularly lung cancer. It is also the major cause of respiratory problems, including emphysema. If you smoke, you are also more likely to develop plaque buildup and clots in the blood vessels of the legs (peripheral artery disease), making it painful to walk. Women who smoke have a higher risk of osteoporosis (bone loss), and they may go through menopause at a younger age than nonsmokers. Smoking is also linked to difficulty getting pregnant and problems during pregnancy, such as having a premature baby.

Section 22.7

Illegal Substance Use and Stroke

"Amphetamine, cocaine usage increase risk of stroke among young adults," April 2, 2007. Reprinted with permission from the University of Texas Southwestern Medical Center News Bureau, www .utsoutwestern.edu/newsroom. © University of Texas Southwestern Medical Center. All rights reserved. Reviewed by David A. Cooke, MD, FACP, January 24, 2013.

Increasing rates of amphetamine and cocaine usage by young adults significantly boost their risk of stroke, with amphetamine abuse associated with the greatest risk, researchers at UT Southwestern Medical Center report.

In the study, available in the [April 1, 2007] *Archives of General Psychiatry*, UT Southwestern physicians examined more than 8,300 stroke patients—ranging in age from 18 to 44—at over 400 Texas hospitals in the years 2000 through 2003.

An analysis of risk factors and trends among stroke victims in this age group pointed to an increase in substance abuse as a major danger, particularly in the abuse of methamphetamines, which are produced in illegal drug labs or illegally imported into the country.

Amphetamines are stimulants, often prescribed for various medical uses as well as used illegally as drugs of choice or as performance enhancers. Methamphetamines (meth) produce more potent, longer lasting, and more harmful effects to the central nervous system than other members of the amphetamine drug class at comparable doses, according to the National Institute of Drug Abuse.

"Using amphetamines or cocaine significantly increases an individual's risk for a stroke," said Dr. Arthur Westover, an instructor of psychiatry at UT Southwestern and the study's lead author. "If we decrease the number of people who are using these substances, then we likely can decrease the number of strokes in this younger population. The implication is that it's preventable."

Dr. Westover is a National Institutes of Health Multidisciplinary Clinical Research Scholar.

The study focused on two kinds of strokes: Hemorrhagic and ischemic. Most strokes—which involve a sudden interruption in the blood supply of the brain—are ischemic, caused by an abrupt blockage of arteries leading to the brain. Hemorrhagic strokes, on the other hand, result from bleeding into brain tissue when a blood vessel bursts.

An evaluation of patient study data from 2003, the first year that U.S. hospitals were required to make a distinction between the two types of strokes in their diagnoses of stroke victims, showed that young people who abuse amphetamines are five times more likely to have a hemorrhagic stroke than non-abusers. If cocaine is abused, the person's likelihood of having either a hemorrhagic or an ischemic stroke more than doubles.

In addition, the 2003 data showed that more than 14 percent of hemorrhagic strokes and 14 percent of ischemic strokes were caused by abuse of drugs, including amphetamines, cocaine, cannabis (marijuana), and tobacco.

"Basically, speed kills," said Dr. Robert Haley, the study's senior author and chief of epidemiology at UT Southwestern. "And meth seems to be increasing as the preferred drug of abuse among the youngest population— people who don't always know its dangers, often thinking it's fairly safe.

"This is the first study large enough to confirm the link that meth kills by causing strokes. We hope that our findings will lead to getting the word out to young people who are tempted to use meth, explaining that the drug is extremely dangerous and can kill them."

Also involved in the study was Dr. Susan McBride from the Dallas-Fort Worth Hospital Council in Irving. The study was supported in part by a grant from the National Institute of Mental Health.

Section 22.8

Trauma and Stroke

Excerpted from "Traumatic Brain Injury: Hope through Research," by the National Institute of Neurological Disorders and Stroke (NINDS, www.ninds.nih.gov), part of the National Institutes of Health, June 14, 2012.

Introduction

Traumatic brain injury (TBI) is a major public health problem, especially among male adolescents and young adults ages 15 to 24, and among elderly people of both sexes 75 years and older. Children aged 5 and younger are also at high risk for TBI.

Perhaps the most famous TBI patient in the history of medicine was Phineas Gage. In 1848, Gage was a 25-year-old railway construction foreman working on the Rutland and Burlington Railroad in Vermont. In the 19th century, little was understood about the brain and even less was known about how to treat injury to it. Most serious injuries to the brain resulted in death due to bleeding or infection. Gage was working with explosive powder and a packing rod, called a tamping iron, when a spark caused an explosion that propelled the 3-foot long, pointed rod through his head. It penetrated his skull at the top of his head, passed through his brain, and exited the skull by his temple. Amazingly, he survived the accident with the help of physician John Harlow who treated Gage for 73 days. Before the accident Gage was a quiet, mild-mannered man; after his injuries he became an obscene, obstinate, self-absorbed man. He continued to suffer personality and behavioral problems until his death in 1861.

Today, we understand a great deal more about the healthy brain and its response to trauma, although science still has much to learn about how to reverse damage resulting from head injuries.

TBI costs the country more than $56 billion a year, and more than 5 million Americans alive today have had a TBI resulting in a permanent need for help in performing daily activities. Survivors of TBI are often left with significant cognitive, behavioral, and communicative disabilities, and some patients develop long-term medical complications, such as epilepsy.

Other statistics dramatically tell the story of head injury in the United States. Each year:

- approximately 1.4 million people experience a TBI;
- approximately 50,000 people die from head injury;
- approximately 1 million head-injured people are treated in hospital emergency rooms; and
- approximately 230,000 people are hospitalized for TBI and survive.

What Is a Traumatic Brain Injury?

TBI, a form of acquired brain injury, occurs when a sudden trauma causes damage to the brain. The damage can be focal—confined to one area of the brain—or diffuse—involving more than one area of the brain. TBI can result from a closed head injury or a penetrating head injury. A closed injury occurs when the head suddenly and violently hits an object but the object does not break through the skull. A penetrating injury occurs when an object pierces the skull and enters brain tissue.

Signs and Symptoms of TBI

Symptoms of a TBI can be mild, moderate, or severe, depending on the extent of the damage to the brain. Some symptoms are evident immediately, while others do not surface until several days or weeks after the injury. A person with a mild TBI may remain conscious or may experience a loss of consciousness for a few seconds or minutes. The person may also feel dazed or not like himself for several days or weeks after the initial injury. Other symptoms of mild TBI include headache, confusion, lightheadedness, dizziness, blurred vision or tired eyes, ringing in the ears, bad taste in the mouth, fatigue or lethargy, a change in sleep patterns, behavioral or mood changes, and trouble with memory, concentration, attention, or thinking.

A person with a moderate or severe TBI may show these same symptoms, but may also have a headache that gets worse or does not go away, repeated vomiting or nausea, convulsions or seizures, inability to awaken from sleep, dilation of one or both pupils of the eyes, slurred speech, weakness or numbness in the extremities, loss of coordination, and/or increased confusion, restlessness, or agitation. Small children with moderate to severe TBI may show some of these signs as well as signs specific to young children, such as persistent crying, inability to be consoled, and/or refusal to nurse or eat. Anyone with signs of moderate or severe TBI should receive medical attention as soon as possible.

Causes of and Risk Factors for TBI

Half of all TBIs are due to transportation accidents involving automobiles, motorcycles, bicycles, and pedestrians. These accidents are the major cause of TBI in people under age 75. For those 75 and older, falls cause the majority of TBIs. Approximately 20 percent of TBIs are due to violence, such as firearm assaults and child abuse, and about 3 percent are due to sports injuries. Fully half of TBI incidents involve alcohol use.

The cause of the TBI plays a role in determining the patient's outcome. For example, approximately 91 percent of firearm TBIs (two-thirds of which may be suicidal in intent) result in death, while only 11 percent of TBIs from falls result in death.

Different Types of TBI

Concussion is the most minor and the most common type of TBI. Technically, a concussion is a short loss of consciousness in response to a head injury, but in common language the term has come to mean any minor injury to the head or brain.

Other injuries are more severe. As the first line of defense, the skull is particularly vulnerable to injury. Skull fractures occur when the bone of the skull cracks or breaks. A depressed skull fracture occurs when pieces of the broken skull press into the tissue of the brain. A penetrating skull fracture occurs when something pierces the skull, such as a bullet, leaving a distinct and localized injury to brain tissue.

Skull fractures can cause bruising of brain tissue called a contusion. A contusion is a distinct area of swollen brain tissue mixed with blood released from broken blood vessels. A contusion can also occur in response to shaking of the brain back and forth within the confines of the skull, an injury called contrecoup. This injury often occurs in car accidents after high-speed stops and in shaken baby syndrome, a severe form of head injury that occurs when a baby is shaken forcibly enough to cause the brain to bounce against the skull. In addition, contrecoup can cause diffuse axonal injury, also called shearing, which involves damage to individual nerve cells (neurons) and loss of connections among neurons. This can lead to a breakdown of overall communication among neurons in the brain.

Damage to a major blood vessel in the head can cause a hematoma, or heavy bleeding into or around the brain. Three types of hematomas can cause brain damage. An epidural hematoma involves bleeding into the area between the skull and the dura. With a subdural hematoma, bleeding is confined to the area between the dura and the arachnoid membrane. Bleeding within the brain itself is called intracerebral hematoma.

Another insult to the brain that can cause injury is anoxia. Anoxia is a condition in which there is an absence of oxygen supply to an organ's tissues, even if there is adequate blood flow to the tissue. Hypoxia refers to a decrease in oxygen supply rather than a complete absence of oxygen. Without oxygen, the cells of the brain die within several minutes. This type of injury is often seen in near-drowning victims, in heart attack patients, or in people who suffer significant blood loss from other injuries that decrease blood flow to the brain.

Medical Care a TBI Patient Should Receive

Medical care usually begins when paramedics or emergency medical technicians arrive on the scene of an accident or when a TBI patient arrives at the emergency department of a hospital. Because little can be done to reverse the initial brain damage caused by trauma, medical personnel try to stabilize the patient and focus on preventing further injury. Primary concerns include insuring proper oxygen supply to the brain and the rest of the body, maintaining adequate blood flow, and controlling blood pressure. Emergency medical personnel may have to open the patient's airway or perform other procedures to make sure the patient is breathing. They may also perform CPR to help the heart pump blood to the body, and they may treat other injuries to control or stop bleeding. Because many head-injured patients may also have spinal cord injuries, medical professionals take great care in moving and transporting the patient. Ideally, the patient is placed on a backboard and in a neck restraint. These devices immobilize the patient and prevent further injury to the head and spinal cord.

As soon as medical personnel have stabilized the head-injured patient, they assess the patient's condition by measuring vital signs and reflexes and by performing a neurological examination. They check the patient's temperature, blood pressure, pulse, breathing rate, and pupil size in response to light. They assess the patient's level of consciousness and neurological functioning using the Glasgow Coma Scale, a standardized, 15-point test that uses three measures—eye opening, best verbal response, and best motor response—to determine the severity of the patient's brain injury.

Imaging tests help in determining the diagnosis and prognosis of a TBI patient. Patients with mild to moderate injuries may receive skull and neck X-rays to check for bone fractures or spinal instability. The patient should remain immobilized in a neck and back restraint until medical personnel are certain that there is no risk of spinal cord injury. For moderate to severe cases, the gold standard imaging test is a computed tomography (CT) scan. The CT scan creates a series of cross-sectional X-ray images of the head and brain and can show bone fractures as well as the presence of hemorrhage, hematomas, contusions, brain tissue swelling, and tumors. Magnetic resonance imaging (MRI) may be used after the initial assessment and treatment of the TBI patient. MRI uses magnetic fields to detect subtle changes in brain tissue content and can show more detail than X-rays or CT. Unfortunately, MRI is not ideal for routine emergency imaging of TBI patients because it is time-consuming and is not available in all hospitals.

Approximately half of severely head-injured patients will need surgery to remove or repair hematomas or contusions. Patients may also need surgery to treat injuries in other parts of the body. These patients usually go to the intensive care unit after surgery.

Sometimes when the brain is injured swelling occurs and fluids accumulate within the brain space. It is normal for bodily injuries to cause swelling and disruptions in fluid balance. But when an injury occurs inside the skull-encased brain, there is no place for swollen tissues to expand and no adjoining tissues to absorb excess fluid. This increased pressure is called intracranial pressure (ICP).

Medical personnel measure patients' ICP using a probe or catheter. The instrument is inserted through the skull to the subarachnoid level and is connected to a monitor that registers the patient's ICP. If a patient has high ICP, he or she may undergo a ventriculostomy, a procedure that drains cerebrospinal fluid (CSF) from the brain to bring the pressure down. Drugs that can be used to decrease ICP include mannitol or barbiturates, although the safety and effectiveness of the latter are unknown.

How Does a TBI Affect Consciousness?

A TBI can cause problems with arousal, consciousness, awareness, alertness, and responsiveness. Generally, there are five abnormal states of consciousness that can result from a TBI: stupor, coma, persistent vegetative state, locked-in syndrome, and brain death.

Stupor is a state in which the patient is unresponsive but can be aroused briefly by a strong stimulus, such as sharp pain. Coma is a state in which the patient is totally unconscious, unresponsive, unaware, and unarousable. Patients in a coma do not respond to external stimuli, such as pain or light, and do not have sleep-wake cycles. Coma results from widespread and diffuse trauma to the brain, including the cerebral hemispheres of the upper brain and the lower brain or brainstem. Coma generally is of short duration, lasting a few days to a few weeks. After this time, some patients gradually come out of the coma, some progress to a vegetative state, and others die.

Patients in a vegetative state are unconscious and unaware of their surroundings, but they continue to have a sleep-wake cycle and can have periods of alertness. Unlike coma, where the patients eyes are closed, patients in a vegetative state often open their eyes and may move, groan, or show reflex responses. A vegetative state can result from diffuse injury to the cerebral hemispheres of the brain without damage to the lower brain and brainstem. Anoxia, or lack of oxygen to the brain, which is a common complication of cardiac arrest, can also bring about a vegetative state.

Many patients emerge from a vegetative state within a few weeks, but those who do not recover within 30 days are said to be in a persistent vegetative state (PVS). The chances of recovery depend on the extent of injury to the brain and the patient's age, with younger patients having a better chance of recovery than older patients. Generally adults have a 50 percent chance and children a 60 percent chance of recovering consciousness from a PVS within the first 6 months. After a year, the chances that a PVS patient will regain consciousness are very low and most patients who do recover consciousness experience significant disability. The longer a patient is in a PVS, the more severe the resulting disabilities will be. Rehabilitation can contribute to recovery, but many patients never progress to the point of being able to take care of themselves.

Locked-in syndrome is a condition in which a patient is aware and awake, but cannot move or communicate due to complete paralysis of the body.

Advances in imaging and other technologies have led to devices that help differentiate among the variety of unconscious states.

Unlike PVS, in which the upper portions of the brain are damaged and the lower portions are spared, locked-in syndrome is caused by damage to specific portions of the lower brain and brainstem with no damage to the upper brain. Most locked-in syndrome patients can communicate through movements and blinking of their eyes, which are not affected by the paralysis. Some patients may have the ability to move certain facial muscles as well. The majority of locked-in syndrome patients do not regain motor control, but several devices are available to help patients communicate.

With the development over the last half-century of assistive devices that can artificially maintain blood flow and breathing, the term brain death has come into use. Brain death is the lack of measurable brain function due to diffuse damage to the cerebral hemispheres and the brainstem, with loss of any integrated activity among distinct areas of the brain. Brain death is irreversible. Removal of assistive devices will result in immediate cardiac arrest and cessation of breathing.

Advances in imaging and other technologies have led to devices that help differentiate among the variety of unconscious states. For example, an imaging test that shows activity in the brainstem but little or no activity in the upper brain would lead a physician to a diagnosis of vegetative state and exclude diagnoses of brain death and locked-in syndrome. On the other hand, an imaging test that shows activity in the upper brain with little activity in the brainstem would confirm a diagnosis of locked-in syndrome, while invalidating a diagnosis of brain death or vegetative state. The use of CT and MRI is standard in TBI treatment, but other imaging and diagnostic techniques that may be used to confirm a particular diagnosis include cerebral angiography, electroencephalography (EEG), transcranial Doppler ultrasound, and single photon emission computed tomography (SPECT).

Immediate Post-Injury Complications

Sometimes, health complications occur in the period immediately following a TBI. These complications are not types of TBI, but are distinct medical problems that arise as a result of the injury. Although complications are rare, the risk increases with the severity of the trauma. Complications of TBI include immediate seizures, hydrocephalus or post-traumatic ventricular enlargement, CSF leaks, infections, vascular injuries, cranial nerve injuries, pain, bed sores, multiple organ system failure in unconscious patients, and polytrauma (trauma to other parts of the body in addition to the brain).

About 25 percent of patients with brain contusions or hematomas and about 50 percent of patients with penetrating head injuries will develop immediate seizures, seizures that occur within the first 24 hours of the injury. These immediate seizures increase the risk of early seizures— defined as seizures occurring within one week after injury—but do not seem to be linked to the development of post-traumatic epilepsy (recurrent seizures occurring more than one week after the initial trauma). Generally, medical professionals use anticonvulsant medications to treat seizures in TBI patients only if the seizures persist.

Hydrocephalus or post-traumatic ventricular enlargement occurs when CSF accumulates in the brain resulting in dilation of the cerebral ventricles (cavities in the brain filled with CSF) and an increase in ICP. This condition can develop during the acute stage of TBI or may not appear until later. Generally it occurs within the first year of the injury and is characterized by worsening neurological outcome, impaired consciousness, behavioral changes, ataxia (lack of coordination or balance), incontinence, or signs of elevated ICP. The condition may develop as a result of meningitis, subarachnoid hemorrhage, intracranial hematoma, or other injuries. Treatment includes shunting and draining of CSF as well as any other appropriate treatment for the root cause of the condition.

Skull fractures can tear the membranes that cover the brain, leading to CSF leaks. A tear between the dura and the arachnoid membranes, called a CSF fistula, can cause CSF to leak out of the subarachnoid space into the subdural space; this is called a subdural hygroma. CSF can also leak from the nose and the ear. These tears that let CSF out of the brain cavity can also allow air and bacteria into the cavity, possibly causing infections such as meningitis. Pneumocephalus occurs when air enters the intracranial cavity and becomes trapped in the subarachnoid space.

Infections within the intracranial cavity are a dangerous complication of TBI. They may occur outside of the dura, below the dura, below the arachnoid (meningitis), or within the space of the brain itself (abscess). Most of these injuries develop within a few weeks of the initial trauma and result from skull fractures or penetrating injuries. Standard treatment involves antibiotics and sometimes surgery to remove the infected tissue. Meningitis may be especially dangerous, with the potential to spread to the rest of the brain and nervous system.

Any damage to the head or brain usually results in some damage to the vascular system, which provides blood to the cells of the brain. The body's immune system can repair damage to small blood vessels, but damage to larger vessels can result in serious complications. Damage to one of the major arteries leading to the brain can cause a stroke, either through bleeding from the artery (hemorrhagic stroke) or through the formation of a clot at the site of injury, called a thrombus or thrombosis, blocking blood flow to the brain (ischemic stroke). Blood clots also can develop in other parts of the head. Symptoms such as headache, vomiting, seizures, paralysis on one side of the body, and semi-consciousness developing within several days of a head injury may be caused by a blood clot that forms in the tissue of one of the sinuses, or cavities, adjacent to the brain. Thrombotic-ischemic strokes are treated with anticoagulants, while surgery is the preferred treatment for hemorrhagic stroke. Other types of vascular injuries include vasospasm and the formation of aneurysms.

Skull fractures, especially at the base of the skull, can cause cranial nerve injuries that result in compressive cranial neuropathies. All but three of the 12 cranial nerves project out from the brainstem to the head and face. The seventh cranial nerve, called the facial nerve, is the most commonly injured cranial nerve in TBI and damage to it can result in paralysis of facial muscles.

Pain is a common symptom of TBI and can be a significant complication for conscious patients in the period immediately following a TBI. Headache is the most common form of pain experienced by TBI patients, but other forms of pain can also be problematic. Serious complications for patients who are unconscious, in a coma, or in a vegetative state include bed or pressure sores of the skin, recurrent bladder infections, pneumonia or other life-threatening infections, and progressive multiple organ failure.

General Trauma

Most TBI patients have injuries to other parts of the body in addition to the head and brain. Physicians call this polytrauma. These injuries require immediate and specialized care and can complicate treatment of and recovery from the TBI. Other medical complications that may accompany a TBI include pulmonary (lung) dysfunction; cardiovascular (heart) dysfunction from blunt chest trauma; gastrointestinal dysfunction; fluid and hormonal imbalances; and other isolated complications, such as fractures, nerve injuries, deep vein thrombosis, excessive blood clotting, and infections.

Trauma victims often develop hypermetabolism or an increased metabolic rate, which leads to an increase in the amount of heat the body produces. The body redirects into heat the energy needed to keep organ systems functioning, causing muscle wasting and the starvation of other tissues. Complications related to pulmonary dysfunction can include neurogenic pulmonary edema (excess fluid in lung tissue), aspiration pneumonia (pneumonia caused by foreign matter in the lungs), and fat and blood clots in the blood vessels of the lungs.

Fluid and hormonal imbalances can complicate the treatment of hypermetabolism and high ICP. Hormonal problems can result from dysfunction of the pituitary, the thyroid, and other glands throughout the body. Two common hormonal complications of TBI are syndrome of inappropriate secretion of antidiuretic hormone (SIADH) and hypothyroidism.

Blunt trauma to the chest can also cause cardiovascular problems, including damage to blood vessels and internal bleeding, and problems with heart rate and blood flow. Blunt trauma to the abdomen can cause damage to or dysfunction of the stomach, large or small intestines, and pancreas. A serious and common complication of TBI is erosive gastritis, or inflammation and degeneration of stomach tissue. This syndrome can cause bacterial growth in the stomach, increasing the risk of aspiration pneumonia. Standard care of TBI patients includes administration of prophylactic gastric acid inhibitors to prevent the buildup of stomach acids and bacteria.

What Disabilities Can Result from a TBI?

Disabilities resulting from a TBI depend upon the severity of the injury, the location of the injury, and the age and general health of the patient. Some common disabilities include problems with cognition (thinking, memory, and reasoning), sensory processing (sight, hearing, touch, taste, and smell), communication (expression and understanding), and behavior or mental health (depression, anxiety, personality changes, aggression, acting out, and social inappropriateness).

Within days to weeks of the head injury approximately 40 percent of TBI patients develop a host of troubling symptoms collectively called postconcussion syndrome (PCS). A patient need not have suffered a concussion or loss of consciousness to develop the syndrome and many patients with mild TBI suffer from PCS. Symptoms include headache, dizziness, vertigo (a sensation of spinning around or of objects spinning around the patient), memory problems, trouble concentrating, sleeping problems, restlessness, irritability, apathy, depression, and anxiety. These symptoms may last for a few weeks after the head injury. The syndrome is more prevalent in patients who had psychiatric symptoms, such as depression or anxiety, before the injury. Treatment for PCS may include medicines for pain and psychiatric conditions, and psychotherapy and occupational therapy to develop coping skills.

Cognition is a term used to describe the processes of thinking, reasoning, problem solving, information processing, and memory. Most patients with severe TBI, if they recover consciousness, suffer from cognitive disabilities, including the loss of many higher level mental skills. The most common cognitive impairment among severely head-injured patients is memory loss, characterized by some loss of specific memories and the partial inability to form or store new ones. Some of these patients may experience post-traumatic amnesia (PTA), either anterograde or retrograde. Anterograde PTA is impaired memory of events that happened after the TBI, while retrograde PTA is impaired memory of events that happened before the TBI.

Many patients with mild to moderate head injuries who experience cognitive deficits become easily confused or distracted and have problems with concentration and attention. They also have problems with higher level, so-called executive functions, such as planning, organizing, abstract reasoning, problem solving, and making judgments, which may make it difficult to resume pre-injury work-related activities. Recovery from cognitive deficits is greatest within the first 6 months after the injury and more gradual after that.

The most common cognitive impairment among severely head-injured patients is memory loss, characterized by some loss of specific memories and the partial inability to form or store new ones.

Patients with moderate to severe TBI have more problems with cognitive deficits than patients with mild TBI, but a history of several mild TBIs may have an additive effect, causing cognitive deficits equal to a moderate or severe injury.

Many TBI patients have sensory problems, especially problems with vision. Patients may not be able to register what they are seeing or may be slow to recognize objects. Also, TBI patients often have difficulty with hand-eye coordination. Because of this, TBI patients may be prone to bumping into or dropping objects, or may seem generally unsteady. TBI patients may have difficulty driving a car, working complex machinery, or playing sports. Other sensory deficits may include problems with hearing, smell, taste, or touch. Some TBI patients develop tinnitus, a ringing or roaring in the ears. A person with damage to the part of the brain that processes taste or smell may develop a persistent bitter taste in the mouth or perceive a persistent noxious smell. Damage to the part of the brain that controls the sense of touch may cause a TBI patient to develop persistent skin tingling, itching, or pain. Although rare, these conditions are hard to treat.

Language and communication problems are common disabilities in TBI patients. Some may experience aphasia, defined as difficulty with understanding and producing spoken and written language; others may have difficulty with the more subtle aspects of communication, such as body language and emotional, non-verbal signals.

In non-fluent aphasia, also called Broca aphasia or motor aphasia, TBI patients often have trouble recalling words and speaking in complete sentences. They may speak in broken phrases and pause frequently. Most patients are aware of these deficits and may become extremely frustrated. Patients with fluent aphasia, also called Wernicke aphasia or sensory aphasia, display little meaning in their speech, even though they speak in complete sentences and use correct grammar. Instead, they speak in flowing gibberish, drawing out their sentences with non-essential and invented words. Many patients with fluent aphasia are unaware that they make little sense and become angry with others for not understanding them. Patients with global aphasia have extensive damage to the portions of the brain responsible for language and often suffer severe communication disabilities.

TBI patients may have problems with spoken language if the part of the brain that controls speech muscles is damaged. In this disorder, called dysarthria, the patient can think of the appropriate language, but cannot easily speak the words because they are unable to use the muscles needed to form the words and produce the sounds. Speech is often slow, slurred, and garbled. Some may have problems with intonation or inflection, called prosodic dysfunction. An important aspect of speech, inflection conveys emotional meaning and is necessary for certain aspects of language, such as irony.

These language deficits can lead to miscommunication, confusion, and frustration for the patient as well as those interacting with him or her.

Most TBI patients have emotional or behavioral problems that fit under the broad category of psychiatric health. Family members of TBI patients often find that personality changes and behavioral problems are the most difficult disabilities to handle. Psychiatric problems that may surface include depression, apathy, anxiety, irritability, anger, paranoia, confusion, frustration, agitation, insomnia or other sleep problems, and mood swings. Problem behaviors may include aggression and violence, impulsivity, disinhibition, acting out, noncompliance, social inappropriateness, emotional outbursts, childish behavior, impaired self-control, impaired self-awareness, inability to take responsibility or accept criticism, egocentrism, inappropriate sexual activity, and alcohol or drug abuse/addiction. Some patients' personality problems may be so severe that they are diagnosed with borderline personality disorder, a psychiatric condition characterized by many of the problems mentioned above. Sometimes TBI patients suffer from developmental stagnation, meaning that they fail to mature emotionally, socially, or psychologically after the trauma. This is a serious problem for children and young adults who suffer from a TBI. Attitudes and behaviors that are appropriate for a child or teenager become inappropriate in adulthood. Many TBI patients who show psychiatric or behavioral problems can be helped with medication and psychotherapy.

Long-Term Problems Associated with a TBI

In addition to the immediate post-injury complications discussed on page 13, other long-term problems can develop after a TBI. These include Parkinson disease and other motor problems, Alzheimer disease, dementia pugilistica, and post-traumatic dementia.

Alzheimer disease (AD): AD is a progressive, neurodegenerative disease characterized by dementia, memory loss, and deteriorating cognitive abilities. Recent research suggests an association between head injury in early adulthood and the development of AD later in life; the more severe the head injury, the greater the risk of developing AD. Some evidence indicates that a head injury may interact with other factors to trigger the disease and may hasten the onset of the disease in individuals already at risk. For example, people who have a particular form of the protein apolipoprotein E (apoE4) and suffer a head injury fall into this increased risk category. (ApoE4 is a naturally occurring protein that helps transport cholesterol through the bloodstream.)

Parkinson disease and other motor problems: Movement disorders as a result of TBI are rare but can occur. Parkinson disease may develop years after TBI as a result of damage to the basal ganglia. Symptoms of Parkinson disease include tremor or trembling, rigidity or stiffness, slow movement (bradykinesia), inability to move (akinesia), shuffling walk, and stooped posture. Despite many scientific advances in recent years, Parkinson disease remains a chronic and progressive disorder, meaning that it is incurable and will progress in severity until the end of life. Other movement disorders that may develop after TBI include tremor, ataxia (uncoordinated muscle movements), and myoclonus (shock-like contractions of muscles).

Dementia pugilistica: Also called chronic traumatic encephalopathy, dementia pugilistica primarily affects career boxers. The most common symptoms of the condition are dementia and parkinsonism caused by repetitive blows to the head over a long period of time. Symptoms begin anywhere between 6 and 40 years after the start of a boxing career, with an average onset of about 16 years.

Post-traumatic dementia: The symptoms of post-traumatic dementia are very similar to those of dementia pugilistica, except that post-traumatic dementia is also characterized by long-term memory problems and is caused by a single, severe TBI that results in a coma.

What Kinds of Rehabilitation Should a TBI Patient Receive?

Rehabilitation is an important part of the recovery process for a TBI patient. During the acute stage, moderately to severely injured patients may receive treatment and care in an intensive care unit of a hospital. Once stable, the patient may be transferred to a subacute unit of the medical center or to an independent rehabilitation hospital. At this point, patients follow many diverse paths toward recovery because there are a wide variety of options for rehabilitation.

Testing by a trained neuropsychologist can assess the individual's cognitive, language, behavioral, motor, and executive functions and provide information regarding the need for rehabilitative services.

In 1998, the NIH held a Consensus Development Conference on Rehabilitation of Persons with Traumatic Brain Injury. The Consensus Development Panel recommended that TBI patients receive an individualized rehabilitation program based upon the patient's strengths and capacities and that rehabilitation services should be modified over time to adapt to the patient's changing needs. The panel also recommended that moderately to severely injured patients receive rehabilitation treatment that draws on the skills of many specialists. This involves individually tailored treatment programs in the areas of physical therapy, occupational therapy, speech/language therapy, physiatry (physical medicine), psychology/psychiatry, and social support. Medical personnel who provide this care include rehabilitation specialists, such as rehabilitation nurses, psychologists, speech/language pathologists, physical and occupational therapists, physiatrists (physical medicine specialists), social workers, and a team coordinator or administrator.

The overall goal of rehabilitation after a TBI is to improve the patient's ability to function at home and in society. Therapists help the patient adapt to disabilities or change the patient's living space, called environmental modification, to make everyday activities easier.

Some patients may need medication for psychiatric and physical problems resulting from the TBI. Great care must be taken in prescribing medications because TBI patients are more susceptible to side effects and may react adversely to some pharmacological agents. It is important for the family to provide social support for the patient by being involved in the rehabilitation program. Family members may also benefit from psychotherapy.

It is important for TBI patients and their families to select the most appropriate setting for rehabilitation. There are several options, including home-based rehabilitation, hospital outpatient rehabilitation, inpatient rehabilitation centers, comprehensive day programs at rehabilitation centers, supportive living programs, independent living centers, club-house programs, school based programs for children, and others. The TBI patient, the family, and the rehabilitation team members should work together to find the best place for the patient to recover.

How Can TBI Be Prevented?

Unlike most neurological disorders, head injuries can be prevented. The Centers for Disease Control and Prevention (CDC) have issued the following safety tips for reducing the risk of suffering a TBI.

- Wear a seatbelt every time you drive or ride in a car.

- Buckle your child into a child safety seat, booster seat, or seatbelt (depending on the child's age) every time the child rides in a car.

- Wear a helmet and make sure your children wear helmets when riding a bike or motorcycle; playing a contact sport such as football or ice hockey; using in-line skates or riding a skateboard; batting and running bases in baseball or softball; riding a horse; skiing or snowboarding.

- Keep firearms and bullets stored in a locked cabinet when not in use.

- Avoid falls by using a step-stool with a grab bar to reach objects on high shelves; installing handrails on stairways; installing window guards to keep young children from falling out of open windows; using safety gates at the top and bottom of stairs when young children are around.

- Make sure the surface on your child's playground is made of shock-absorbing material (e.g., hardwood mulch, sand).

What Research Is the NINDS Conducting?

The National Institute of Neurological Disorders and Stroke (NINDS) conducts and supports research to better understand CNS injury and the biological mechanisms underlying damage to the brain, to develop strategies and interventions to limit the primary and secondary brain damage that occurs within days of a head trauma, and to devise therapies to treat brain injury and help in long-term recovery of function.

On a microscopic scale, the brain is made up of billions of cells that interconnect and communicate.

The neuron is the main functional cell of the brain and nervous system, consisting of a cell body (soma), a tail or long nerve fiber (axon), and projections of the cell body called dendrites. The axons travel in tracts or clusters throughout the brain, providing extensive interconnections between brain areas.

One of the most pervasive types of injury following even a minor trauma is damage to the nerve cell's axon through shearing; this is referred to as diffuse axonal injury. This damage causes a series of reactions that eventually lead to swelling of the axon and disconnection from the cell body of the neuron. In addition, the part of the neuron that communicates with other neurons degenerates and releases toxic levels of chemical messengers called neurotransmitters into the synapse or space between neurons, damaging neighboring neurons through a secondary neuroexcitatory cascade. Therefore, neurons that were unharmed from the primary trauma suffer damage from this secondary insult. Many of these cells cannot survive the toxicity of the chemical onslaught and initiate programmed cell death, or apoptosis. This process usually takes place within the first 24 to 48 hours after the initial injury, but can be prolonged.

One area of research that shows promise is the study of the role of calcium ion influx into the damaged neuron as a cause of cell death and general brain tissue swelling. Calcium enters nerve cells through damaged channels in the axon's membrane. The excess calcium inside the cell causes the axon to swell and also activates chemicals, called proteases, that break down proteins. One family of proteases, the calpains, are especially damaging to nerve cells because they break down proteins that maintain the structure of the axon. Excess calcium within the cell is also destructive to the cell's mitochondria, structures that produce the cell's energy. Mitochondria soak up excess calcium until they swell and stop functioning. If enough mitochondria are damaged, the nerve cell degenerates. Calcium influx has other damaging effects: it activates destructive enzymes, such as caspases that damage the DNA in the cell and trigger programmed cell death, and it damages sodium channels in the cell membrane, allowing sodium ions to flood the cell as well. Sodium influx exacerbates swelling of the cell body and axon.

NINDS researchers have shown, in both cell and animal studies, that giving specialized chemicals can reduce cell death caused by calcium ion influx. Other researchers have shown that the use of cyclosporin A, which blocks mitochondrial membrane permeability, protects axons from calcium influx. Another avenue of therapeutic intervention is the use of hypothermia (an induced state of low body temperature) to slow the progression of cell death and axon swelling.

In the healthy brain, the chemical glutamate functions as a neurotransmitter, but an excess amount of glutamate in the brain causes neurons to quickly overload from too much excitation, releasing toxic chemicals. These substances poison the chemical environment of surrounding cells, initiating degeneration and programmed cell death. Studies have shown that a group of enzymes called matrix metallo-proteinases contribute to the toxicity by breaking down proteins that maintain the structure and order of the extracellular environment. Other research shows that glutamate reacts with calcium and sodium ion channels on the cell membrane, leading to an influx of calcium and sodium ions into the cell. Investigators are looking for ways to decrease the toxic effects of glutamate and other excitatory neurotransmitters.

The brain attempts to repair itself after a trauma, and is more successful after mild to moderate injury than after severe injury. Scientists have shown that after diffuse axonal injury neurons can spontaneously adapt and recover by sprouting some of the remaining healthy fibers of the neuron into the spaces once occupied by the degenerated axon. These fibers can develop in such a way that the neuron can resume communication with neighboring neurons. This is a very delicate process and can be disrupted by any of a number of factors, such as neuroexcitation, hypoxia (low oxygen levels), and hypotension (low blood flow). Following trauma, excessive neuroexcitation, that is the electrical activation of nerve cells or fibers, especially disrupts this natural recovery process and can cause sprouting fibers to lose direction and connect with the wrong terminals.

Scientists suspect that these misconnections may contribute to some long-term disabilities, such as pain, spasticity, seizures, and memory problems. NINDS researchers are trying to learn more about the brain's natural recovery process and what factors or triggers control it. They hope that through manipulation of these triggers they can increase repair while decreasing misconnections.

NINDS investigators are also looking at larger, tissue-specific changes within the brain after a TBI. Researchers have shown that trauma to the frontal lobes of the brain can damage specific chemical messenger systems, specifically the dopaminergic system, the collection of neurons in the brain that uses the neurotransmitter dopamine. Dopamine is an important chemical messenger—for example, degeneration of dopamine-producing neurons is the primary cause of Parkinson disease. NINDS researchers are studying how the dopaminergic system responds after a TBI and its relationship to neurodegeneration and Parkinson disease.

The use of stem cells to repair or replace damaged brain tissue is a new and exciting avenue of research. A neural stem cell is a special kind of cell that can multiply and give rise to other more specialized cell types. These cells are found in adult neural tissue and normally develop into several different cell types found within the central nervous system. NINDS researchers are investigating the ability of stem cells to develop into neurotransmitter-producing neurons, specifically dopamine-producing cells. Researchers are also looking at the power of stem cells to develop into oligodendrocytes, a type of brain cell that produces myelin, the fatty sheath that surrounds and insulates axons. One study in mice has shown that bone marrow stem cells can develop into neurons, demonstrating that neural stem cells are not the only type of stem cell that could be beneficial in the treatment of brain and nervous system disorders. At the moment, stem cell research for TBI is in its infancy, but future research may lead to advances for treatment and rehabilitation.

In addition to the basic research described above, NINDS scientists also conduct broader based clinical research involving patients. One area of study focuses on the plasticity of the brain after injury. In the strictest sense, plasticity means the ability to be formed or molded. When speaking of the brain, plasticity means the ability of the brain to adapt to deficits and injury. NINDS researchers are investigating the extent of brain plasticity after injury and developing therapies to enhance plasticity as a means of restoring function.

The plasticity of the brain and the rewiring of neural connections make it possible for one part of the brain to take up the functions of a disabled part. Scientists have long known that the immature brain is generally more plastic than the mature brain, and that the brains of children are better able to adapt and recover from injury than the brains of adults. NINDS researchers are investigating the mechanisms underlying this difference and theorize that children have an overabundance of hard-wired neural networks, many of which naturally decrease through a process called pruning. When an injury destroys an important neural network in children, another less useful neural network that would have eventually died takes over the responsibilities of the damaged network. Some researchers are looking at the role of plasticity in memory, while others are using imaging technologies, such as functional MRI, to map regions of the brain and record evidence of plasticity.

In the strictest sense, plasticity means the ability to be formed or molded. When speaking of the brain, plasticity means the ability of the brain to adapt to deficits and injury.

Another important area of research involves the development of improved rehabilitation programs for those who have disabilities from a TBI. The Congressional Children's Health Act of 2000 authorized the NINDS to conduct and support research related to TBI with the goal of designing therapies to restore normal functioning in cognition and behavior.

Chapter 23

Stroke Prevention

Chapter Contents

Section 23.1

Preventing and Managing Diabetes

"Prevent Diabetes," from the Centers for Disease Control
and Prevention (CDC, www.cdc.gov), May 14, 2012.

Research studies have found that moderate weight loss and exercise can prevent or delay type 2 diabetes among adults at high risk of diabetes. Find out more about the risk factors for type 2 diabetes, what it means to have prediabetes, and what you can do to prevent or delay diabetes.

What are the most important things to do to prevent diabetes?

The Diabetes Prevention Program (DPP), a major federally funded study of 3,234 people at high risk for diabetes, showed that people can delay and possibly prevent the disease by losing a small amount of weight (5 to 7 percent of total body weight) through 30 minutes of physical activity 5 days a week and healthier eating.

When should I be tested for diabetes?

Anyone aged 45 years or older should consider getting tested for diabetes, especially if you are overweight. If you are younger than 45, but are overweight and have one or more additional risk factors, you should consider getting tested.

What are the risk factors which increase the likelihood of developing diabetes?

- Being overweight or obese

- Having a parent, brother, or sister with diabetes

- Being African American, American Indian, Asian American, Pacific Islander, or Hispanic American/Latino heritage

- Having a prior history of gestational diabetes or birth of at least one baby weighing more than nine pounds

- Having high blood pressure measuring 140/90 or higher

- Having abnormal cholesterol with HDL (high density lipoprotein, or good) cholesterol 35 or lower or a triglyceride level 250 or higher

- Being physically inactive/exercising fewer than three times a week

How does body weight affect the likelihood of developing diabetes?

Being overweight or obese is a leading risk factor for type 2 diabetes. Being overweight can keep your body from making and using insulin properly, and can also cause high blood pressure. The Diabetes Prevention Program showed that moderate diet and exercise of about 30 minutes or more, 5 or more days per week, or of 150 or more minutes per week, resulted in a 5% to 7% weight loss and can delay and possibly prevent type 2 diabetes.

What is prediabetes?

People with blood glucose levels that are higher than normal but not yet in the diabetic range have "prediabetes." Doctors sometimes call this condition impaired fasting glucose (IFG) or impaired glucose tolerance (IGT), depending on the test used to diagnose it. Insulin resistance and prediabetes usually have no symptoms. You may have one or both conditions for several years without noticing anything.

If you have prediabetes, you have a higher risk of developing type 2 diabetes. In addition, people with prediabetes also have a higher risk of heart disease.

Progression to diabetes among those with prediabetes is not inevitable. Studies suggest that weight loss and increased physical activity among people with prediabetes prevent or delay diabetes and may return blood glucose levels to normal.

Can vaccines cause diabetes?

No. Carefully performed scientific studies show that vaccines do not cause diabetes or increase a person's risk of developing diabetes. In 2002, the Institute of Medicine reviewed the existing studies and released a report concluding that the scientific evidence favors rejection of the theory that immunizations cause diabetes. The only evidence suggesting a relationship between vaccination and diabetes comes from Dr. John B. Classen, who has suggested that certain vaccines if given at birth may decrease the occurrence of diabetes, whereas if initial vaccination is performed after 2 months of age the occurrence of diabetes increases. Dr. Classen's studies have a number of limitations and have not been verified by other researchers.

Section 23.2

Preventing and Managing High Blood Pressure

Excerpted from "How to Prevent High Blood Pressure," by the Centers for Disease Control and Prevention (CDC, www.cdc.gov), February 1, 2010.

Increases in blood pressure increases your risk for heart disease. People at any age can take steps each day to keep blood pressure levels normal.

- **Eat a healthy diet.** Eating healthfully can help keep your blood pressure down. Eat lots of fresh fruits and vegetables, which provide nutrients such as potassium and fiber. Also, eat foods that are low in saturated fat and cholesterol.

- **Avoid sodium by limiting the amount of salt you add to your food.** Be aware that many processed foods and restaurant meals are high in sodium.

- **Maintain a healthy weight.** Being overweight can raise your blood pressure. Losing weight can help you lower your blood pressure. To find out whether your weight is healthy, doctors often calculate a number called the body mass index (BMI). Doctors sometimes also use waist and hip measurements to measure a person's excess body fat.

- **Be physically active.** Physical activity can help lower blood pressure. The Surgeon General recommends that adults should engage in moderate physical activities for at least 30 minutes on most days of the week.

- **Don't smoke.** Smoking injures blood vessels and speeds up the hardening of the arteries. Further, smoking is a major risk for heart disease and stroke. If you don't smoke, don't start. If you do smoke, quitting will lower your risk for heart disease and stroke. Your doctor can suggest programs to help you quit.

- **Limit alcohol use.** Drinking too much alcohol is associated with high blood pressure. If you drink alcohol, you should do so in moderation—no more than one drink per day for women or two drinks per day for men.

- **Check your blood pressure.** Getting your blood pressure checked is important because high blood pressure often has no symptoms. Your doctor can measure your blood pressure, or you can use a machine available at many pharmacies. You can also use a home monitoring device to measure your blood pressure.

- **Treat high blood pressure.** If you already have high blood pressure, your doctor may prescribe medications in addition to lifestyle changes. All drugs may have side effects, so talk with your doctor on a regular basis. As your blood pressure improves, your doctor will want to monitor it often.

- **Prevent and manage diabetes.** You can reduce your risk of diabetes by eating a healthy diet, maintaining a healthy weight, and being physically active. About 60% of people who have diabetes also have high blood pressure.

Lifestyle changes are just as important as taking medications.

Section 23.3

Preventing and Managing High Cholesterol

Excerpted from "Cholesterol," by the Centers for Disease Control and Prevention (CDC, www.cdc.gov), March 14, 2012.

High cholesterol increases your risk for heart disease. People at any age can take steps to keep cholesterol levels normal.

Get a Blood Test

High cholesterol usually has no signs or symptoms. Only a doctor's check will reveal it.

Your doctor can do a simple blood test to check your cholesterol levels. The test is called a lipoprotein profile. It measures several kinds of cholesterol as well as triglycerides. Some doctors do a simpler blood test that just checks total and HDL [high-density lipoprotein] cholesterol.

The National Cholesterol Education Program recommends that healthy adults get their cholesterol levels checked every five years. See Table 23.1.

Eat a Healthy Diet

A healthy diet can help keep blood cholesterol levels down. Avoid saturated fat, trans fats, and dietary cholesterol, which tend to raise cholesterol levels. Other types of fats, such as monounsaturated and polyunsaturated fats, can actually lower blood cholesterol levels. Eating fiber can also help lower cholesterol.

For some people, eating too many carbohydrates can lower HDL (good cholesterol) and raise triglycerides. Drinking alcohol can also raise triglycerides. Too much alcohol can cause high blood pressure, which increases the risk for heart disease and stroke.

Maintain a Healthy Weight

Being overweight or obese can raise your bad cholesterol levels. Losing weight can help lower your cholesterol.

Table 23.1. Desirable Cholesterol Levels

Total cholesterol	Less than 200 mg/dL
LDL (bad cholesterol)	Less than 100 mg/dL*
HDL (good cholesterol)	40 mg/dL or higher
Triglycerides	Less than 150 mg/dL

*Note: Optimal level.

To determine whether your weight is in a healthy range, doctors often calculate a number called the body mass index (BMI). Doctors sometimes also use waist and hip measurements to measure a person's excess body fat.

Exercise Regularly

Physical activity can help maintain a healthy weight and lower cholesterol. The Surgeon General recommends that adults should engage in moderate-intensity exercise for at least 30 minutes on most days of the week.

Don't Smoke

Smoking injures blood vessels and speeds up the hardening of the arteries. Smoking greatly increases a person's risk for heart disease and stroke.

If you don't smoke, don't start. If you do smoke, quitting will lower your risk for heart disease and stroke. Your doctor can suggest programs to help you stop smoking.

Breathing secondhand smoke increases a person's risk for a heart attack and other heart conditions.

Treat High Cholesterol

If you have high cholesterol, your doctor may prescribe medications in addition to lifestyle changes. Controlling LDL [low-density lipoprotein] cholesterol is the primary focus of treatment.

Your treatment plan will depend on your current LDL level and risk for heart disease and stroke. Your risk for heart disease and stroke depends on other risk factors including high blood pressure, smoking status, age, HDL level, and family history of early heart disease. In addition, people with existing cardiovascular disease or diabetes are at high risk.

Section 23.4

Quitting Smoking Reduces Stroke Risk

"Five Keys for Quitting Smoking," by the Centers for Disease Control and Prevention (CDC, www.cdc.gov), January 26, 2011.

Studies have shown that these five steps will help you quit and quit for good. You have the best chances of quitting if you use them together.

Get Ready

- Set a quit date.

- Change your environment.

- Get rid of all cigarettes and ashtrays in your home, car, and place of work.

- Don't let people smoke in your home.

- Review your past attempts to quit. Think about what worked and what did not.

- Once you quit, don't smoke—not even a puff!

Get Support and Encouragement

Studies have shown that you have a better chance of being successful if you have help. You can get support in many ways:

- Tell your family, friends, and co-workers that you are going to quit and want their support. Ask them not to smoke around you or leave cigarettes out where you can see them.

- Talk to your health care provider (e.g., doctor, dentist, nurse, pharmacist, psychologist, or smoking cessation coach or counselor).

- Get individual, group, or telephone counseling. Counseling doubles your chances of success.

- The more help you have, the better your chances are of quitting. Free programs are available at local hospitals and health centers. Call your local health department for information about programs in your area.

- Telephone counseling is available at 800-QUIT-NOW.

Learn New Skills and Behaviors

- Try to distract yourself from urges to smoke. Talk to someone, go for a walk, or get busy with a task.
- When you first try to quit, change your routine. Use a different route to work. Drink tea instead of coffee. Eat breakfast in a different place.
- Do something to reduce your stress. Take a hot bath, exercise, or read a book.
- Plan something enjoyable to do every day.
- Drink a lot of water and other fluids.

Get Medication and Use It Correctly

Medications can help you stop smoking and lessen the urge to smoke. The U.S. Food and Drug Administration (FDA) has approved seven medications to help you quit smoking:

- Bupropion SR—Available by prescription
- Nicotine gum—Available over-the-counter
- Nicotine inhaler—Available by prescription
- Nicotine nasal spray—Available by prescription
- Nicotine patch—Available by prescription and over-the-counter
- Nicotine lozenge—Available over-the-counter
- Varenicline tartrate—Available by prescription

Ask your health care provider for advice and carefully read the information on the package.

All of these medications will at least double your chances of quitting and quitting for good.

Nearly everyone who is trying to quit can benefit from using a medication. However, if you are pregnant or trying to become pregnant, nursing, younger than 18 years of age, smoking fewer than 10 cigarettes per day, or have a medical condition, talk to your doctor or other health care provider before taking medications.

Be Prepared for Relapse or Difficult Situations

Most relapses occur within the first three months after quitting. Don't be discouraged if you start smoking again. Remember, most people try several times before they finally quit. The following are some difficult situations you may encounter:

- Alcohol: Avoid drinking alcohol. Drinking lowers your chances of success.

- Other smokers: Being around smoking can make you want to smoke.

- Weight gain: Many smokers will gain some weight when they quit, usually less than 10 pounds. Eat a healthy diet and stay active. Don't let weight gain distract you from your main goal— quitting smoking. Some quit-smoking medications may help delay weight gain.

- Bad mood or depression: There are a lot of ways to improve your mood other than smoking. Some smoking cessation medications also lessen depression.

If you are having problems with any of these situations, talk to your doctor or other health care provider.

For more information on quitting, call 800-QUIT-NOW or visit www.smokefree.gov.

Section 23.5

Even Modest Weight Loss Produces Health Benefits

This section contains text from "Losing Weight," by the Centers for Disease Control and Prevention (CDC, www.cdc.gov), August 17, 2011, and text excerpted from "Keeping It Off," by the Centers for Disease Control and Prevention (CDC, www.cdc.gov), September 13, 2011.

Losing Weight

It's natural for anyone trying to lose weight to want to lose it very quickly. But evidence shows that people who lose weight gradually and steadily (about one to two pounds per week) are more successful at keeping weight off. Healthy weight loss isn't just about a diet or program. It's about an ongoing lifestyle that includes long-term changes in daily eating and exercise habits.

To lose weight, you must use up more calories than you take in. Since one pound equals 3,500 calories, you need to reduce your caloric intake by 500–1000 calories per day to lose about 1 to 2 pounds per week.

Once you've achieved a healthy weight, by relying on healthful eating and physical activity most days of the week (about 60–90 minutes, moderate intensity), you are more likely to be successful at keeping the weight off over the long term.

Losing weight is not easy, and it takes commitment. But if you're ready to get started, we've got a step-by-step guide to help get you on the road to weight loss and better health.

Even Modest Weight Loss Can Mean Big Benefits

The good news is that no matter what your weight loss goal is, even a modest weight loss, such as 5 to 10 percent of your total body weight, is likely to produce health benefits, such as improvements in blood pressure, blood cholesterol, and blood sugars.

For example, if you weigh 200 pounds, a 5 percent weight loss equals 10 pounds, bringing your weight down to 190 pounds. While this weight may still be in the overweight or obese range, this modest weight loss can decrease your risk factors for chronic diseases related to obesity.

So even if the overall goal seems large, see it as a journey rather than just a final destination. You'll learn new eating and physical activity habits that will help you live a healthier lifestyle. These habits may help you maintain your weight loss over time.

In addition to improving your health, maintaining a weight loss is likely to improve your life in other ways. For example, a study of participants in the National Weight Control Registry found that those who had maintained a significant weight loss reported improvements in not only their physical health, but also their energy levels, physical mobility, general mood, and self-confidence.

Keeping It Off

If you've recently lost excess weight, congratulations. It's an accomplishment that will likely benefit your health now and in the future. Now that you've lost weight, here are some ways to maintain that success.

The following tips are some of the common characteristics among people who have successfully lost weight and maintained that loss over time.

- **Follow a healthy and realistic eating pattern.** You have embarked on a healthier lifestyle, now the challenge is maintaining the positive eating habits you've developed along the way. In studies of people who have lost weight and kept it off for at least a year, most continued to eat a diet lower in calories as compared to their pre-weight loss diet.

- **Keep your eating patterns consistent.** Follow a healthy eating pattern regardless of changes in your routine. Plan ahead for weekends, vacations, and special occasions. By making a plan, it is more likely you'll have healthy foods on hand for when your routine changes.

- **Eat breakfast every day.** Eating breakfast is a common trait among people who have lost weight and kept it off. Eating a healthful breakfast may help you avoid getting "over-hungry" and then overeating later in the day.

- **Get daily physical activity.** People who have lost weight and kept it off typically engage in 60–90 minutes of moderate intensity physical activity most days of the week while not exceeding calorie needs. This doesn't necessarily mean 60–90 minutes at one time. It might mean 20–30 minutes of physical activity three times a day. For example, a brisk walk in the morning, at lunch time, and in the evening. Some people may need to talk to their healthcare provider before participating in this level of physical activity.

- **Monitor your diet and activity.** Keeping a food and physical activity journal can help you track your progress and spot trends. For example, you might notice that your weight creeps up during periods when you have a lot of business travel or when you have to work overtime. Recognizing this tendency can be a signal to try different behaviors, such as packing your own healthful food for the plane and making time to use your hotel's exercise facility when you are traveling. Or if working overtime, maybe you can use your breaks for quick walks around the building.

- **Monitor your weight.** Check your weight regularly. When managing your weight loss, it's a good idea to keep track of your weight so you can plan accordingly and adjust your diet and exercise plan as necessary. If you have gained a few pounds, get back on track quickly.

- **Get support from family, friends, and others.** People who have successfully lost weight and kept it off often rely on support from others to help them stay on course and get over any bumps. Sometimes having a friend or partner who is also losing weight or maintaining a weight loss can help you stay motivated.

Part Four

Diagnosis and Treatment of Stroke

Chapter 24

After a Stroke:
The First 24 Hours

What Happens at the Hospital after Someone Has a Stroke?

It's a frightening time when someone close to you has a stroke. But you can help him get the best treatment possible—and have the best chance of recovery—by being his advocate in the emergency room. Here's what will happen in the ER and what you can do to assist.

First Stop after a Stroke: The Emergency Room

The first stop after a stroke will be the hospital emergency room. If you've ever been in an ER waiting room, you're probably familiar with the crowds and chaos that characterize them. Doctors and nurses are spread thin, and the intake nurse usually does triage (figures out who needs to be seen first).

However, a stroke is a major medical emergency, so be assertive about having the person you're caring for seen right away. Ideally, he was transported to the ER by paramedics, who normally tell hospital staff about the patient's condition—but if not, you'll need to make sure staff know immediately.

Treatment and Testing in the Emergency Room

The doctors have two main goals while a patient is in the ER: Determine what type of stroke he's having, and treat him to minimize brain damage and prevent more strokes.

Strokes are categorized as either ischemic or hemorrhagic. Ischemic strokes (also called white strokes) occur when a blood vessel to the brain is blocked, preventing blood from flowing to part of the brain. Hemorrhagic strokes (also called red strokes) are caused by a broken or torn blood vessel bleeding into or around the brain.

To determine what kind of stroke or medical event someone is having, ER staff will:

- monitor vital signs (blood pressure, heart rate, breathing, and body temperature);

- draw blood to determine if he has a clotting disorder that might preclude treatment with the clot-busting drug tPA (tissue plasminogen activator);

- check heart function (with an electrocardiogram, or EKG);

- perform a CT [computed tomography] scan to detect bleeding in or around the brain;

- run additional tests, such as an MRI [magnetic resonance imaging], if the CT scan doesn't show what's causing the stroke;

- possibly perform a spinal tap if bleeding still isn't detected but doctors suspect an aneurysm;

- insert an intravenous (IV) line into one of his veins so the staff can deliver fluids and medications.

Doctors will treat your friend or relative to minimize brain damage and the chance of more strokes. If he's having an ischemic stroke that began less than three hours ago, he will probably be given tPA. However, tPA is not used for transient ischemic attacks (TIA), whose symptoms will clear up on their own. If tPA isn't used, he'll probably be given a different drug to minimize the risk of more clots forming. Ultimately, the cause of the original clot will need to be determined, but this can be done later.

If the person you're caring for is having a hemorrhagic stroke, he'll be admitted to a special stroke unit or intensive care unit (ICU) as quickly as possible.

If the patient was transported to the hospital by ambulance, the ER staff should already know the nature of his emergency. Still, he needs you to serve as his advocate, which you can do in a number of ways:

- **Speak up!** Don't be shy or embarrassed to advocate for your good friend or relative. In his book *Stroke for Dummies*, John Marler says that something is wrong if someone who's had a stroke has been in the ER for more than five minutes without attention. You're not being pushy if you insist on his being seen immediately; stroke treatment is a race against time. Your job is to make sure the doctors and nurses understand that he's had a stroke.

- **Report events accurately.** Tell the ER staff exactly what happened and when it happened. For many strokes, treatment with intravenous clot-busting drugs can greatly reduce brain damage and increase the chances of recovery. But these drugs need to be administered within three hours of the onset of stroke symptoms—and the sooner treatment starts, the better the outcome. So if his stroke began less than three hours before his arrival at the ER, it's even more critical that he be evaluated right away.

- **Provide medical background.** The ER staff will need to know important medical information about him, in addition to the details about this particular event. Has he had a stroke before? If so, when and what kind was it? What medications is he taking—and does he actually take them as prescribed?

- **Ask questions.** Does the hospital have a stroke team? If so, is that who's treating the person you're caring for? If not, why not? Can his stroke be treated with drugs that dissolve blood clots? If so, has the treatment been started yet? If not, why not?

- **Consider yourself part of the treatment team.** Although you are his advocate, try not to be adversarial about it. James Frank, ICU [intensive care unit] director at the San Francisco Medical Center, spends much of his time talking to families of critically ill patients. "The best way you can advocate for someone is by working with the doctors and nurses," says Frank. He also recommends appointing a single spokesperson for the entire family so the ER staff isn't bombarded with questions and demands from different people. It's best if this spokesperson has durable power of attorney or has been appointed as the stroke survivor's agent in an advanced health care directive.

But your role doesn't end once you're comfortable with how your loved one is being cared for in the ER. Next he'll be moved into a hospital bed, where you can continue to be his staunch supporter and learn how to deal with the aftereffects of the stroke.

Chapter 25

Working with a Neurologist

What Is a Neurologist?

A neurologist is a medical doctor with specialized training in diagnosing, treating, and managing disorders of the brain and nervous system. Neurologists do not perform surgery.

A neurologist's training includes an undergraduate degree, four years of medical school, a one-year internship, and at least three years of specialized training. Many neurologists also have additional training in other areas—or subspecialties—of neurology such as stroke, epilepsy, neuromuscular disease, and movement disorders. These are some of the more common subspecialties within the field of neurology.

What Does a Neurologist Treat?

Common neurologic disorders include:

- amyotrophic lateral sclerosis (ALS, also called Lou Gehrig's disease);

- Alzheimer's disease;

- brain and spinal cord injuries;

- brain tumors;

- epilepsy;

"Working with Your Doctor," © 2010 American Academy of Neurology. Reprinted with permission.

- hoadache;
- pain;
- multiple sclerosis;
- Parkinson's disease;
- stroke;
- tremor.

What Is the Role of a Neurologist?

Neurologists are principal care providers, consultants to other doctors, or both. When a person has a neurologic disorder that requires frequent care, a neurologist is often the principal care provider. People with disorders, such as Parkinson's disease, Alzheimer's disease, seizure disorders, or multiple sclerosis may use a neurologist as their principal care doctor.

In a consulting role, a neurologist will diagnose and treat a neurologic disorder and then advise the primary care doctor managing the person's overall health. For example, a neurologist may act in a consulting role for conditions such as stroke, concussion, or headache.

Neurologists can recommend surgical treatment, but they do not perform surgery. When treatment includes surgery, neurologists may monitor the patients and supervise their continuing treatment. Neurosurgeons are medical doctors who specialize in performing surgical treatments of the brain or nervous system.

Diagnosis and Treatment of Neurologic Disorders

An accurate diagnosis is the first step toward effective treatment. Diagnosis involves getting a detailed health history of the patient, and neurologic tests for mental status, vision, strength, coordination, reflexes, and sensation. Sometimes, further tests are needed to reach a diagnosis.

Some common neurologic tests are:

- computerized tomography or computer-assisted tomography (CT or CAT scan);
- magnetic resonance imaging (MRI);
- transcranial Doppler (TCD);
- neurosonography;
- electroencephalogram (EEG);

- electromyogram including nerve conduction study (EMG);

- evoked potentials;

- sleep studies;

- cerebral spinal fluid analysis (spinal tap or lumbar puncture).

Computerized tomography or computer assisted tomography (CT or CAT scan): This test uses X-rays and computers to create multidimensional images of selected body parts. Dye may be injected into a patient's vein to obtain a clearer view. Other than needle insertion for the dye, this test is painless.

Magnetic resonance imaging (MRI): An MRI is an advanced way of taking pictures of the inner brain. It is harmless and involves magnetic fields and radio waves. It is performed when a patient is lying in a small chamber for about 30 minutes. It is painless, but may be stressful for individuals with claustrophobia (fear of closed areas). A physician can offer options to help you relax.

Transcranial Doppler (TCD): This test uses sound waves to measure blood flow in the vessels of the brain. A microphone is placed on different parts of the head to view the blood vessels. This test is painless.

Neurosonography: This test uses ultra-high frequency sound wave to analyze blood flow and blockage in the blood vessels in or leading to the brain. This test is painless.

Electroencephalogram (EEG): The EEG records the brain's continuous electrical activity through electrodes attached to the scalp. It is used to help diagnose structural diseases of the brain and episodes such as seizures, fainting, or blacking out. This test is painless.

Electromyogram (EMG): An EMG measures and records electrical activity in the muscles and nerves. This may be helpful in determining the cause of pain, numbness, tingling, or weakness in the muscles or nerves. Small needles are inserted into the muscle and mild electrical shocks are given to stimulate the nerve (nerve conduction study). Discomfort may be associated with this test.

Evoked potentials: This test records the brain's electrical response to visual, auditory, and sensory stimulation. This test is useful in evaluating and diagnosing symptoms of dizziness, numbness, and tingling, as well as visual disorders. Discomfort may be associated with this test.

Sleep studies: These tests are used to diagnose specific causes of sleep problems. To perform the tests, it is often necessary for a patient to spend the night in a sleep laboratory. Brain wave activity, heart rate, electrical activity of the heart, breathing, and oxygen in the blood are all measured during the sleep test. These tests are painless.

Cerebrospinal fluid analysis (spinal tap or lumbar puncture): This test is used to check for bleeding, hemorrhage, infection, or other disorder of the brain, spinal cord, and nerves. In this test, the lower back is numbed with local anesthesia and a thin needle is placed into the space that contains the spinal fluid. The amount of spinal fluid that is needed for the tests is removed and the needle is withdrawn. Discomfort may be associated with this test.

Chapter 26

Diagnosing Stroke

Chapter Contents

Section 26.1

How a Stroke Is Diagnosed

If you have had a stroke, or have had stroke warning signs or risk factors, it is very important to seek prompt medical attention. Your doctor will work with you to find the cause of your problem and determine the best treatment. Even if your symptoms resolve without treatment, you should still discuss them with your doctor. Don't assume that a problem is unimportant if it goes away on its own. Never try to make a diagnosis by yourself.

Important: If you or someone you know is having stroke symptoms now, call 911. Stroke is a medical emergency.

The first step in understanding your problem is to obtain a careful medical history. Your doctor or health care provider will ask questions about your situation. If you can't communicate, a family member or friend will be asked to provide this information. Your doctor will ask about the symptoms you are having now and have had in the past, previous medical problems or operations, and any illnesses which run in your family. Be sure to bring a current list of all the medicines you take (prescription and non-prescription.) If your symptoms lasted only a while, your doctor might also want to talk with someone else who was with you at the time.

The next step is a thorough physical examination. Your doctor will check your pulse and blood pressure, and examine the rest of your body (heart, lungs, etc). The neurologic examination includes detailed tests of your muscles and nerves. The doctor will check your strength, sensation, coordination, and reflexes. In addition, you will be asked questions to check your memory, speech, and thinking.

Depending on the results of your evaluation, your doctor may need additional tests to fully understand your problem. You may also be referred to a medical specialist in brain disorders (neurologist), brain surgery (neurosurgery), or another area. Be patient. Sometimes it takes a while to discover the cause of stroke symptoms, and sometimes the cause of a stroke cannot be determined. Be sure to discuss any questions or concerns with your doctor or health care provider.

Section 26.2

Overview of Lab Tests and Neurological Procedures

Excerpted from "Neurological Diagnostic Tests and Procedures," by the National Institute of Neurological Disorders and Stroke (NINDS, www.ninds .nih.gov), part of the National Institutes of Health, August 4, 2011.

Diagnostic tests and procedures are vital tools that help physicians confirm or rule out the presence of a neurological disorder or other medical condition. A century ago, the only way to make a positive diagnosis for many neurological disorders was by performing an autopsy after a patient had died. But decades of basic research into the characteristics of disease, and the development of techniques that allow scientists to see inside the living brain and monitor nervous system activity as it occurs, have given doctors powerful and accurate tools to diagnose disease and to test how well a particular therapy may be working.

Perhaps the most significant changes in diagnostic imaging over the past 20 years are improvements in spatial resolution (size, intensity, and clarity) of anatomical images and reductions in the time needed to send signals to and receive data from the area being imaged. These advances allow physicians to simultaneously see the structure of the brain and the changes in brain activity as they occur. Scientists continue to improve methods that will provide sharper anatomical images and more detailed functional information.

Researchers and physicians use a variety of diagnostic imaging techniques and chemical and metabolic analyses to detect, manage, and treat neurological disease. Some procedures are performed in specialized settings, conducted to determine the presence of a particular disorder or abnormality. Many tests that were previously conducted in a hospital are now performed in a physician's office or at an outpatient testing facility, with little if any risk to the patient. Depending on the type of procedure, results are either immediate or may take several hours to process.

What are some of the more common screening tests?

Laboratory screening tests of blood, urine, or other substances are used to help diagnose disease, better understand the disease process, and monitor levels of therapeutic drugs. Certain tests, ordered by the physician as part of a regular check-up, provide general information, while others are used to identify specific health concerns. For example, blood and blood product tests can detect brain and/or spinal cord infection, bone marrow disease, hemorrhage, blood vessel damage, toxins that affect the nervous system, and the presence of antibodies that signal the presence of an autoimmune disease. Blood tests are also used to monitor levels of therapeutic drugs used to treat epilepsy and other neurological disorders. Genetic testing of DNA extracted from white cells in the blood can help diagnose Huntington disease and other congenital diseases. Analysis of the fluid that surrounds the brain and spinal cord can detect meningitis, acute and chronic inflammation, rare infections, and some cases of multiple sclerosis. Chemical and metabolic testing of the blood can indicate protein disorders, some forms of muscular dystrophy and other muscle disorders, and diabetes. Urinalysis can reveal abnormal substances in the urine or the presence or absence of certain proteins that cause diseases including the mucopolysaccharidoses.

Genetic testing or counseling can help parents who have a family history of a neurological disease determine if they are carrying one of the known genes that cause the disorder or find out if their child is affected. Genetic testing can identify many neurological disorders, including spina bifida, in utero (while the child is inside the mother's womb).

What is a neurological examination?

A neurological examination assesses motor and sensory skills, the functioning of one or more cranial nerves, hearing and speech, vision, coordination and balance, mental status, and changes in mood or behavior, among other abilities. Items including a tuning fork, flashlight, reflex hammer, ophthalmoscope, and needles are used to help diagnose brain tumors, infections such as encephalitis and meningitis, and diseases such as Parkinson disease, Huntington disease, amyotrophic lateral sclerosis (ALS), and epilepsy. Some tests require the services of a specialist to perform and analyze results.

X-rays of the patient's chest and skull are often taken as part of a neurological work-up. X-rays can be used to view any part of the body, such as a joint or major organ system. In a conventional X-ray, also called a radiograph, a technician passes a concentrated burst of low-dose ionized radiation through the body and onto a photographic plate. Since calcium in bones absorbs X-rays more easily than soft tissue or muscle, the bony structure appears white on the film. Any vertebral misalignment or fractures can be seen within minutes. Tissue masses such as injured ligaments or a bulging disk are not visible on conventional X-rays. This fast, noninvasive, painless procedure is usually performed in a doctor's office or at a clinic.

Fluoroscopy is a type of X-ray that uses a continuous or pulsed beam of low-dose radiation to produce continuous images of a body part in motion. The fluoroscope (X-ray tube) is focused on the area of interest and pictures are either videotaped or sent to a monitor for viewing. A contrast medium may be used to highlight the images. Fluoroscopy can be used to evaluate the flow of blood through arteries.

What are some diagnostic tests used to diagnose neurological disorders?

Based on the result of a neurological exam, physical exam, patient history, X-rays of the patient's chest and skull, and any previous screening or testing, physicians may order one or more of the following diagnostic tests to determine the specific nature of a suspected neurological disorder or injury. These diagnostics generally involve either nuclear medicine imaging, in which very small amounts of radioactive materials are used to study organ function and structure, or diagnostic imaging, which uses magnets and electrical charges to study human anatomy.

The following list of available procedures—in alphabetical rather than sequential order—includes some of the more common tests used to help diagnose a neurological condition.

Angiography is a test used to detect blockages of the arteries or veins. A cerebral angiogram can detect the degree of narrowing or obstruction of an artery or blood vessel in the brain, head, or neck. It is used to diagnose stroke and to determine the location and size of a brain tumor, aneurysm, or vascular malformation. This test is usually performed in a hospital outpatient setting and takes up to 3 hours, followed by a 6- to 8-hour resting period. The patient, wearing a hospital or imaging gown, lies on a table that is wheeled into the imaging area. While the patient is awake, a physician anesthetizes a small area of the leg near the groin and then inserts a catheter into a major artery located there. The catheter is threaded through the body and into an artery in the neck. Once the catheter is in place, the needle is removed and a guide wire is inserted. A small capsule containing a radiopaquo dyo (one that is highlighted on X-rays) is passed over the guide wire to the site of release. The dye is released and travels through the bloodstream into the head and neck. A series of X-rays is taken and any obstruction is noted. Patients may feel a warm to hot sensation or slight discomfort as the dye is released.

Biopsy involves the removal and examination of a small piece of tissue from the body. Muscle or nerve biopsies are used to diagnose neuromuscular disorders and may also reveal if a person is a carrier of a defective gene that could be passed on to children. A small sample of muscle or nerve is removed under local anesthetic and studied under a microscope. The sample may be removed either surgically, through a slit made in the skin, or by needle biopsy, in which a thin hollow needle is inserted through the skin and into the muscle. A small piece of muscle or nerve remains in the hollow needle when it is removed from the body. The biopsy is usually performed at an outpatient testing facility. A brain biopsy, used to determine tumor type, requires surgery to remove a small piece of the brain or tumor. Performed in a hospital, this operation is riskier than a muscle biopsy and involves a longer recovery period.

Brain scans are imaging techniques used to diagnose tumors, blood vessel malformations, or hemorrhage in the brain. These scans are used to study organ function or injury or disease to tissue or muscle. Types of brain scans include computed tomography, magnetic resonance imaging, and positron emission tomography.

Cerebrospinal fluid analysis involves the removal of a small amount of the fluid that protects the brain and spinal cord. The fluid is tested to detect any bleeding or brain hemorrhage, diagnose infection to the brain and/or spinal cord, identify some cases of multiple sclerosis and other neurological conditions, and measure intracranial pressure.

The procedure is usually done in a hospital. The sample of fluid is commonly removed by a procedure known as a lumbar puncture, or spinal tap. The patient is asked to either lie on one side, in a ball position with knees close to the chest, or lean forward while sitting on a table or bed. The doctor will locate a puncture site in the lower back, between two vertebrae, then clean the area and inject a local anesthetic. The patient may feel a slight stinging sensation from this injection. Once the anesthetic has taken effect, the doctor will insert a special needle into the spinal sac and remove a small amount of fluid (usually about three teaspoons) for testing. Most patients will feel a sensation of pressure only as the needle is inserted.

A common after-effect of a lumbar puncture is headache, which can be lessened by having the patient lie flat. Risk of nerve root injury or infection from the puncture can occur but it is rare. The entire procedure takes about 45 minutes.

Computed tomography, also known as a CT scan, is a noninvasive, painless process used to produce rapid, clear two-dimensional images of organs, bones, and tissues. Neurological CT scans are used to view the brain and spine. They can detect bone and vascular irregularities, certain brain tumors and cysts, herniated disks, epilepsy, encephalitis, spinal stenosis (narrowing of the spinal canal), a blood clot or intracranial bleeding in patients with stroke, brain damage from head injury, and other disorders. Many neurological disorders share certain characteristics and a CT scan can aid in proper diagnosis by differentiating the area of the brain affected by the disorder.

Scanning takes about 20 minutes (a CT of the brain or head may take slightly longer) and is usually done at an imaging center or hospital on an outpatient basis. The patient lies on a special table that slides into a narrow chamber. A sound system built into the chamber allows the patient to communicate with the physician or technician. As the patient lies still, X-rays are passed through the body at various angles and are detected by a computerized scanner. The data is processed and displayed as cross-sectional images, or slices, of the internal structure of the body or organ. A light sedative may be given to patients who are unable to lie still and pillows may be used to support and stabilize the head and body. Persons who are claustrophobic may have difficulty taking this imaging test.

Occasionally a contrast dye is injected into the bloodstream to highlight the different tissues in the brain. Patients may feel a warm or cool sensation as the dye circulates through the bloodstream or they may experience a slight metallic taste.

Although very little radiation is used in CT, pregnant women should avoid the test because of potential harm to the fetus from ionizing radiation.

Diskography is often suggested for patients who are considering lumbar surgery or whose lower back pain has not responded to conventional treatments. This outpatient procedure is usually performed at a testing facility or a hospital. The patient is asked to put on a metal-free hospital gown and lie on an imaging table. The physician numbs the skin with anesthetic and inserts a thin needle, using X-ray guidance, into the spinal disk. Once the needle is in place, a small amount of contrast dye is injected and CT scans are taken. The contrast dye outlines any damaged areas. More than one disk may be imaged at the same time. Patient recovery usually takes about an hour. Pain medicine may be prescribed for any resulting discomfort.

An intrathecal contrast-enhanced CT scan (also called cisternography) is used to detect problems with the spine and spinal nerve roots. This test is most often performed at an imaging center. The patient is asked to put on a hospital or imaging gown. Following application of a topical anesthetic, the physician removes a small sample of the spinal fluid via lumbar puncture. The sample is mixed with a contrast dye and injected into the spinal sac located at the base of the lower back. The patient is then asked to move to a position that will allow the contrast fluid to travel to the area to be studied. The dye allows the spinal canal and nerve roots to be seen more clearly on a CT scan. The scan may take up to an hour to complete. Following the test, patients may experience some discomfort and/or headache that may be caused by the removal of spinal fluid.

Electroencephalography, or EEG, monitors brain activity through the skull. EEG is used to help diagnose certain seizure disorders, brain tumors, brain damage from head injuries, inflammation of the brain and/or spinal cord, alcoholism, certain psychiatric disorders, and metabolic and degenerative disorders that affect the brain. EEGs are also used to evaluate sleep disorders, monitor brain activity when a patient has been fully anesthetized or loses consciousness, and confirm brain death.

This painless, risk-free test can be performed in a doctor's office or at a hospital or testing facility. Prior to taking an EEG, the person must avoid caffeine intake and prescription drugs that affect the nervous system. A series of cup-like electrodes are attached to the patient's scalp, either with a special conducting paste or with extremely fine needles. The electrodes (also called leads) are small devices that are attached to wires and carry the electrical energy of the brain to a machine for reading. A very low electrical current is sent through the electrodes and the baseline brain energy is recorded. Patients are then exposed to a variety of external stimuli—including bright or flashing light, noise or certain drugs—or are asked to open and close the eyes, or to change breathing patterns. The electrodes transmit the resulting changes in brain wave patterns. Since movement and nervousness can change brain wave patterns, patients usually recline in a chair or on a bed during the test, which takes up to an hour. Testing for certain disorders requires performing an EEG during sleep, which takes at least three hours.

In order to learn more about brain wave activity, electrodes may be inserted through a surgical opening in the skull and into the brain to reduce signal interference from the skull.

Electromyography, or EMG, is used to diagnose nerve and muscle dysfunction and spinal cord disease. It records the electrical activity from the brain and/or spinal cord to a peripheral nerve root (found in the arms and legs) that controls muscles during contraction and at rest.

During an EMG, very fine wire electrodes are inserted into a muscle to assess changes in electrical voltage that occur during movement and when the muscle is at rest. The electrodes are attached through a series of wires to a recording instrument. Testing usually takes place at a testing facility and lasts about an hour but may take longer, depending on the number of muscles and nerves to be tested. Most patients find this test to be somewhat uncomfortable.

An EMG is usually done in conjunction with a nerve conduction velocity (NCV) test, which measures electrical energy by assessing the nerve's ability to send a signal. This two-part test is conducted most often in a hospital. A technician tapes two sets of flat electrodes on the skin over the muscles. The first set of electrodes is used to send small pulses of electricity (similar to the sensation of static electricity) to stimulate the nerve that directs a particular muscle. The second set of electrodes transmits the responding electrical signal to a recording machine. The physician then reviews the response to verify any nerve damage or muscle disease. Patients who are preparing to take an EMG or NCV test may be asked to avoid caffeine and not smoke for 2 to 3 hours prior to the test, as well as to avoid aspirin and non-steroidal anti-inflammatory drugs for 24 hours before the EMG. There is no discomfort or risk associated with this test.

Electronystagmography (ENG) describes a group of tests used to diagnose involuntary eye movement, dizziness, and balance disorders, and to evaluate some brain functions. The test is performed at an imaging center. Small electrodes are taped around the eyes to record eye movements. If infrared photography is used in place of electrodes, the patient wears special goggles that help record the information. Both versions of the test are painless and risk-free.

Evoked potentials (also called evoked response) measure the electrical signals to the brain generated by hearing, touch, or sight. These tests are used to assess sensory nerve problems and confirm neurological conditions including multiple sclerosis, brain tumor, acoustic neuroma (small tumors of the inner ear), and spinal cord injury. Evoked potentials are also used to test sight and hearing (especially in infants and young children), monitor brain activity among coma patients, and confirm brain death.

Testing may take place in a doctor's office or hospital setting. It is painless and risk-free. Two sets of needle electrodes are used to test for nerve damage. One set of electrodes, which will be used to measure the electrophysiological response to stimuli, is attached to the patient's scalp using conducting paste. The second set of electrodes is attached to the part of the body to be tested. The physician then records the amount of time it takes for the impulse generated by stimuli to reach the brain. Under normal circumstances, the process of signal transmission is instantaneous.

Auditory evoked potentials (also called brain stem auditory evoked response) are used to assess high-frequency hearing loss, diagnose any damage to the acoustic nerve and auditory pathways in the brainstem, and detect acoustic neuromas. The patient sits in a soundproof room and wears headphones. Clicking sounds are delivered one at a time to one ear while a masking sound is sent to the other ear. Each ear is usually tested twice, and the entire procedure takes about 45 minutes.

Visual evoked potentials detect loss of vision from optic nerve damage (in particular, damage caused by multiple sclerosis). The patient sits close to a screen and is asked to focus on the center of a shifting checkerboard pattern. Only one eye is tested at a time; the other eye is either kept closed or covered with a patch. Each eye is usually tested twice. Testing takes 30–45 minutes.

Somatosensory evoked potentials measure response from stimuli to the peripheral nerves and can detect nerve or spinal cord damage or nerve degeneration from multiple sclerosis and other degenerating diseases. Tiny electrical shocks are delivered by electrode to a nerve in an arm or leg. Responses to the shocks, which may be delivered for more than a minute at a time, are recorded. This test usually lasts less than an hour.

Magnetic resonance imaging (MRI) uses computer-generated radio waves and a powerful magnetic field to produce detailed images of body structures including tissues, organs, bones, and nerves. Neurological uses include the diagnosis of brain and spinal cord tumors, eye disease, inflammation, infection, and vascular irregularities that may lead to stroke. MRI can also detect and monitor degenerative disorders such as multiple sclerosis and can document brain injury from trauma.

The equipment houses a hollow tube that is surrounded by a very large cylindrical magnet. The patient, who must remain still during the test, lies on a special table that is slid into the tube. The patient will be asked to remove jewelry, eyeglasses, removable dental work, or other items that might interfere with the magnetic imaging. The patient should wear a sweat shirt and sweat pants or other clothing free of metal eyelets or buckles. MRI scanning equipment creates a magnetic field around the body strong enough to temporarily realign water molecules in the tissues. Radio waves are then passed through the body to detect the relaxation of the molecules back to a random alignment and trigger a resonance signal at different angles within the body. A computer processes this resonance into either a three-dimensional picture or a two-dimensional slice of the tissue being scanned, and differentiates between bone, soft tissues, and fluid-filled spaces by their water content and structural properties. A contrast dye may be used to enhance visibility of certain areas or tissues. The patient may hear grating or knocking noises when the magnetic field is turned on and off. (Patients may wear special earphones to block out the sounds.) Unlike CT scanning, MRI does not use ionizing radiation to produce images. Depending on the part(s) of the body to be scanned, MRI can take up to an hour to complete. The test is painless and risk-free, although persons who are obese or claustrophobic may find it somewhat uncomfortable. (Some centers also use open MRI machines that do not completely surround the person being tested and are less confining. However, open MRI does not currently provide the same picture quality as standard MRI and some tests may not be available using this equipment). Due to the incredibly strong magnetic field generated by an MRI, patients with implanted medical devices such as a pacemaker should avoid the test.

Functional MRI (fMRI) uses the blood's magnetic properties to produce real-time images of blood flow to particular areas of the brain. An fMRI can pinpoint areas of the brain that become active and note how long they stay active. It can also tell if brain activity within a region occurs simultaneously or sequentially. This imaging process is used to assess brain damage from head injury or degenerative disorders such as Alzheimer disease and to identify and monitor other neurological disorders, including multiple sclerosis, stroke, and brain tumors.

Myelography involves the injection of a water- or oil-based contrast dye into the spinal canal to enhance X-ray imaging of the spine. Myelograms are used to diagnose spinal nerve injury, herniated disks, fractures, back or leg pain, and spinal tumors.

The procedure takes about 30 minutes and is usually performed in a hospital. Following an injection of anesthesia to a site between two vertebrae in the lower back, a small amount of the cerebrospinal fluid is removed by spinal tap and the contrast dye is injected into the spinal canal. After a series of X-rays is taken, most or all of the contrast dye is removed by aspiration. Patients may experience some pain during the spinal tap and when the dye is injected and removed. Patients may also experience headache following the spinal tap. The risk of fluid leakage or allergic reaction to the dye is slight.

Positron emission tomography (PET) scans provide two- and three-dimensional pictures of brain activity by measuring radioactive isotopes that are injected into the bloodstream. PET scans of the brain are used to detect or highlight tumors and diseased tissue, measure cellular and/or tissue metabolism, show blood flow, evaluate patients who have seizure disorders that do not respond to medical therapy and patients with certain memory disorders, and determine brain changes following injury or drug abuse, among other uses. PET may be ordered as a follow-up to a CT or MRI scan to give the physician a greater understanding of specific areas of the brain that may be involved with certain problems. Scans are conducted in a hospital or at a testing facility, on an outpatient basis. A low-level radioactive isotope, which binds to chemicals that flow to the brain, is injected into the bloodstream and can be traced as the brain performs different functions. The patient lies still while overhead sensors detect gamma rays in the body's tissues. A computer processes the information and displays it on a video monitor or on film. Using different compounds, more than one brain function can be traced simultaneously. PET is painless and relatively risk-free. Length of test time depends on the part of the body to be scanned. PET scans are performed by skilled technicians at highly sophisticated medical facilities.

A polysomnogram measures brain and body activity during sleep. It is performed over one or more nights at a sleep center. Electrodes are pasted or taped to the patient's scalp, eyelids, and/or chin. Throughout the night and during the various wake/sleep cycles, the electrodes record brain waves, eye movement, breathing, leg and skeletal muscle activity, blood pressure, and heart rate. The patient may be videotaped to note any movement during sleep. Results are then used to identify any characteristic patterns of sleep disorders, including restless legs syndrome, periodic limb movement disorder, insomnia, and breathing disorders such as obstructive sleep apnea. Polysomnograms are non-invasive, painless, and risk-free.

Single photon emission computed tomography (SPECT), a nuclear imaging test involving blood flow to tissue, is used to evaluate certain brain functions. The test may be ordered as a follow-up to an MRI to diagnose tumors, infections, degenerative spinal disease, and stress fractures. As with a PET scan, a radioactive isotope, which binds to chemicals that flow to the brain, is injected intravenously into the body. Areas of increased blood flow will collect more of the isotope. As the patient lies on a table, a gamma camera rotates around the head and records where the radioisotope has traveled. That information is converted by computer into cross-sectional slices that are stacked to produce a detailed three-dimensional image of blood flow and activity within the brain. The test is performed at either an imaging center or a hospital.

Thermography uses infrared sensing devices to measure small temperature changes between the two sides of the body or within a specific organ. Also known as digital infrared thermal imaging, thermography may be used to detect vascular disease of the head and neck, soft tissue injury, various neuromusculoskeletal disorders, and the presence or absence of nerve root compression. It is performed at an imaging center, using infrared light recorders to take thousands of pictures of the body from a distance of 5 to 8 feet. The information is converted into electrical signals which results in a computer-generated two-dimensional picture of abnormally cold or hot areas indicated by color or shades of black and white. Thermography does not use radiation and is safe, risk-free, and noninvasive.

Ultrasound imaging, also called ultrasound scanning or sonography, uses high-frequency sound waves to obtain images inside the body. Neurosonography (ultrasound of the brain and spinal column) analyzes blood flow in the brain and can diagnose stroke, brain tumors, hydrocephalus (build-up of cerebrospinal fluid in the brain), and vascular problems. It can also identify or rule out inflammatory processes causing pain. It is more effective than an X-ray in displaying soft tissue masses and can show tears in ligaments, muscles, tendons, and other soft tissue masses in the back. Transcranial Doppler ultrasound is used to view arteries and blood vessels in the neck and determine blood flow and risk of stroke.

During ultrasound, the patient lies on an imaging table and removes clothing around the area of the body to be scanned. A jelly-like lubricant is applied and a transducer, which both sends and receives high-frequency sound waves, is passed over the body. The sound wave echoes are recorded and displayed as a computer-generated real-time visual image of the structure or tissue being examined. Ultrasound is painless, noninvasive, and risk-free. The test is performed on an outpatient basis and takes between 15 and 30 minutes to complete.

Section 26.3

Blood Tests
for Stroke

If you are being evaluated for stroke, it is likely that your doctor will order some blood tests. Stroke cannot be diagnosed by a blood test alone. However, these tests can provide information about stroke risk factors and other medical problems which may be important.

Please note that the first set of tests are commonly used for routine or emergency evaluation of stroke, while the others are used only in very specific situations. Unless otherwise noted, each of these tests require just one tube of blood (a few teaspoons) drawn from a vein.

Commonly Used Blood Tests

CBC (Complete Blood Count)

This is a routine test to determine the number of red blood cells, white blood cells, and platelets in your blood. Hematocrit and hemoglobin are measures of the number of red blood cells. A complete blood count might be used to diagnose anemia (too little blood) or infection (shown by too many white blood cells).

Coagulation Tests: PT (Prothrombin Time), PTT (Partial Thromboplastin Time), and INR (International Normalized Ratio)

These tests measure how quickly your blood clots. An abnormality could result in excessive bleeding or excessive clotting (which is difficult to measure). If you have been prescribed a blood-thinning medicine such as warfarin (Coumadin or similar drugs), the INR is used to be sure that you receive the correct dose. It is very important that you obtain regular checks. If you are taking heparin, the PTT (or a PTT) test is used to determine the correct dose.

Blood Chemistry Tests

These tests measure the levels of normal chemical substances in your blood. The most important test in emergency stroke evaluation is glucose (or blood sugar), because levels of blood glucose which are too high or too low can cause symptoms which may be mistaken for stroke. A fasting blood glucose is used to help in the diagnosis of diabetes, which is a risk factor for stroke. Other blood chemistry tests measure serum electrolytes, the normal ions in your blood (sodium, potassium, calcium) or check the function of your liver or kidneys.

Blood Lipid Tests: Cholesterol, Total Lipids, HDL, and LDL

Elevated cholesterol (particularly bad cholesterol, or LDL [low-density lipoprotein]) is a risk factor for heart disease and stroke. More information about cholesterol and cardiovascular risks is available from the National Institutes of Health.

Blood Tests for Specific Situations

This is a partial list of less common blood tests sometimes ordered for specific stroke situations, or where the cause of stroke is unclear (for example, in a young person without known stroke risk factors). Abnormal results may suggest a cause for the stroke.

- Antinuclear antibodies (ANA)
- Antiphospholipid antibodies (APL), Anticardiolipin antibodies (ACL), Lupus anticoagulant (LA)
- Blood culture
- Cardiac enzymes: Troponin, Creatine kinase (CPK, CK), LDH isoenzymes
- Coagulation factors: Antithrombin III, Protein C, Protein S; Factor VIII; activated Protein C resistance (Factor V Leiden)
- Erythrocyte sedimentation rate (ESR)
- Hemoglobin electrophoresis
- Homocysteine
- Syphilis serology (VDRL, FTA, others)
- Toxicology screen (serum or urine)

Please note that this list applies only to the use of these tests for stroke diagnosis. Be sure to discuss any questions or concerns with your doctor or health care provider.

Section 26.4

Angiography

Cerebral angiography is a procedure that uses a special dye (contrast material) and X-rays to see how blood flows through the brain.

How the Test Is Performed

Cerebral angiography is done in the hospital or large radiology center. You will be asked to lie on an X-ray table. Your head is positioned and held still using a strap, tape, or sandbags, so you do not move during the procedure. The health care provider will attach electrocardiogram (ECG) leads to your arms and legs, which monitor your heart activity during the test.

Before the test starts, you will be given a mild sedative to help you relax.

An area of your body, usually the groin, is cleaned and numbed with a local numbing medicine (anesthetic). A thin, hollow tube called a catheter is placed through an artery and carefully moved up through the main blood vessels in the belly area and chest and into an artery in the neck. Moving X-ray images help the doctor position the catheter.

Once the catheter is in place, a special dye (contrast material) is injected into catheter. X-ray images are taken to see how the dye moves through the artery and blood vessels of the brain. The dye helps highlight any blockages in blood flow.

After the X-rays are taken, the needle and catheter are withdrawn. Pressure is immediately applied on the leg at the site of insertion for 10–15 minutes to stop the bleeding. After that time, the area is checked and a tight bandage is applied. Your leg should be kept straight for four to six hours after the procedure. Watch the area for bleeding for at least the next 12 hours.

Digital subtraction angiography (DSA) uses a computer to "subtract" or take out the bones and tissues in the area viewed, so that only the blood vessels filled with the contrast dye are seen.

How to Prepare for the Test

You must sign a consent form. Your health care provider will explain the procedure and its risks.

Routine blood tests and examination of the nervous system will be done before the procedure.

Tell the health care provider if you:

- are allergic to shellfish or iodine substances;

- have a history of bleeding problems;

- have had an allergic reaction to X-ray contrast dye or any iodine substance;

- may be pregnant.

You may be told not to eat or drink anything for four to eight hours before the test.

When you arrive at the testing site, you will be given a hospital gown to wear. You must remove all jewelry.

How the Test Will Feel

The X-ray table may feel hard and cold. You may wish to ask for a blanket or pillow.

Some people feel a sting when the numbing medicine (anesthetic) is given. You will feel a brief, sharp pain as the catheter is inserted. There is a feeling of pressure as the catheter is moved into the body.

Some people feel a warm or burning sensation of the skin of the face or head when the contrast dye is injected.

You may have slight tenderness and bruising at the site of the injection after the test.

Why the Test Is Performed

Cerebral angiography is most frequently used to identify or confirm problems with the blood vessels in the brain.

Your doctor may order this test if you have symptoms or signs of:

- abnormal blood vessels (vascular malformation);

- aneurysm;

- narrowing of the arteries in the brain;

- vasculitis.

It is sometimes used to:

- confirm a brain tumor;

- evaluate the arteries of the head and neck before surgery;

- find a clot that may have caused a stroke.

In some cases, this procedure may be used to get more detailed information after something abnormal has been detected by an MRI [magnetic resonance imaging] or CT [computed tomography] scan of the head.

This test may also be done in preparation for medical treatment (interventional radiology procedures) by way of certain blood vessels.

What Abnormal Results Mean

Contrast dye flowing out of the blood vessel may be a sign of internal bleeding.

Narrowed arteries may suggest cholesterol deposits, a spasm, or inherited disorders.

Out of place blood vessels may be due to brain tumors, bleeding within the skull, aneurysm (bulging of the artery walls), or arteriovenous malformation.

Abnormal results may also be due to:

- intracerebral hemorrhage;

- metastatic brain tumor;

- neurosyphilis;

- optic glioma;

- pituitary tumor;

- primary brain tumors.

Risks

There is the possibility of significant complications, including:

- allergic reaction to the contrast dye;

- blood clot or bleeding at the needle stick site, which could partly block blood flow to the leg;

- damage to an artery or artery wall from the catheter, which can block blood flow and cause a stroke (rare).

Considerations

Tell your health care provider immediately if you have:

- facial weakness;
- numbness in your leg during or after the procedure;
- slurred speech;
- vision problems.

Section 26.5

Echocardiogram

Excerpted from "Echocardiogram," by the National Heart, Lung,
and Blood Institute (NHLBI, www.nhlbi.nih.gov), part of the
National Institutes of Health, October 31, 2011.

Echocardiography, or echo, is a painless test that uses sound waves to create moving pictures of your heart. The pictures show the size and shape of your heart. They also show how well your heart's chambers and valves are working.

Echo also can pinpoint areas of heart muscle that aren't contracting well because of poor blood flow or injury from a previous heart attack. A type of echo called Doppler ultrasound shows how well blood flows through your heart's chambers and valves.

Echo can detect possible blood clots inside the heart, fluid buildup in the pericardium (the sac around the heart), and problems with the aorta. The aorta is the main artery that carries oxygen-rich blood from your heart to your body.

Doctors also use echo to detect heart problems in infants and children.

Who Needs Echocardiography?

Your doctor may recommend echocardiography if you have signs or symptoms of heart problems.

For example, shortness of breath and swelling in the legs are possible signs of heart failure. Heart failure is a condition in which your heart can't pump enough oxygen-rich blood to meet your body's needs. Echo can show how well your heart is pumping blood.

Echo also can help your doctor find the cause of abnormal heart sounds, such as heart murmurs. Heart murmurs are extra or unusual sounds heard during the heartbeat. Some heart murmurs are harmless, whereas others are signs of heart problems.

Types of Echocardiography

There are several types of echocardiography (echo)—all use sound waves to create moving pictures of your heart. This is the same technology that allows doctors to see an unborn baby inside a pregnant woman.

Unlike X-rays and some other tests, echo doesn't involve radiation.

Transthoracic echocardiography: Transthoracic echo is the most common type of echocardiogram test. It's painless and noninvasive. Noninvasive means that no surgery is done and no instruments are inserted into your body.

This type of echo involves placing a device called a transducer on your chest. The device sends special sound waves, called ultrasound, through your chest wall to your heart. The human ear can't hear ultrasound waves.

As the ultrasound waves bounce off the structures of your heart, a computer in the echo machine converts them into pictures on a screen.

Stress echocardiography: Stress echo is done as part of a stress test. During a stress test, you exercise or take medicine (given by your doctor) to make your heart work hard and beat fast. A technician will use echo to create pictures of your heart before you exercise and as soon as you finish.

Some heart problems, such as coronary heart disease, are easier to diagnose when the heart is working hard and beating fast.

Transesophageal echocardiography: Your doctor may have a hard time seeing the aorta and other parts of your heart using a standard transthoracic echo. Thus, he or she may recommend transesophageal echo, or TEE.

During this test, the transducer is attached to the end of a flexible tube. The tube is guided down your throat and into your esophagus (the passage leading from your mouth to your stomach). This allows your doctor to get more detailed pictures of your heart.

Fetal echocardiography: Fetal echo is used to look at an unborn baby's heart. A doctor may recommend this test to check a baby for heart problems. When recommended, the test is commonly done at about 18 to 22 weeks of pregnancy. For this test, the transducer is moved over the pregnant woman's belly.

Three-dimensional echocardiography: A three-dimensional (3D) echo creates 3D images of your heart. These detailed images show how your heart looks and works.

During transthoracic echo or TEE, 3D images can be taken as part of the process used to do these types of echo.

Doctors may use 3D echo to diagnose heart problems in children. They also may use 3D echo for planning and overseeing heart valve surgery.

Researchers continue to study new ways to use 3D echo.

What to Expect before Echocardiography

Echocardiography is done in a doctor's office or a hospital. No special preparations are needed for most types of echo. You usually can eat, drink, and take any medicines as you normally would.

The exception is if you're having a transesophageal echo. This test usually requires that you don't eat or drink for eight hours prior to the test.

If you're having a stress echo, you may need to take steps to prepare for the stress test. Your doctor will let you know what steps you need to take.

What to Expect during Echocardiography

Echocardiography is painless; the test usually takes less than an hour to do. For some types of echo, your doctor will need to inject saline or a special dye into one of your veins. The substance makes your heart show up more clearly on the echo pictures.

The dye used for echo is different from the dye used during angiography (a test used to examine the body's blood vessels).

For most types of echo, you will remove your clothing from the waist up. Women will be given a gown to wear during the test. You'll lie on your back or left side on an exam table or stretcher.

Soft, sticky patches called electrodes will be attached to your chest to allow an EKG (electrocardiogram) to be done. An EKG is a test that records the heart's electrical activity.

A doctor or sonographer (a person specially trained to do ultrasounds) will apply gel to your chest. The gel helps the sound waves reach your heart. A wand-like device called a transducer will then be moved around on your chest.

The transducer transmits ultrasound waves into your chest. A computer will convert echoes from the sound waves into pictures of your heart on a screen. During the test, the lights in the room will be dimmed so the computer screen is easier to see.

The sonographer will record pictures of various parts of your heart. He or she will put the recordings on a computer disc for a cardiologist (heart specialist) to review.

During the test, you may be asked to change positions or hold your breath for a short time. This allows the sonographer to get better pictures of your heart.

At times, the sonographer may apply a bit of pressure to your chest with the transducer. You may find this pressure a little uncomfortable, but it helps get the best picture of your heart. You should let the sonographer know if you feel too uncomfortable.

Transesophageal Echocardiography

Transesophageal echo (TEE) is used if your doctor needs a more detailed view of your heart. For example, your doctor may use TEE to look for blood clots in your heart. A doctor, not a sonographer, will perform this type of echo.

TEE uses the same technology as transthoracic echo, but the transducer is attached to the end of a flexible tube.

Your doctor will guide the tube down your throat and into your esophagus (the passage leading from your mouth to your stomach). From this angle, your doctor can get a more detailed image of the heart and major blood vessels leading to and from the heart.

For TEE, you'll likely be given medicine to help you relax during the test. The medicine will be injected into one of your veins.

Your blood pressure, the oxygen content of your blood, and other vital signs will be checked during the test. You'll be given oxygen through a tube in your nose. If you wear dentures or partials, you'll have to remove them.

The back of your mouth will be numbed with gel or spray. Your doctor will gently place the tube with the transducer in your throat and guide it down until it's in place behind your heart.

The pictures of your heart are then recorded as your doctor moves the transducer around in your esophagus and stomach. You shouldn't feel any discomfort as this happens.

Although the imaging usually takes less than an hour, you may be watched for a few hours at the doctor's office or hospital after the test.

Stress Echocardiography

Stress echo is a transthoracic echo combined with either an exercise or pharmacological stress test.

For an exercise stress test, you'll walk or run on a treadmill or pedal a stationary bike to make your heart work hard and beat fast. For a pharmacological stress test, you'll be given medicine to increase your heart rate.

A technician will take pictures of your heart using echo before you exercise and as soon as you finish.

What You May See and Hear during Echocardiography

As the doctor or sonographer moves the transducer around, you will see different views of your heart on the screen of the echo machine. The structures of your heart will appear as white objects, while any fluid or blood will appear black on the screen.

Doppler ultrasound often is used during echo tests. Doppler ultrasound is a special ultrasound that shows how blood is flowing through the blood vessels.

This test allows the sonographer to see blood flowing at different speeds and in different directions. The speed and direction of blood flow appear as different colors moving within the black and white images.

The human ear is unable to hear the sound waves used in echo. If you have a Doppler ultrasound, you may be able to hear whooshing sounds. Your doctor can use these sounds to learn about blood flow through your heart.

What to Expect after Echocardiography

You usually can go back to your normal activities right after having echocardiography (echo).

If you have a transesophageal echo (TEE), you may be watched for a few hours at the doctor's office or hospital after the test. Your throat might be sore for a few hours after the test.

You also may not be able to drive for a short time after having TEE. Your doctor will let you know whether you need to arrange for a ride home.

What Does Echocardiography Show?

Echocardiography shows the size, structure, and movement of various parts of your heart. These parts include the heart valves, the septum (the wall separating the right and left heart chambers), and the walls of the heart chambers. Doppler ultrasound shows the movement of blood through your heart.

Your doctor may use echo to do the following:

- Diagnose heart problems

- Guide or determine next steps for treatment

- Monitor changes and improvement

- Determine the need for more tests

Echo can detect many heart problems. Some might be minor and pose no risk to you. Others can be signs of serious heart disease or other heart conditions. Your doctor may use echo to learn about:

- The size of your heart: An enlarged heart might be the result of high blood pressure, leaky heart valves, or heart failure. Echo also can detect increased thickness of the ventricles (the heart's lower chambers). Increased thickness may be due to high blood pressure, heart valve disease, or congenital heart defects.

- Heart muscles that are weak and aren't pumping well: Damage from a heart attack may cause weak areas of heart muscle. Weakening also might mean that the area isn't getting enough blood supply, a sign of coronary heart disease.

- Heart valve problems: Echo can show whether any of your heart valves don't open normally or close tightly.

- Problems with your heart's structure: Echo can detect congenital heart defects, such as holes in the heart. Congenital heart defects are structural problems present at birth. Infants and children may have echo to detect these heart defects.

- Blood clots or tumors: If you've had a stroke, you may have echo to check for blood clots or tumors that could have caused the stroke.

What Are the Risks of Echocardiography?

Transthoracic and fetal echocardiography have no risks. These tests are safe for adults, children, and infants.

If you have a transesophageal echo (TEE), some risks are associated with the medicine given to help you relax. For example, you may have a bad reaction to the medicine, problems breathing, and nausea (feeling sick to your stomach).

Your throat also might be sore for a few hours after the test. Rarely, the tube used during TEE causes minor throat injuries.

Stress echo has some risks, but they're related to the exercise or medicine used to raise your heart rate, not the echo. Serious complications from stress tests are very uncommon. Go to the Health Topics Stress Testing article for more information about the risks of that test.

Clinical Trials

The National Heart, Lung, and Blood Institute (NHLBI) is strongly committed to supporting research aimed at preventing and treating heart, lung, and blood diseases and conditions and sleep disorders.

NHLBI-supported research has led to many advances in medical knowledge and care. For example, this research has helped look for better ways to diagnose and evaluate heart problems using tests such as echocardiography.

The NHLBI continues to support research on various testing methods, including echo. For example, the NHLBI currently sponsors a study to explore how three-dimensional (3D) echo can help assess mitral valve backflow (a heart valve problem).

Much of the NHLBI's research depends on the willingness of volunteers to take part in clinical trials. Clinical trials test new ways to prevent, diagnose, or treat various diseases and conditions.

For example, new treatments for a disease or condition (such as medicines, medical devices, surgeries, or procedures) are tested in volunteers who have the illness. Testing shows whether a treatment is safe and effective in humans before it is made available for widespread use.

By taking part in a clinical trial, you can gain access to new treatments before they're widely available. You also will have the support of a team of health care providers, who will likely monitor your health closely. Even if you don't directly benefit from the results of a clinical trial, the information gathered can help others and add to scientific knowledge.

If you volunteer for a clinical trial, the research will be explained to you in detail. You'll learn about treatments and tests you may receive, and the benefits and risks they may pose. You'll also be given a chance to ask questions about the research. This process is called informed consent.

If you agree to take part in the trial, you'll be asked to sign an informed consent form. This form is not a contract. You have the right to withdraw from a study at any time, for any reason. Also, you have the right to learn about new risks or findings that emerge during the trial.

Section 26.6

Electrocardiogram

Excerpted from "Electrocardiogram," by the National Heart,
Lung, and Blood Institute (NHLBI, www.nhlbi.nih.gov), part of the
National Institutes of Health, October 1, 2010.

An electrocardiogram, also called an EKG or ECG, is a simple, pain-less test that records the heart's electrical activity. To understand this test, it helps to understand how the heart works.

With each heartbeat, an electrical signal spreads from the top of the heart to the bottom. As it travels, the signal causes the heart to contract and pump blood. The process repeats with each new heartbeat.

The heart's electrical signals set the rhythm of the heartbeat.

An EKG shows the following:

• How fast your heart is beating

• Whether the rhythm of your heartbeat is steady or irregular

• The strength and timing of electrical signals as they pass through each part of your heart

Doctors use EKGs to detect and study many heart problems, such as heart attacks, arrhythmias, and heart failure. The test's results also can suggest other disorders that affect heart function.

Who Needs an Electrocardiogram?

Your doctor may recommend an electrocardiogram if you have signs or symptoms that suggest a heart problem. Examples of such signs and symptoms include the following:

• Chest pain

• Heart pounding, racing, or fluttering, or the sense that your heart is beating unevenly

• Breathing problems

• Tiredness and weakness

- Unusual heart sounds when your doctor listens to your heartbeat

You may need to have more than one EKG so your doctor can diagnose certain heart conditions.

An EKG also may be done as part of a routine health exam. The test can screen for early heart disease that has no symptoms. Your doctor is more likely to look for early heart disease if your mother, father, brother, or sister had heart disease—especially early in life.

You may have an EKG so your doctor can check how well heart medicine or a medical device, such as a pacemaker, is working. The test also may be used for routine screening before major surgery.

Your doctor also may use EKG results to help plan your treatment for a heart condition.

What to Expect before an Electrocardiogram

You don't need to take any special steps before having an electrocardiogram. However, tell your doctor or his or her staff about the medicines you're taking. Some medicines can affect EKG results.

What to Expect during an Electrocardiogram

An electrocardiogram is painless and harmless. A nurse or technician will attach soft, sticky patches called electrodes to the skin of your chest, arms, and legs. The patches are about the size of a quarter.

Often, 12 patches are attached to your body. This helps detect your heart's electrical activity from many areas at the same time. The nurse may have to shave areas of your skin to help the patches stick.

After the patches are placed on your skin, you'll lie still on a table while the patches detect your heart's electrical signals. A machine will record these signals on graph paper or display them on a screen.

The entire test will take about 10 minutes.

What to Expect after an Electrocardiogram

After an electrocardiogram, the nurse or technician will remove the electrodes (soft patches) from your skin. You may develop a rash or redness where the EKG patches were attached. This mild rash often goes away without treatment.

You usually can go back to your normal daily routine after an EKG.

What Does an Electrocardiogram Show?

Many heart problems change the heart's electrical activity in distinct ways. An electrocardiogram can help detect these heart problems.

EKG recordings can help doctors diagnose heart attacks that are in progress or have happened in the past. This is especially true if doctors can compare a current EKG recording to an older one.

An EKG also can show the following:

- Lack of blood flow to the heart muscle (coronary heart disease)

- A heartbeat that's too fast, too slow, or irregular (arrhythmia)

- A heart that doesn't pump forcefully enough (heart failure)

- Heart muscle that's too thick or parts of the heart that are too big (cardiomyopathy)

- Birth defects in the heart (congenital heart defects)

- Problems with the heart valves (heart valve disease)

- Inflammation of the sac that surrounds the heart (pericarditis)

An EKG can reveal whether the heartbeat starts in the correct place in the heart. The test also shows how long it takes for electrical signals to travel through the heart. Delays in signal travel time may suggest heart block or long QT syndrome.

What Are the Risks of an Electrocardiogram?

An electrocardiogram has no serious risks. It's a harmless, painless test that detects the heart's electrical activity. EKGs don't give off electrical charges, such as shocks.

You may develop a mild rash where the electrodes (soft patches) were attached. This rash often goes away without treatment.

Section 26.7

CT Scan

A cranial computed tomography (CT) scan uses many X-rays to create pictures of the head, including the skull, brain, eye sockets, and sinuses.

How the Test Is Performed

You will be asked to lie on a narrow table that slides into the center of the CT scanner.

Once you are inside the scanner, the machine's X-ray beam rotates around you. (Modern "spiral" scanners can perform the exam without stopping.)

A computer creates separate images of the body area, called slices. These images can be stored, viewed on a monitor, or printed on film. Three-dimensional models of the head area can be created by stacking the slices together.

You must be still during the exam, because movement causes blurred images. You may be told to hold your breath for short periods of time.

Generally, complete scans take only a few minutes. The newest scanners can image your entire body, head to toe, in less than 30 seconds.

How to Prepare for the Test

Certain exams require a special dye, called contrast, to be delivered into the body before the test starts. Contrast helps certain areas show up better on the X-rays.

- Contrast can be given through a vein (IV) in your hand or forearm. If contrast is used, you may also be asked not to eat or drink anything for four to six hours before the test.

- Let your doctor know if you have ever had a reaction to contrast. You may need to take medications before the test in order to safely receive this substance.

- Before receiving the contrast, tell your health care provider if you take the diabetes medication metformin (Glucophage) because you may need to take extra precautions.

If you weigh more than 300 pounds, find out if the CT machine has a weight limit. Too much weight can cause damage to the scanner's working parts.

You will be asked to remove jewelry and wear a hospital gown during the study.

How the Test Will Feel

The X-rays produced by the CT scan are painless. Some people may have discomfort from lying on the hard table.

Contrast given through a vein may cause a slight burning sensation, a metallic taste in the mouth, and a warm flushing of the body. These sensations are normal and usually go away within a few seconds.

Why the Test Is Performed

A cranial CT scan is recommended to help diagnose or monitor the following conditions:

- Birth (congenital) defect of the head or brain
- Brain infection
- Brain tumor
- Buildup of fluid inside the skull (hydrocephalus)
- Craniosynostosis
- Injury (trauma) to the head and face
- Stroke or bleeding in the brain

A cranial CT may also be done to look for the cause of:

- changes in thinking or behavior;
- fainting;
- headache, when certain other signs or symptoms are present;
- hearing loss (in some patients);
- symptoms of damage to part of the brain, such as vision problems, muscle weakness, numbness and tingling, hearing loss, speaking difficulties, or swallowing problems.

What Abnormal Results Mean

Abnormal results may be due to:

- abnormal blood vessels (arteriovenous malformation);
- aneurysm in the brain;
- bleeding (for example, chronic subdural hematoma or intracranial hemorrhage);
- bone infection;
- brain abscess or infection;
- brain damage due to injury;
- brain tissue swelling or injury;
- brain tumor or other growth (mass);
- cerebral atrophy (loss of brain tissue);
- hydrocephalus (fluid collecting in the skull);
- problems with the hearing nerve;
- stroke or transient ischemic attack (TIA).

Risks

Risks of CT scans include:

- being exposed to radiation;
- allergic reaction to contrast dye.

CT scans do expose you to more radiation than regular X-rays. Having many X-rays or CT scans over time may increase your risk for cancer. However, the risk from any one scan is small. You and your doctor should weigh this risk against the benefits of getting a correct diagnosis for a medical problem.

Some people have allergies to contrast dye. Let your doctor know if you have ever had an allergic reaction to injected contrast dye.

- The most common type of contrast given into a vein contains iodine. If a person with an iodine allergy is given this type of contrast, nausea or vomiting, sneezing, itching, or hives may occur.

- If you absolutely must be given such contrast, your doctor may give you antihistamines (such as Benadryl) or steroids before the test.

• The kidneys help remove iodine out of the body. Those with kidney disease or diabetes may need to receive extra fluids after the test to help flush the iodine out of the body.

Rarely, the dye may cause a life-threatening allergic response called anaphylaxis. If you have any trouble breathing during the test, you should notify the scanner operator immediately. Scanners come with an intercom and speakers, so the operator can hear you at all times.

Considerations

A CT scan can reduce or avoid the need for invasive procedures to diagnose problems in the skull. This is one of the safest ways to study the head and neck.

Other tests that may be done instead of cranial CT scan include:

• MRI [magnetic resonance imaging] of the head

• Positron emission tomography (PET) scan of the head

• Skull X-ray

Section 26.8

MRI

A head MRI (magnetic resonance imaging) scan of the head is an imaging test that uses powerful magnets and radio waves to create pictures of the brain and surrounding nerve tissues.

It does not use radiation.

How the Test Is Performed

You may be asked to wear a hospital gown or clothing without metal fasteners (such as sweatpants and a t-shirt). Certain types of metal can cause blurry images.

You will lie on a narrow table, which slides into a large tunnel-shaped scanner.

Some exams require a special dye (contrast). The dye is usually given before the test through a vein (IV, or intravenously) in your hand or forearm. The dye helps the radiologist see certain areas more clearly.

During the MRI, the person who operates the machine will watch you from another room. The test most often lasts 30–60 minutes, but it may take longer.

How to Prepare for the Test

You may be asked not to eat or drink anything for 4–6 hours before the scan.

Tell your doctor if you are afraid of close spaces (have claustrophobia). You may receive medicine to help you feel sleepy and less anxious, or your doctor may suggest an "open" MRI, in which the machine is not as close to the body.

Before the test, tell your health care provider if you have:

- brain aneurysm clips;
- certain types of artificial heart valves;
- heart defibrillator or pacemaker;

- inner ear (cochlear) implants;

- kidney disease or dialysis (you may not be able to receive contrast);

- recently placed artificial joints;

- certain types of vascular stents;

- worked with sheet metal in the past (you may need tests to check for metal pieces in your eyes).

Because the MRI contains strong magnets, metal objects are not allowed into the room with the MRI scanner:

- Pens, pocketknives, and eyeglasses may fly across the room.

- Items such as jewelry, watches, credit cards, and hearing aids can be damaged.

- Pins, hairpins, metal zippers, and similar metallic items can distort the images.

- Removable dental work should be taken out just before the scan.

How the Test Will Feel

An MRI exam causes no pain. If you have difficulty lying still or are very nervous, you may be given a medicine to relax you. Too much movement can blur MRI images and cause errors.

The table may be hard or cold, but you can request a blanket or pillow. The machine produces loud thumping and humming noises when turned on. You can wear ear plugs to help reduce the noise.

An intercom in the room allows you to speak to someone at any time. Some MRIs have televisions and special headphones that you can use to help the time pass.

There is no recovery time, unless you were given a medicine to relax. After an MRI scan, you can resume your normal diet, activity, and medications.

Why the Test Is Performed

MRI provides detailed pictures of the brain and nerve tissues. It also provides clear pictures of parts of the brain that are difficult to see clearly on CT [computed tomography] scans.

A brain MRI can be used to diagnose and monitor many diseases and disorders that affect the brain, including:

- birth defect of the brain;

- bleeding in the brain (subarachnoid or intracranial hemorrhage);

- brain infection;

- brain tumors;

- hormonal disorders (such as acromegaly, galactorrhea, and Cushing syndrome);

- multiple sclerosis;

- stroke.

An MRI scan of the head can also determine the cause of:

- muscle weakness or numbness and tingling;

- changes in thinking or behavior;

- hearing loss;

- headaches when certain other symptoms or signs are present;

- speaking difficulties;

- vision problems.

A special type of MRI (called MRA, or magnetic resonance angiography) may be done to look at blood vessels in the brain.

What Abnormal Results Mean

Abnormal results may be due to:

- abnormal blood vessels in the brain (arteriovenous malformations of the head);

- acoustic neuroma;

- bleeding in the brain;

- brain abscess;

- brain aneurysms;

- brain tissue swelling;

- brain tumors;

- damage to the brain from an injury;

- hydrocephalus (fluid collecting around the brain);

- infection of the bones (osteomyelitis);

- loss of brain tissue;

- multiple sclerosis;

- optic glioma;

- pituitary tumor;

- stroke or transient ischemic attack (TIA);

- structural problems in the brain, blood vessels, or pituitary gland.

Risks

MRI uses no radiation. To date, no side effects from the magnetic fields and radio waves have been reported.

The most common type of contrast (dye) used is gadolinium. It is very safe. Allergic reactions to the substance rarely occur. However, gadolinium can be harmful to patients with kidney problems who require dialysis. If you have kidney problems, please tell your health care provider before the test.

The strong magnetic fields created during an MRI can make heart pacemakers and other implants not work as well. It can also cause a piece of metal inside your body to move or shift.

Considerations

Tests that may be done instead of an MRI of the head include:

- cranial CT scan;

- positron emission tomography (PET) scan of the brain;

- skull X-ray.

A CT scan may be preferred in the following cases, since it is faster and usually available right in the emergency room:

- Acute trauma of the head and face

- Bleeding in the brain (within the first 24–48 hours)

- Early symptoms of stroke

- Skull bone disorders and disorders involving the bones of the ear

Section 26.9

Ultrasound

Excerpted from "Carotid Ultrasound," by the National Heart, Lung, and Blood Institute (NHLBI, www.nhlbi.nih.gov), part of the National Institutes of Health, February 3, 2012.

Carotid ultrasound is a painless and harmless test that uses high-frequency sound waves to create pictures of the insides of your carotid arteries.

You have two common carotid arteries, one on each side of your neck. They each divide into internal and external carotid arteries.

The internal carotid arteries supply oxygen-rich blood to your brain. The external carotid arteries supply oxygen-rich blood to your face, scalp, and neck.

Overview

Carotid ultrasound shows whether a waxy substance called plaque has built up in your carotid arteries. The buildup of plaque in the carotid arteries is called carotid artery disease.

Over time, plaque can harden or rupture (break open). Hardened plaque narrows the carotid arteries and reduces the flow of oxygen-rich blood to the brain.

If the plaque ruptures, a blood clot can form on its surface. A clot can mostly or completely block blood flow through a carotid artery, which can cause a stroke.

A piece of plaque or a blood clot also can break away from the wall of the carotid artery. The plaque or clot can travel through the bloodstream and get stuck in one of the brain's smaller arteries. This can block blood flow in the artery and cause a stroke.

A standard carotid ultrasound shows the structure of your carotid arteries. Your carotid ultrasound test might include a Doppler ultrasound. Doppler ultrasound is a special test that shows the movement of blood through your blood vessels.

Your doctor might need results from both types of ultrasound to fully assess whether you have a blood flow problem in your carotid arteries.

Who Needs Carotid Ultrasound?

A carotid ultrasound shows whether you have plaque buildup in your carotid arteries. Over time, plaque can harden or rupture (break open). This can reduce or block the flow of oxygen-rich blood to your brain and cause a stroke.

Your doctor may recommend a carotid ultrasound if you had the following:

- A stroke or mini-stroke recently: During a mini-stroke, you may have some or all of the symptoms of a stroke. However, the symptoms usually go away on their own within 24 hours.

- An abnormal sound called a carotid bruit in one of your carotid arteries: Your doctor can hear a carotid bruit using a stethoscope. A bruit might suggest a partial blockage in your carotid artery, which could lead to a stroke.

Your doctor also may recommend a carotid ultrasound if he or she thinks you have blood clots in one of your carotid arteries or a split between the layers of your carotid artery wall. The split can weaken the wall or reduce blood flow to your brain.

A carotid ultrasound also might be done to see whether carotid artery surgery, also called carotid endarterectomy, has restored normal blood flow through a carotid artery.

If you had a procedure called carotid stenting, your doctor might use carotid ultrasound afterward to check the position of the stent in your carotid artery. (The stent, a small mesh tube, supports the inner artery wall.)

Carotid ultrasound sometimes is used as a preventive screening test in people at increased risk of stroke, such as those who have high blood pressure and diabetes.

What to Expect before Carotid Ultrasound

Carotid ultrasound is a painless test. Typically, there is little to do in advance of the test. Your doctor will tell you how to prepare for your carotid ultrasound.

What to Expect during Carotid Ultrasound

Carotid ultrasound usually is done in a doctor's office or hospital. The test is painless and often doesn't take more than 30 minutes.

The ultrasound machine includes a computer, a screen, and a transducer. The transducer is a hand-held device that sends and receives ultrasound waves.

You will lie on your back on an exam table for the test. Your technician or doctor will put gel on your neck where your carotid arteries are located. The gel helps the ultrasound waves reach the arteries.

Your technician or doctor will put the transducer against different spots on your neck and move it back and forth. The transducer gives off ultrasound waves and detects their echoes as they bounce off the artery walls and blood cells. Ultrasound waves can't be heard by the human ear.

The computer uses the echoes to create and record pictures of the insides of the carotid arteries. These pictures usually appear in black and white. The screen displays these live images for your doctor to review.

Your carotid ultrasound test might include a Doppler ultrasound. Doppler ultrasound is a special test that shows the movement of blood through your arteries. Blood flow through the arteries usually appears in color on the ultrasound pictures.

What to Expect after Carotid Ultrasound

You usually can return to your normal activities as soon as the carotid ultrasound is over. Your doctor will likely be able to tell you the results of the carotid ultrasound when it occurs or soon afterward.

What Does a Carotid Ultrasound Show?

A carotid ultrasound can show whether plaque buildup has narrowed one or both of your carotid arteries. If so, you might be at risk of having a stroke. The risk depends on the extent of the blockage and how much it has reduced blood flow to your brain.

To lower your risk of stroke, your doctor may recommend medical or surgical treatments to reduce or remove plaque from your carotid arteries.

What Are the Risks of Carotid Ultrasound?

Carotid ultrasound has no risks because the test uses harmless sound waves. They are the same type of sound waves that doctors use to record pictures of fetuses in pregnant women.

Chapter 27

Stroke Prognosis and Treatment

Chapter Contents

Section 27.1

What You Should Know about Stroke Prognosis

Understanding a Stroke Prognosis

No two strokes are exactly alike, but they all have one thing in common: A stroke almost always causes some brain damage. How much damage depends on the type, location, duration, and severity of the stroke. And the extent and location of damage is what largely determines the stroke prognosis—the chance for survival or quality of life down the road.

When someone survives a stroke, the big question on everyone's mind is what the stroke survivor's life will be like. What types of physical problems will she have? How seriously disabled will she be? Will she be able to speak? Walk? Live on her own?

It's important to keep in mind that there's no magic formula for predicting the outcome, nor is there a set timeline for recovery. But there's reason for hope: Although up to 30 percent of stroke survivors suffer some permanent disability, more than half recover functional independence after a stroke.

Ischemic Versus Hemorrhagic Stroke

When considering stroke prognosis, in general, people who have ischemic strokes (caused by a blood clot) have a better chance of surviving than those who have hemorrhagic strokes (caused by a ruptured blood vessel). That's because hemorrhagic strokes have the potential to cause more damage to the brain. When a blood vessel ruptures inside the brain, the bleeding not only destroys brain cells but it can result in other serious complications, including increased pressure on the brain and spasms of other blood vessels.

But there's good news for hemorrhagic stroke survivors: Studies suggest that people who survive hemorrhagic strokes have a greater chance of recovering function than those who have survived ischemic stroke.

Evaluating a Stroke by National Institutes of Health (NIH) Guidelines

The NIH has developed a scoring system called a stroke scale that helps predict the severity and outcome of stroke. It's a complicated formula that includes 11 different factors measured during a neurological exam:

- Level of consciousness
- Gaze
- Visual field
- Facial movement
- Motor function in arms
- Motor function in legs
- Coordination
- Sensory loss
- Language problems
- Ability to articulate
- Attention

Each impairment noted during the exam is assigned a certain number of points, so the higher the score, the worse the stroke:

- 0 No stroke
- 1–4 Minor stroke
- 5–15 Moderate stroke
- 15–20 Moderate to severe stroke
- 21–42 Severe stroke

Up to 70 percent of stroke patients who score less than 10 have a favorable outlook after a year, while less than 16 percent who score more than 20 do well.

Avoiding Another Stroke and Dealing with Uncertainty

Probably the most important factor affecting a person's future after a stroke is whether she has another stroke. There are two important factors to consider:

- Having already had one stroke increases the risk of having another.
- The risk for another stroke is highest within the first few weeks and months.
- It's always important to do everything possible to prevent a future stroke.

The future after a stroke isn't always clear. There are many things that affect stroke prognosis, including impossible-to-measure factors such as how the brain heals and rewires itself. One of your most challenging tasks as a caregiver looking at stroke prognosis will be coming to terms with uncertainty about the future—and helping the person in your care do the same.

Section 27.2

How Is Stroke Treated?

"How Is a Stroke Treated?" by the National Heart, Lung,
and Blood Institute (NHLBI, www.nhlbi.nih.gov), part of the
National Institutes of Health, February 1, 2011.

Treatment for a stroke depends on whether it is ischemic or hemorrhagic. Treatment for a transient ischemic attack (TIA) depends on its cause, how much time has passed since symptoms began, and whether you have other medical conditions.

Strokes and TIAs are medical emergencies. If you have stroke symptoms, call 911 right away. Do not drive to the hospital or let someone else drive you. Call an ambulance so that medical personnel can begin life-saving treatment on the way to the emergency room. During a stroke, every minute counts.

Once you receive initial treatment, your doctor will try to treat your stroke risk factors and prevent complications.

Treating Ischemic Stroke and Transient Ischemic Attack

An ischemic stroke or TIA occurs if an artery that supplies oxygen-rich blood to the brain becomes blocked. Often, blood clots cause the blockages that lead to ischemic strokes and TIAs.

Treatment for an ischemic stroke or TIA may include medicines and medical procedures.

Medicines

A medicine called tissue plasminogen activator (tPA) can break up blood clots in the arteries of the brain. A doctor will inject tPA into a vein in your arm. This medicine must be given within four hours of the start of symptoms to work. Ideally, it should be given as soon as possible.

If, for medical reasons, your doctor can't give you tPA, you may get an antiplatelet medicine. For example, aspirin may be given within 48 hours of a stroke. Antiplatelet medicines help stop platelets from clumping together to form blood clots.

313

Your doctor also may prescribe anticoagulants, or blood thinners. These medicines can keep blood clots from getting larger and prevent new blood clots from forming.

Medical Procedures

If you have carotid artery disease, your doctor may recommend a carotid endarterectomy or carotid artery angioplasty. Both procedures open blocked carotid arteries.

Researchers are testing other treatments for ischemic stroke, such as intra-arterial thrombolysis and mechanical clot (embolus) removal in cerebral ischemia (MERCI).

In intra-arterial thrombolysis, a long flexible tube called a catheter is put into your groin (upper thigh) and threaded to the tiny arteries of the brain. Your doctor can deliver medicine through this catheter to break up a blood clot in the brain.

MERCI is a device that can remove blood clots from an artery. During the procedure, a catheter is threaded through a carotid artery to the affected artery in the brain. The device is then used to pull the blood clot out through the catheter.

Treating Hemorrhagic Stroke

A hemorrhagic stroke occurs if an artery in the brain leaks blood or ruptures (breaks open). The first steps in treating a hemorrhagic stroke are to find the cause of bleeding in the brain and then control it.

Unlike ischemic strokes, hemorrhagic strokes aren't treated with antiplatelet medicines and blood thinners. This is because these medicines can make bleeding worse.

If you're taking antiplatelet medicines or blood thinners and have a hemorrhagic stroke, you'll be taken off the medicine.

If high blood pressure is the cause of bleeding in the brain, your doctor may prescribe medicines to lower your blood pressure. This can help prevent further bleeding.

Surgery also may be needed to treat a hemorrhagic stroke. The types of surgery used include aneurysm clipping, coil embolization, and arteriovenous malformation (AVM) repair.

Aneurysm Clipping and Coil Embolization

If an aneurysm (a balloon-like bulge in an artery) is the cause of a stroke, your doctor may recommend aneurysm clipping or coil embolization.

Aneurysm clipping is done to block off the aneurysm from the blood vessels in the brain. This surgery helps prevent further leaking of blood from the aneurysm. It also can help prevent the aneurysm from bursting again.

During the procedure, a surgeon will make an incision (cut) in the brain and place a tiny clamp at the base of the aneurysm. You'll be given medicine to make you sleep during the surgery. After the surgery, you'll need to stay in the hospital's intensive care unit for a few days.

Coil embolization is a less complex procedure for treating an aneurysm. The surgeon will insert a tube called a catheter into an artery in the groin. He or she will thread the tube to the site of the aneurysm.

Then, a tiny coil will be pushed through the tube and into the aneurysm. The coil will cause a blood clot to form, which will block blood flow through the aneurysm and prevent it from bursting again.

Coil embolization is done in a hospital. You'll be given medicine to make you sleep during the surgery.

Arteriovenous Malformation Repair

If an AVM is the cause of a stroke, your doctor may recommend an AVM repair. (An AVM is a tangle of faulty arteries and veins that can rupture within the brain.) AVM repair helps prevent further bleeding in the brain.

Doctors use several methods to repair AVMs. These methods include:

- surgery to remove the AVM;

- injecting a substance into the blood vessels of the AVM to block blood flow;

- using radiation to shrink the blood vessels of the AVM.

Treating Stroke Risk Factors

After initial treatment for a stroke or TIA, your doctor will treat your risk factors. He or she may recommend lifestyle changes to help control your risk factors.

Lifestyle changes may include quitting smoking, following a healthy diet, maintaining a healthy weight, and being physically active.

If lifestyle changes aren't enough, you may need medicine to control your risk factors.

Quitting Smoking

If you smoke or use tobacco, quit. Smoking can damage your blood vessels and raise your risk of stroke and other health problems. Talk with your doctor about programs and products that can help you quit. Also, try to avoid secondhand smoke. Secondhand smoke also can damage the blood vessels.

Following a Healthy Diet

A healthy diet is an important part of a healthy lifestyle. Choose a variety of fruits, vegetables, and grains; half of your grains should come from whole-grain products.

Choose foods that are low in saturated fat, trans fat, and cholesterol. Healthy choices include lean meats, poultry without skin, fish, beans, and fat-free or low-fat milk and milk products.

Choose and prepare foods with little sodium (salt). Too much salt can raise your risk of high blood pressure. Studies show that following the Dietary Approaches to Stop Hypertension (DASH) eating plan can lower blood pressure.

Choose foods and beverages that are low in added sugar. If you drink alcoholic beverages, do so in moderation.

Maintaining a Healthy Weight

Maintaining a healthy weight can lower your risk of stroke. A general goal to aim for is a body mass index (BMI) of less than 25.

BMI measures your weight in relation to your height and gives an estimate of your total body fat. You can measure your BMI using the NHLBI's online calculator [nhlbisupport.com/bmi/], or your health care provider can measure your BMI.

A BMI between 25 and 29.9 is considered overweight. A BMI of 30 or more is considered obese. A BMI of less than 25 is the goal for preventing a stroke.

Being Physically Active

Regular physical activity can help control many stroke risk factors, such as high blood pressure, unhealthy cholesterol levels, and excess weight.

Talk with your doctor before you start a new exercise plan. Ask him or her how much and what kinds of physical activity are safe for you.

People gain health benefits from as little as 60 minutes of moderate-intensity aerobic activity per week. The more active you are, the more you will benefit.

Chapter 28

Surgical Procedures Used in the Treatment of Stroke

Chapter Contents

Section 28.1

Brain Aneurysm Repair

Brain aneurysm repair is a surgical procedure to correct an aneurysm, a weak area in a blood vessel wall that causes the blood vessel to bulge or balloon out and sometimes burst (rupture). It may cause:

- bleeding into an area around the brain (also called a subarachnoid hemorrhage);

- bleeding in the brain that forms a collection of blood (hematoma).

Description

You and your health care provider will decide the best way to perform surgery on your aneurysm. There are two common methods used to repair an aneurysm:

- Clipping used to be the most common way to repair an aneurysm. This is done during an open craniotomy.

- Endovascular repair, most often using a coil or coiling and stenting (mesh tubes), is a less invasive way to treat some aneurysms. It is now done in more than half of patients.

During aneurysm clipping:

- You are given general anesthesia and a breathing tube.

- Your scalp, skull, and the coverings of the brain are opened up.

- A metal clip is placed at the base (neck) of the aneurysm to prevent it from breaking open (bursting).

During endovascular repair of an aneurysm:

- The procedure is usually done in the radiology section of the hospital.

- You may have general anesthesia and a breathing tube. Or, you may be given medicine to relax you, but not enough to put you to sleep.

- A catheter is guided through a small cut in your groin to an artery and then to the small blood vessels in your brain where the aneurysm is located.

- Thin metal wires or glue are put into the aneurysm. They then coil up into a mesh ball. Blood clots that form around this coil prevent the aneurysm from breaking open and bleeding. Sometimes stents (mesh tubes) are also put in to hold the coils in place.

During and right after this procedure, you may be given a blood thinner called heparin.

Why the Procedure Is Performed

If an aneurysm in the brain ruptures, it is an emergency that needs medical treatment, often surgery. Endovascular repair is more often used when this happens.

A person may have an aneurysm but have no symptoms. This kind of aneurysm may be found when an MRI [magnetic resonance imaging] or CT [computed tomography] scan of the brain is done for another reason.

Not all aneurysms need to be treated right away. Aneurysms that have never bled and are very small (less than 7 mm at their largest point) do not need to be treated right away. These aneurysms are less likely to break open.

Your doctor will help you decide whether it is safer to have surgery to block off the aneurysm before it can break open (rupture).

Risks

Risks for any anesthesia are:

- breathing problems;

- reactions to medications.

Possible risks of brain surgery are:

- blood clot or bleeding in the brain;

- brain swelling;

- infection in the brain, or parts around the brain such as the skull or scalp;

- seizures;

- stroke.

Surgery on any one area of the brain may cause problems with speech, memory, muscle weakness, balance, vision, coordination, and other functions. These problems may be mild or severe, and they may last a short while or they may not go away.

Signs of brain and nervous system (neurological) problems include:

- behavior changes;
- confusion;
- loss of balance or coordination;
- numbness;
- problems noticing things around you;
- speech problems;
- vision problems (from blindness to problems with side vision);
- weakness.

Before the Procedure

This procedure is often performed on an emergency basis. If it is not an emergency:

- Tell your doctor or nurse what drugs or herbs you are taking and if you have been drinking a lot of alcohol.
- Ask your doctor which drugs you should still take on the day of the surgery.
- Always try to stop smoking.

You will usually be asked not to eat or drink anything for eight hours before the surgery.

Take the drugs your doctor told you to take with a small sip of water. Your doctor or nurse will tell you when to arrive.

After the Procedure

A hospital stay for endovascular repair of an aneurysm may be as short as one to two days if there was no bleeding beforehand.

The hospital stay after craniotomy and aneurysm clipping is usually four to six days. When bleeding or other complications occur before or during surgery, the hospital stay can be one to two weeks, or more.

You will probably have an X-ray test of the blood vessels in the brain (angiogram) before you are sent home.

Ask your doctor if it will be safe for you to have MRI scans in the future.

Outlook (Prognosis)

After successful surgery for a bleeding aneurysm, it is uncommon for it to bleed again.

The outlook also depends on whether any brain damage occurred from bleeding before, during, or after the surgery.

Most of the time, open surgery or endovascular repair can prevent a brain aneurysm that has not caused symptoms from becoming larger and breaking open.

You may have more than one aneurysm. After endovascular treatment (coiling), you will need to be seen by your health care provider every year.

Section 28.2

Carotid Artery Angioplasty and Stent Placement

"Stents," by the National Heart, Lung, and Blood Institute (NHLBI, www.nhlbi.nih.gov), part of the National Institutes of Health, November 8, 2011.

A stent is a small mesh tube that's used to treat narrow or weak arteries. Arteries are blood vessels that carry blood away from your heart to other parts of your body.

A stent is placed in an artery as part of a procedure called angioplasty. Angioplasty restores blood flow through narrow or blocked arteries. A stent helps support the inner wall of the artery in the months or years after angioplasty.

Doctors also may place stents in weak arteries to improve blood flow and help prevent the arteries from bursting.

Stents usually are made of metal mesh, but sometimes they're made of fabric. Fabric stents, also called stent grafts, are used in larger arteries.

Some stents are coated with medicine that is slowly and continuously released into the artery. These stents are called drug-eluting stents. The medicine helps prevent the artery from becoming blocked again.

How Are Stents Used?

For the Coronary Arteries

Doctors may use stents to treat coronary heart disease (CHD). CHD is a disease in which a waxy substance called plaque builds up inside the coronary arteries. These arteries supply your heart muscle with oxygen-rich blood.

When plaque builds up in the arteries, the condition is called atherosclerosis.

Plaque narrows the coronary arteries, reducing the flow of oxygen-rich blood to your heart. This can lead to chest pain or discomfort called angina.

The buildup of plaque also makes it more likely that blood clots will form in your coronary arteries. If blood clots block a coronary artery, a heart attack will occur.

Doctors may use angioplasty and stents to treat CHD. During angioplasty, a thin, flexible tube with a balloon or other device on the end is threaded through a blood vessel to the narrow or blocked coronary artery.

Once in place, the balloon is inflated to compress the plaque against the wall of the artery. This restores blood flow through the artery, which reduces angina and other CHD symptoms.

Unless an artery is too small, a stent usually is placed in the treated portion of the artery during angioplasty. The stent supports the artery's inner wall. It also reduces the chance that the artery will become narrow or blocked again. A stent also can support an artery that was torn or injured during angioplasty.

Even with a stent, there's about a 10–20 percent chance that an artery will become narrow or blocked again in the first year after angioplasty. When a stent isn't used, the risk can be twice as high.

For the Carotid Arteries

Doctors also may use stents to treat carotid artery disease. This is a disease in which plaque builds up in the arteries that run along each side of your neck. These arteries, called carotid arteries, supply oxygen-rich blood to your brain.

The buildup of plaque in the carotid arteries limits blood flow to your brain and puts you at risk for a stroke.

Doctors use stents to help support the carotid arteries after they're widened with angioplasty. How well this treatment works in the long term still isn't known. Researchers continue to explore the risks and benefits of carotid artery stenting.

For Other Arteries

Plaque also can narrow other arteries, such as those in the kidneys and limbs. Narrow kidney arteries can affect kidney function and lead to severe high blood pressure.

Narrow arteries in the limbs, a condition called peripheral arterial disease (PAD), can cause pain and cramping in the affected arm or leg. Severe narrowing can completely cut off blood flow to a limb, which could require surgery.

To relieve these problems, doctors may do angioplasty on a narrow kidney, arm, or leg artery. They often will place a stent in the affected artery during the procedure. The stent helps support the artery and keep it open.

For the Aorta in the Abdomen or Chest

The aorta is a major artery that carries oxygen-rich blood from the left side of the heart to the body. This artery runs through the chest and down into the abdomen.

Over time, some areas of the aorta's walls can weaken. These weak areas can cause a bulge in the artery called an aneurysm. An aneurysm in the aorta can burst, leading to serious internal bleeding. When aneurysms occur, they're usually in the abdominal aorta.

To help avoid a burst, doctors may place a fabric stent in the weak area of the abdominal aorta. The stent creates a stronger inner lining for the artery.

Aneurysms also can develop in the part of the aorta that runs through the chest. Doctors also use stents to treat these aneurysms. How well the stents work over the long term still isn't known.

To Close off Aortic Tears

Another problem that can occur in the aorta is a tear in its inner wall. If blood is forced into the tear, it will widen.

The tear can reduce blood flow to the tissues that the aorta serves. Over time, the tear can block blood flow through the artery or burst. If this happens, it usually occurs in the chest portion of the aorta.

Researchers are developing and testing fabric stents that will prevent blood from flowing into aortic tears. A fabric stent placed within the torn area of the aorta might help restore normal blood flow and reduce the risk of a burst aorta.

How Are Stents Placed?

Doctors place stents in arteries as part of a procedure called angioplasty. To place a stent, your doctor will make a small opening in a blood vessel in your groin (upper thigh), arm, or neck.

Through this opening, your doctor will thread a thin, flexible tube called a catheter. The catheter will have a deflated balloon at its tip.

A stent is placed around the deflated balloon. Your doctor will move the tip of the catheter to the narrow section of the artery or to the aneurysm or aortic tear site.

Special X-ray movies will be taken of the tube as it's threaded through your blood vessel. These movies will help your doctor position the catheter.

For Arteries Narrowed by Plaque

Your doctor will use special dye to help show narrow or blocked areas in the artery. He or she will then move the catheter to the area and inflate the balloon.

As the balloon inflates, it pushes the plaque against the artery wall. This widens the artery and helps restore blood flow. The fully extended balloon also expands the stent, pushing it into place in the artery.

The balloon is deflated and pulled out along with the catheter. The stent remains in your artery. Over time, cells in your artery grow to cover the mesh of the stent. They create an inner layer that looks like the inside of a normal blood vessel.

Coronary Artery Stent Placement

A very narrow artery, or one that's hard to reach with a catheter, may require more steps to place a stent. At first, your doctor may use a small balloon to expand the artery. He or she then removes the balloon.

The small balloon is replaced with a larger balloon that has a collapsed stent around it. At this point, your doctor can follow the standard process of compressing the plaque and placing the stent.

Doctors use a special filter device when doing angioplasty and stent placement on the carotid arteries. The filter helps keep blood clots and loose pieces of plaque from traveling to the brain during the procedure.

For Aortic Aneurysms

The procedure to place a stent in an artery with an aneurysm is very similar to the one described in the preceding text. However, the stent used to treat an aneurysm is different. It's made out of pleated fabric instead of metal mesh, and it often has one or more tiny hooks.

The stent is expanded to fit tight against the artery wall. The hooks latch on to the wall of the artery, holding the stent in place.

The stent creates a new inner lining for that portion of the artery. Over time, cells in the artery grow to cover the fabric. They create an inner layer that looks like the inside of a normal blood vessel.

What to Expect before a Stent Procedure

Most stent procedures require an overnight stay in a hospital and someone to take you home. Talk with your doctor about the following:

- When to stop eating and drinking before coming to the hospital

- What medicines you should or shouldn't take on the day of the procedure

- When to come to the hospital and where to go

If you have diabetes, kidney disease, or other conditions, ask your doctor whether you need to take any extra steps during or after the procedure to avoid complications.

Before the procedure, your doctor may talk to you about medicines you'll likely need to take after the stent is placed. These medicines help prevent blood clots from forming in the stent.

You'll need to know how long you should take these medicines and why they're important.

What to Expect during a Stent Procedure

For Arteries Narrowed by Plaque

This procedure usually takes about an hour. It might take longer if stents are inserted into more than one artery during the procedure.

Before the procedure starts, you'll get medicine to help you relax. You'll be on your back and awake during the procedure. This allows you to follow your doctor's instructions.

Your doctor will numb the area where the catheter will be inserted. You won't feel the doctor threading the catheter, balloon, or stent inside the artery. You may feel some pain when the balloon is expanded to push the stent into place.

For Aortic Aneurysms

Although this procedure takes only a few hours, it often requires a two- to three-day hospital stay.

Before the procedure, you'll be given medicine to help you relax. If your doctor is placing the stent in your abdominal aorta, you may receive medicine to numb your stomach area. However, you'll be awake during the procedure.

If your doctor is placing the stent in the chest portion of your aorta, you'll likely receive medicine to make you sleep during the procedure.

Once you're numb or asleep, your doctor will make a small cut in your groin (upper thigh). He or she will insert a catheter into the blood vessel through this cut.

Sometimes two cuts (one in the groin area of each leg) are needed to place fabric stents that come in two parts. You will not feel the doctor threading the catheter, balloon, or stent into the artery.

What to Expect after a Stent Procedure

Recovery

After either type of stent procedure (for arteries narrowed by plaque or aortic aneurysms), your doctor will remove the catheter from your artery. The site where the catheter was inserted will be bandaged.

A small sandbag or other type of weight may be put on top of the bandage to apply pressure and help prevent bleeding. You'll recover in a special care area, where your movement will be limited.

While you're in recovery, a nurse will check your heart rate and blood pressure regularly. The nurse also will look to see whether you're bleeding from the insertion site.

Eventually, a small bruise and sometimes a small, hard knot will appear at the insertion site. This area may feel sore or tender for about a week.

You should let your doctor know if any of the following are true:

- You have a constant or large amount of bleeding at the insertion site that can't be stopped with a small bandage.

- You have any unusual pain, swelling, redness, or other signs of infection at or near the insertion site.

Common Precautions after a Stent Procedure

Blood Clotting Precautions

After a stent procedure, your doctor will likely recommend that you take aspirin and another anticlotting medicine. These medicines help prevent blood clots from forming in the stent. A blood clot can lead to a heart attack, stroke, or other serious problems.

If you have a metal stent, your doctor may recommend aspirin and another anticlotting medicine for at least one month. If your stent is coated with medicine, your doctor may recommend aspirin and another anticlotting medicine for 12 months or more. Your doctor will work with you to decide the best course of treatment.

Your risk of blood clots significantly increases if you stop taking the anticlotting medicine too early. Taking these medicines for as long as your doctor recommends is important. He or she may recommend lifelong treatment with aspirin.

If you're considering surgery for some other reason while you're on these medicines, talk to your doctor about whether it can wait until after you've stopped the medicine. Anticlotting medicines may increase the risk of bleeding.

Also, anticlotting medicines can cause side effects, such as an allergic rash. Talk to your doctor about how to reduce the risk of these side effects.

Other Precautions

You should avoid vigorous exercise and heavy lifting for a short time after the stent procedure. Your doctor will let you know when you can go back to your normal activities.

If you have a metal stent, you shouldn't have a magnetic resonance imaging (MRI) test for a couple of months after the procedure. Metal detectors used in airports and other screening areas don't affect stents. Your stent shouldn't cause metal detectors to go off.

If you have an aortic fabric stent, your doctor will likely recommend followup imaging tests (for example, chest X-ray) within the first year of having the procedure. After the first year, he or she may recommend yearly imaging tests.

Lifestyle Changes

Stents help prevent arteries from becoming narrow or blocked again in the months or years after angioplasty. However, stents aren't a cure for atherosclerosis or its risk factors.

Making lifestyle changes can help prevent plaque from building up in your arteries again. Talk with your doctor about your risk factors for atherosclerosis and the lifestyle changes you'll need to make.

Lifestyle changes may include changing your diet, quitting smoking, being physically active, losing weight, and reducing stress. You also should take all medicines as your doctor prescribes.

What Are the Risks of Having a Stent?

Risks Related to Angioplasty

Angioplasty, the procedure used to place stents, is a common medical procedure. Angioplasty carries a small risk of serious complications, such as the following:

- Bleeding from the site where the catheter was inserted into the skin

- Damage to the blood vessel from the catheter

- Arrhythmias (irregular heartbeats)

- Damage to the kidneys caused by the dye used during the procedure

- An allergic reaction to the dye used during the procedure

- Infection

Another problem that can occur after angioplasty is too much tissue growth within the treated portion of the artery. This can cause the artery to become narrow or blocked again. When this happens, it's called restenosis.

Using drug-eluting stents can help prevent this problem. These stents are coated with medicine to stop excess tissue growth.

Treating the tissue around the stent with radiation also can prevent tissue growth. For this procedure, the doctor threads a wire through a catheter to the stent. The wire releases radiation and stops cells around the stent from growing and blocking the artery.

Risks Related to Stents

About 1–2 percent of people who have stented arteries develop a blood clot at the stent site. Blood clots can cause a heart attack, stroke, or other serious problems. The risk of blood clots is greatest during the first few months after the stent is placed in the artery.

Your doctor will likely recommend that you take aspirin and another anticlotting medicine, such as clopidogrel, for at least one month or up to a year or more after having a stent procedure. These medicines help prevent blood clots.

The length of time you need to take anticlotting medicines depends on the type of stent you have. Your doctor may recommend lifelong treatment with aspirin.

Stents coated with medicine may raise your risk of dangerous blood clots. (These stents often are used to keep clogged heart arteries open.) However, research hasn't proven that these stents increase the chances of having a heart attack or dying, if used as recommended.

Section 28.3

Carotid Endarterectomy

"Questions and Answers about Carotid Endarterectomy," by the National Institute of Neurological Disorders and Stroke (NINDS, www.ninds.nih.gov), part of the National Institutes of Health, July 5, 2012.

What is a carotid endarterectomy?

A carotid endarterectomy is a surgical procedure in which a doctor removes fatty deposits blocking one of the two carotid arteries, the main supply of blood for the brain. Carotid artery problems become more common as people age. The disease process that causes the buildup of fat and other material inside the artery walls is called atherosclerosis, popularly known as hardening of the arteries. The fatty deposit is called plaque; the narrowing of the artery is called stenosis. The degree of stenosis is usually expressed as a percentage of the normal diameter of the opening.

Why is surgery performed?

Carotid endarterectomy is performed to prevent stroke. Two large clinical trials supported by the National Institute of Neurological Disorders and Stroke (NINDS) have identified specific individuals for whom the surgery is beneficial when performed by surgeons and in institutions that can match the standards set in those studies. The surgery has been found highly beneficial for persons who have already had a stroke or experienced the symptoms of a stroke and have a severe stenosis of 70 to 99 percent. In this group, surgery reduces the estimated 2-year risk of stroke or death by more than 80 percent, from greater than 1 in 4 to less than 1 in 10.

For patients who have already had transient or mild stroke symptoms due to moderate carotid stenosis (50 to 69 percent), surgery reduces the 5-year risk of stroke or death by 6.5 percent. The failure rate for ipsilateral stroke or death for the medical group is 22.2 percent, and for the surgery group is 15.7 percent from greater than 1 in 4 to less than 1 in 7. Individuals who have already had stroke symptoms, and who have carotid stenosis greater than 50 percent, may wish to consider surgery to prevent future stroke. Based on findings of the North American Symptomatic Carotid Endarterectomy Trial (NASCET) trial, patients with moderate (50 to 69 percent) stenosis are now better able to make more informed decisions.

In another trial (Asymptomatic Carotid Atherosclerosis Study, or ACAS), the procedure has also been found highly beneficial for persons who are symptom-free but have a carotid stenosis of 60 to 99 percent. In this group, the surgery reduces the estimated 5-year risk of stroke by more than one-half, from about 1 in 10 to less than 1 in 20.

The Carotid Revascularization Endarterectomy vs. Stenting Trial (CREST) compared carotid endarterectomy surgery to carotid artery stenting and found no significance between the procedures regarding the 4-year rate of stroke or death in patients with or without a previous stroke. The pivotal differences were the lower rate of stroke following surgery and the lower rate of heart attack following stenting. The study also found that the age of the patient made a difference with a larger benefit for stenting, the younger the age of the patient. At age 69 and younger, stenting results were slightly better. Conversely, for patients older than 70, surgical benefits were slightly superior to stenting, with larger benefit for surgery, the older the patient.

What is a stroke?

A stroke occurs when blood flow is cut off from part of the brain. In the same way that a person suffering a loss of blood to the heart can be said to be having a heart attack, a person with a loss of blood to the brain can be said to be having a brain attack. There are two kinds of stroke, hemorrhagic and ischemic. Hemorrhagic strokes are caused by bleeding within the brain. Ischemic strokes, which are far more common, are caused by a blockage of blood flow in an artery in the head or neck leading to the brain. Some ischemic strokes are due to stenosis, or narrowing of arteries due to the buildup of plaque, fatty deposits and blood clots along the artery wall. A vascular disease that can cause stenosis is atherosclerosis, in which deposits of plaque build-up along the inner wall of large and medium-sized arteries, decreasing blood flow. Atherosclerosis in the carotid arteries, two large arteries in the neck that carry blood to the brain, is a major risk factor for ischemic stroke.

What are the symptoms of a stroke?

Symptoms of stroke include:

- sudden numbness, weakness, or paralysis of face, arm, or leg, especially on one side of the body;
- sudden confusion, trouble talking, or understanding speech;
- sudden trouble seeing in one or both eyes;
- sudden trouble walking, loss of balance, or coordination;
- sudden severe headache with no known cause (often described as the worst headache in a person's life).

Symptoms may last a few moments and then disappear. When they disappear within 24 hours or less, they are called a transient ischemic attack (TIA).

How important is a blockage as a cause of stroke?

A blockage of a blood vessel is the most frequent cause of stroke and is responsible for about 80 percent of the approximately 700,000 strokes in the United States each year. With nearly 150,000 stroke deaths each year, stroke ranks as the fourth leading killer in the United States. Stroke is the leading cause of adult disability in the United States with 2 million of the 3 million Americans who have survived a stroke sustaining some permanent disability. The overall cost of stroke to the nation is $40 billion a year.

How many carotid endarterectomies are performed each year?

An estimated 140,000 carotid endarterectomies were performed in the United States in 2009, according to the National Hospital Discharge Survey. The procedure was first described in the mid-1950s. It bogan to be used increasingly as a stroke prevention measure in the 1960s and 1970s. Its use peaked in the mid-1980s when more than 100,000 operations were performed each year. At that time, several authorities began to question the trend and the risk-benefit ratio for some groups, and the use of the procedure dropped precipitously. The NINDS-supported NASCET and ACAS trials were launched in the mid-1980s to identify the specific groups of people with carotid artery disease who would clearly benefit from the procedure.

What are the risk factors and how risky is the surgery?

Important risk factors in addition to the degree of stenosis include gender, diabetes, the type of stroke symptoms, and blockage of the carotid artery on the opposite side. Without other complicating illnesses, age alone is not a worrisome risk factor. Risk factors can affect patients in two ways. They can, particularly in combination, greatly increase a person's risk of having a stroke. In addition, these risk factors can increase the likelihood of surgical complications.

How is carotid artery disease diagnosed?

In some cases, the disease can be detected during a normal checkup by a physician. In other cases further testing is needed. Some of the tests a physician can use or order include ultrasound imaging, arteriography, and magnetic resonance angiography (MRA). Frequently these procedures are carried out in a stepwise fashion: From a doctor's evaluation of signs and symptoms to ultrasound, MRA, and arteriography for increasingly difficult cases.

History and physical exam: A doctor will ask about symptoms of a stroke such as numbness or muscle weakness, speech or vision difficulties, or lightheadedness. Using a stethoscope, a doctor may hear a rushing sound, called a bruit, in the carotid artery. Unfortunately, dangerous levels of disease sometimes fail to make a sound, and some blockages with a low risk can make the same sound.

Ultrasound imaging: This is a painless, noninvasive test in which sound waves above the range of human hearing are sent into the neck. Echoes bounce off the moving blood and the tissue in the artery and can be formed into an image. Ultrasound is fast, risk-free, relatively inexpensive, and painless compared to MRA and arteriography.

Arteriography: This can be used to confirm the findings of ultrasound imaging which can be uncertain in some cases. Arteriography is an X-ray of the carotid artery taken when a special dye is injected into the artery. A burning sensation may be felt when the dye is injected. An arteriogram is more expensive and carries its own small risk of causing a stroke.

Magnetic resonance angiography (MRA): This is a new imaging technique that avoids most of the risks associated with arteriography. An MRA is a type of image that uses magnetism instead of X-rays to create an image of the carotid arteries.

What is best medical therapy for stroke prevention?

The mainstay of stroke prevention is risk factor management: Smoking cessation, treatment of high blood pressure, and control of blood sugar levels among persons with diabetes. Additionally, physicians may prescribe aspirin, warfarin, or ticlopidine for some individuals.

Chapter 29

Medications Used to Treat Stroke

Chapter Contents

Section 29.1

Tissue Plasminogen Activator (tPA) and Thrombolytic Therapy

"Thrombolytic Therapy," © 2013 A.D.A.M., Inc.
Reprinted with permission.

Thrombolytic therapy is the use of drugs to break up or dissolve blood clots, which are the main cause of both heart attacks and stroke.

Thrombolytic medications are approved for the immediate treatment of stroke and heart attack. The most commonly used drug for thrombolytic therapy is tissue plasminogen activator (tPA), but other drugs can do the same thing.

According to the American Heart Association, you have a better chance of surviving and recovering from a heart attack if you receive a thrombolytic drug within 12 hours after the heart attack starts.

Ideally, you should receive thrombolytic medications within the first 90 minutes after arriving at the hospital for treatment.

For Heart Attacks

A blood clot can block the arteries to the heart. This can cause a heart attack, when part of the muscle dies due to a lack of oxygen being delivered by the blood.

Thrombolytics work by dissolving a major clot quickly. This helps restart blood flow to the heart and helps prevent damage to the heart muscle. Thrombolytics can stop a heart attack that would otherwise be deadly.

The drug restores some blood flow to the heart in most patients. However, the blood flow may not be completely normal and there may still be a small amount of muscle damaged. Additional therapy, such as cardiac catheterization or angioplasty, may be needed.

Your health care provider will base the decisions about whether to give you a thrombolytic medication for a heart attack on many factors. These factors include your history of chest pain and the results of an ECG [electrocardiogram] test.

Other factors used to determine if you are a good candidate for thrombolytics include:

- age;

- gender;

- medical history (including your history of a previous heart attack, diabetes, low blood pressure, or increased heart rate).

Generally, thrombolytics will not be given if you have:

- a recent head injury;

- bleeding problems;

- bleeding ulcers;

- pregnancy;

- surgery;

- taken blood thinning medications such as Coumadin;

- trauma;

- uncontrolled high blood pressure.

For Strokes

Most strokes are caused when blood clots move to a blood vessel in the brain and block blood flow to that area. For such strokes (ischemic strokes), thrombolytics can be used to help dissolve the clot quickly. Giving thrombolytics within three hours of the first stroke symptoms can help limit stroke damage and disability.

The decision to give the drug is based upon:

- a brain CT [computed tomography] scan to make sure there is no bleeding;

- a physical exam that shows a significant stroke;

- your medical history.

As in heart attacks, a clot-dissolving drug isn't usually given if you have one of the other medical problems listed in the preceding text.

Thrombolytics are not given to someone who is having a hemorrhagic stroke. They could worsen the stroke by causing increased bleeding.

Risks

There are various drugs used for thrombolytic therapy, but thrombolytics are used most often. Others drugs include:

- lanoteplase;

- reteplase;

- Staphylokinase;

- Streptokinase (SK);

- tenecteplase;

- urokinase.

Hemorrhage or bleeding is the most common risk. It can be life-threatening.

Minor bleeding from the gums or nose can occur in approximately 25% of people who receive the drug. Bleeding into the brain occurs approximately 1% of the time. This risk is the same for both stroke and heart attack patients.

Contact a Health Care Provider or Call 911

Heart attacks and strokes are medical emergencies. The sooner treatment with thrombolytics begins, the better the chance for a good outcome.

Section 29.2

Antiplatelets and Anticoagulants

"Let's Talk about Anticoagulants and Antiplatelet Agents," reprinted
with permission from the American Stroke Association, www.stroke
association.org, a division of the American Heart Association. © 2012
American Heart Association, Inc.

What should I know about anticoagulants?

Anticoagulants (or blood thinners) are medicines that delay the
clotting of blood. Examples are heparin, warfarin, and dabigatran.

Anticoagulants make it harder for clots to form or keep existing
clots from growing in your heart, veins, or arteries. Treatment should
be managed by your healthcare provider.

- Follow your doctor's (or other healthcare provider's) instructions.

- If you take warfarin or heparin, have regular blood tests so your
  doctor can tell how the medicine is working.

- The test for people on warfarin is called a prothrombin time (PT)
  or international normalized ratio (INR) test.

- The test for persons on heparin is called an activated partial
  thromboplastin time or a PTT test.

- Never take aspirin with anticoagulants unless your doctor tells
  you to.

- You must tell other healthcare providers that you're taking
  anticoagulants.

- Always check with your doctor before taking other medicines
  or supplements, such as aspirin, vitamins, cold medicine, pain
  medicine, sleeping pills, or antibiotics. These can affect the way
  anticoagulants work by strengthening or weakening them.

- Let your doctor know if you have been started on any new
  medications that might interfere with the action of warfarin.

- Discuss your diet with your healthcare providers. Foods rich in Vitamin K can reduce the effectiveness of anticoagulants. Vitamin K is found in leafy, green vegetables, fish, liver, lentils, soybeans, and some vegetable oils.

- Tell your family that you take anticoagulant medicine and carry your emergency medical ID card with you.

Could anticoagulants cause problems?

Yes. Tell your doctor if [the following occur]:

- Your urine turns pink or red.

- Your stools turn red, dark brown, or black. Anticoagulants and antiplatelet agents are medicines that reduce blood clotting in an artery, vein, or the heart. They can also block blood blow to your brain, causing a stroke. Doctors use them to help patients prevent strokes caused by a blood clot.

- You bleed more than normal when you have your period.

- Your gums bleed.

- You have a very bad headache or stomach pain that doesn't go away.

- You get sick or feel weak, faint, or dizzy.

- You think you're pregnant.

- You often find bruises or blood blisters.

- You have an accident of any kind.

What should I know about antiplatelet agents?

Antiplatelet medicines keep blood clots from forming by preventing blood platelets from sticking together. They are used to treat patients with atherosclerosis or with increased clotting tendencies. In atherosclerosis deposits of cholesterol form along inner walls of blood vessels, creating the conditions for blood clots to form.

- Antiplatelets are generally prescribed preventively, when atherosclerosis is evident but there is not yet a large blockage in the artery.

- Antiplatelet drugs include aspirin, ticlopidine, clopidogrel, and the combination of aspirin and dipyridamole.

- Aspirin can help prevent an ischemic stroke. It can also help if you have had a TIA [transient ischemic attack] or if you have heart problems.

You must use aspirin just as your doctor tells you.

Section 29.3

Blood Pressure-Lowering Drugs

Excerpted from "High Blood Pressure: Medicines to Help You,"
by the U.S. Food and Drug Administration (FDA, www.fda.gov),
December 5, 2011.

High blood pressure is a serious illness.

High blood pressure is often called a silent killer because many people have it but do not know it. Some people do not feel sick at first. Over time, people who do not get treated for high blood pressure can get very sick or even die.

High blood pressure can cause:

- kidney failure;

- stroke;

- blindness; and

- heart attacks.

There is good news.

There are life-saving medicines people can take every day to help control their high blood pressure. People who eat healthy foods, exercise, and take their medicines every day can control their blood pressure.

It is important to take your blood pressure medicines every day. Take your medicines even when your blood pressure comes down—even when you do not feel bad. Do not stop taking your medicine until your doctor says that it is OK.

Most people who take high blood pressure medicines do not get any side effects. Like all medicines, high blood pressure medicines can sometimes cause side effects. Some people have common problems like headaches, dizziness, or an upset stomach These problems are small compared to what could happen if you do not take your medicine.

High Blood Pressure Medicines

Use this text to help you talk to your doctor about your blood pressure medicines. Ask your doctor about the risks of taking your medicine. This text only talks about some of the risks. Tell your doctor about any problems you are having. Also, tell your doctor if you are pregnant, nursing, or planning to get pregnant. Your doctor will help you find the medicine that is best for you.

The different kinds of blood pressure medicines are listed in the following text.

ACE [Angiotensin-Converting Enzyme] Inhibitors: What You Should Know

Warnings

Women who are pregnant should talk to their doctor about the risks of using these drugs late in pregnancy.

People who have kidney or liver problems, diabetes, or heart problems should talk to their doctor about the risks of using ACE drugs.

People taking diuretics (water pills) should talk to their doctor about the risks of using ACE drugs.

Common Side Effects

- Cough
- Dizziness
- Feeling tired
- Headache
- Problems sleeping
- Fast heartbeat

Warning Signs

Call your doctor if you have any of these signs:

- Chest pain
- Problems breathing or swallowing
- Swelling in the face, eyes, lips, tongue, or legs

Beta-Blockers: What You Should Know

Warnings

Do not use these drugs if you have slow heart rate, heart block, or shock.

Women who are pregnant or nursing should talk to their doctor before they start using beta-blockers.

The elderly and people who have kidney or liver problems, asthma, diabetes, or overactive thyroid should talk to their doctor about the specific risks of using any of these beta-blockers.

Common Side Effects

- Feeling tired

- Upset stomach

- Headache

- Dizziness

- Constipation/diarrhea

- Feeling lightheaded

Warning Signs

Call your doctor if you have any of these signs:

- Chest pain

- Problems breathing

- Slow or irregular heartbeat

- Swelling in the hands, feet, or legs

Calcium Channel Blockers: What You Should Know

Warnings

Do not use calcium channel blockers if you have a heart condition or if you are taking nitrates, quinidine, or fentanyl.

People who have liver or kidney problems should talk to their doctor about the specific risks of using any calcium channel blocker.

Women who are pregnant or nursing should talk to their doctor before they start using these drugs.

Common Side Effects

- Feeling drowsy
- Headache
- Upset stomach
- Ankle swelling
- Feeling flushed (warm)

Warning Signs

Call your doctor if you have any of these signs:

- Chest pain
- Serious rashes
- Swelling of the face, eyes, lips, tongue, arms, or legs
- Fainting
- Irregular heartbeat

Peripherally Acting Alpha-Adrenergic Blockers: What You Should Know

Warnings

The elderly and people who have liver problems should talk to their doctor about the risks of using these drugs.

Common Side Effects

- Dizziness
- Feeling tired
- Feeling lightheaded
- Vision problems
- Swelling of the hands, feet, ankles, or legs
- Decreased sexual ability

Warning Signs

Call your doctor if you have any of these signs:

- Chest pain

- Irregular heartbeat
- Painful erection in men

Vasodilators: What You Should Know

Warnings

Do not use these drugs if you are also taking bisulfates.

Women who are pregnant or nursing should talk to their doctor before they start using these drugs.

People who have diabetes, heart disease, or uremia (buildup of waste in your blood) should talk to their doctor about the risks of using any of these drugs.

People taking diuretics (water pills), insulin, phenytoin, corticosteroids, estrogen, warfarin, or progesterone should talk to their doctor about the risks of using any of these drugs.

Common Side Effects

- Headache
- Upset stomach
- Dizziness
- Growth in body hair

Warning Signs

Call your doctor if you have any of these signs:

- Fever
- Fast heartbeat
- Fainting
- Chest pain
- Problems breathing
- Sudden weight gain

Angiotensin II Antagonists: What You Should Know

Warnings

Do not use these drugs if you are pregnant or nursing

People who have kidney disease, liver disease, low blood volume, or low salt in their blood should talk to their doctor about the risks of taking these drugs.

People taking diuretics (water pills) should talk to their doctor about the risks of taking these drugs.

Common Side Effects

- Sore throat
- Sinus problems
- Heartburn
- Dizziness
- Diarrhea
- Back pain

Warning Signs

Call your doctor if you have any of these signs:

- Problems breathing
- Fainting
- Swelling of the face, throat, lips, eyes, hands, feet, ankles, or legs

Centrally-Acting Alpha Adrenergics: What You Should Know

Warnings

Women who are pregnant or nursing should talk to their doctor before using these drugs.

People with heart disease, recent heart attack, or kidney disease should talk to their doctor before using these drugs.

Drinking alcohol may make side effects worse.

Common Side Effects

- Dizziness
- Dry mouth
- Upset stomach
- Feeling drowsy or tired

Warning Signs

Call your doctor if you have any of these signs:

- Fainting
- Slow or irregular heartbeat
- Fever
- Swollen ankles or feet

Renin Inhibitors: What You Should Know

Warnings

Women who are pregnant or planning to become pregnant should talk to their doctor before using this drug.

People with kidney problems should talk to their doctor before using this drug.

Tell your doctor if you are taking water pills (diuretics), high blood pressure medicines, heart medicines, or medicines to treat a fungus.

Common Side Effects

- Diarrhea

Warning Signs

Call your doctor if you have any of these signs:

- Low blood pressure
- Swelling of the face, throat, lips, eyes, or tongue

Caduet

Caduet is used to treat people who have both high blood pressure and high cholesterol.

Warnings

Do not take Caduet if you are pregnant or planning to become pregnant.

Do not take Caduet if you are breastfeeding.

Do not take Caduet if you have liver problems.

Common Side Effects

- Swelling of the legs or ankles (edema)
- Muscle or joint pain
- Headache
- Diarrhea or constipation
- Feeling dizzy
- Feeling tired or sleepy
- Gas
- Rash
- Nausea
- Stomach pain
- Fast or Irregular heartbeat
- Face feels hot or warm (flushing)

Warning Signs

Call your doctor if you have any of these signs:

- Muscle problems like weakness, tenderness, or pain that happens without a good reason (like exercise or injury)
- Brown or dark-colored urine
- Skin or eyes look yellow (jaundice)
- Feel more tired than usual

Diuretics: What You Should Know

Warnings

Tell your doctor if you are breastfeeding. These medicines may pass into your breast milk.

Do not use these medicines if you have problems making urine.

People with kidney or liver problems, pregnant women, and the elderly should talk to their doctor about the risks of using diuretics.

Common Side Effects

- Dizziness
- Frequent urination

- Headache
- Feeling thirsty
- Muscle cramps
- Upset stomach

Warning Signs

Call your doctor if you have any of these signs:

- Severe rash
- Problems breathing or swallowing
- Hyperuricemia (gout)

Questions to Ask Your Doctor

- What drugs am I taking?
- What are the side effects?
- What other prescription drugs should I avoid while taking my medicines?
- What foods, herbs, or over-the-counter medicines should I avoid?
- When should I take each drug? How many times per day do I take each drug?
- Can I take my medicines if I am pregnant or nursing?

Section 29.4

Taking Statins after Stroke Reduces Risk of Death

A new study suggests that using cholesterol-lowering medications known as statins after having a stroke may increase the likelihood of returning home and lessen the chance of dying in the hospital. The research is published in the May 22, 2012, print issue of *Neurology*, the medical journal of the American Academy of Neurology.

"Statins are known to reduce the risk of further strokes, but the timing of when a statin should be started has been unclear," said study author Alexander C. Flint, MD, PhD, with Kaiser Permanente in Redwood City, California, and a member of the American Academy of Neurology. "Our research suggests that people should be given statins while they are in the hospital."

Researchers examined the records of 12,689 people admitted to a Kaiser Permanente hospital in northern California with an ischemic stroke over a seven-year period.

Electronic medical and pharmacy records were used to determine statin use before and during stroke hospitalization.

Outcomes of hospital visits were identified as discharged to home, discharged to an institution, such as a rehabilitation center or nursing home, or death in the hospital.

The study found that people who used statins before and during their hospital stay were more likely to return home than people who did not use statins, with 57 percent of the statin users returning home compared to 47 percent of the non-users. Six percent of those who used statins before and during the hospital stay died in the hospital, compared to 11 percent of those who did not use statins.

For the study, the authors employed both a previously developed statistical technique known as grouped-treatment analysis and a new technique known as last prior treatment analysis. Together, these methods appear to strengthen the causal relationship between statin use and improved discharge disposition.

"There are a multitude of benefits to returning directly home after experiencing a stroke for the patient and the family, both functionally and financially," said Flint.

The study was supported by the Centers for Disease Control and Prevention and Kaiser Permanente Community Benefits Research Fund.

To learn more about stroke, visit www.aan.com/patients.

Chapter 30

Other Stroke Treatments

Chapter Contents

Section 30.1

Cooling the Body after Stroke Can Save Brain Function

Excerpted from "Your Brain on Ice," by Jamie Talan, *Neurology Now,*
March/April 2009. © 2009 American Academy of Neurology.
Reprinted with permission.

Each year approximately 250,000 people in the United States die of sudden cardiac arrest, in which the heart loses its rhythm, stops pumping blood, and enters into pulseless electrical activity, called ventricular fibrillation. Most of these people die on the spot. Even if emergency medical services arrives quickly and successfully resuscitates the patient—which happens as little as 20 percent of the time—there remains an 80 to 90 percent chance of severe, irreversible brain damage.

In a study published in 2004 in the *New England Journal of Medicine*, only five percent of out-of-hospital cardiac arrest patients were successfully resuscitated and survived to hospital discharge.

Stephan Mayer, MD, first heard about cooling for sudden cardiac arrest from two studies published in 2002 in the *New England Journal of Medicine*. In the larger trial, conducted in Europe, 75 of 136 patients (55 percent) resuscitated from cardiac arrest due to ventricular fibrillation had a favorable neurological outcome with the cooling treatment. In comparison, 55 of 137 patients (39 percent) had a favorable outcome with standard supportive care alone. Standard care includes reviving the patient and keeping his or her blood pressure and heart rhythm in a normal range. A smaller single-center study from Australia showed similar results.

On the heels of the paper, the American Heart Association and the International Liaison Committee on Resuscitation agreed that medical teams ought to be cooling the body following sudden cardiac arrest.

Still, brain cooling after trauma remains controversial. While there may be potential benefits to hypothermia, says Eugene Fu, MD, associate professor of clinical anesthesiology at the University of Miami, the risk for unwanted effects does exist. Hypothermia can expose people to infections and bleeding; and for those with heart disease, it can worsen myocardial ischemia, Dr. Fu observes.

Section 30.2

Gingko Biloba May Reduce Damaging Effects of Stroke

This section contains text excerpted from "Ginkgo," by the National Center for Complementary and Alternative Medicine (NCCAM, nccam.nih.gov), part of the National Institutes of Health, April 2012, and from "Researchers Investigate Effects of Ginkgo Biloba on Stroke-Related Brain Injury in Mice," by the NCCAM, published October 9, 2008, and updated January 20, 2012.

Ginkgo

The ginkgo tree is one of the oldest types of trees in the world. Ginkgo seeds have been used in traditional Chinese medicine for thousands of years, and cooked seeds are occasionally eaten. Historically, ginkgo leaf extract has been used to treat a variety of ailments and conditions, including asthma, bronchitis, fatigue, and tinnitus (ringing or roaring sounds in the ears). Today, folk uses of ginkgo leaf extracts include attempts to improve memory; to treat or help prevent Alzheimer disease and other types of dementia; to decrease intermittent claudication (leg pain caused by narrowing arteries); and to treat sexual dysfunction, multiple sclerosis, tinnitus, and other health conditions.

Extracts are usually taken from the ginkgo leaf and are used to make tablets, capsules, or teas. Occasionally, ginkgo extracts are used in skin products.

What the Science Says

Numerous studies of ginkgo have been done for a variety of conditions. Among the most widely researched are dementia, memory impairment, intermittent claudication, and tinnitus.

An NCCAM-funded study of the well-characterized ginkgo product EGb-761 found it ineffective in lowering the overall incidence of dementia and Alzheimer disease in the elderly. Further analysis of the same data also found ginkgo to be ineffective in slowing cognitive decline, lowering blood pressure, or reducing the incidence of hypertension. In this clinical trial, known as the Ginkgo Evaluation of Memory study, researchers recruited more than 3,000 volunteers age 75 and over who took 240 mg of ginkgo daily. Participants were followed for an average of approximately six years.

Some smaller studies of ginkgo for memory enhancement have had promising results, but a trial sponsored by the National Institute on Aging of more than 200 healthy adults over age 60 found that ginkgo taken for six weeks did not improve memory.

Overall, the evidence on ginkgo for symptoms of intermittent claudication has not yet shown a significant benefit for this condition, although several small studies have found modest improvements. There is conflicting evidence on the efficacy of ginkgo for tinnitus.

Other NCCAM-funded research includes studies of ginkgo for symptoms of multiple sclerosis, intermittent claudication, cognitive decline, sexual dysfunction due to antidepressants, insulin resistance, and short-term memory loss associated with electroconvulsive therapy for depression.

Side Effects and Cautions

Side effects of ginkgo may include headache, nausea, gastrointestinal upset, diarrhea, dizziness, or allergic skin reactions. More severe allergic reactions have occasionally been reported.

There are some data to suggest that ginkgo can increase bleeding risk, so people who take anticoagulant drugs, have bleeding disorders, or have scheduled surgery or dental procedures should use caution and talk to a health care provider if using ginkgo.

Fresh (raw) ginkgo seeds contain large amounts of a chemical called ginkgotoxin, which can cause serious adverse reactions—even seizures and death. Roasted seeds can also be dangerous. Products made from standardized ginkgo leaf extracts contain little ginkgotoxin and appear to be safe when used orally and appropriately.

Tell all your health care providers about any complementary health practices you use. Give them a full picture of what you do to manage your health. This will help ensure coordinated and safe care.

Researchers Investigate Effects of Ginkgo Biloba on Stroke-Related Brain Injury in Mice

Previous animal studies have indicated that an extract from leaves of the Ginkgo biloba tree may protect against stroke-related brain injury. However, the mechanism involved has not been fully understood. In a NCCAM-funded study from 2008, researchers at Johns Hopkins

University investigated whether and how the ginkgo extract EGb-761 alters outcomes in mice with brain injury from stroke.

The researchers gave the mice oral doses of EGb-761 for 7 days before and at 5 minutes and 4.5 hours after inducing strokes in the animals. Compared with controls, the pretreated mice had less neurological dysfunction and smaller areas of brain damage. The mice treated after the stroke also had less brain damage. The protective effects of EGb-761 weren't seen in a separate group of mice lacking the gene that produces the enzyme heme oxygenase-1 (HO-1)—an indication that HO-1 is part of the protective mechanism.

These findings suggest that ginkgo extracts might be useful as a preventive therapy or as a poststroke treatment to reduce the damaging effects of stroke. The researchers at Johns Hopkins are conducting additional studies to further explain the "signaling cascade" involved in ginkgo's protective effects. Although results from this study of ginkgo in mice are promising, at this time the scientific evidence for use of ginkgo to prevent or treat strokes in humans is not sufficient to make a treatment recommendation.

Reference: Saleem S, Zhuang H, Biswal S, et al. Ginkgo biloba extract neuroprotective action is dependent on heme oxygenase 1 in ischemic reperfusion brain injury. *Stroke.* 2008.

Part Five

Post-Stroke Complications and Rehabilitation

Chapter 31

Cognitive Problems Caused by Stroke

Chapter Contents

Section 31.1

Agnosia

"Agnosia Information Page," by the National Institute of Neurological Disorders and Stroke (NINDS, www.ninds.nih.gov), part of the National Institutes of Health, October 2, 2007. Reviewed by David A. Cooke, MD, FACP, January 24, 2013.

What is agnosia?

Agnosia is a rare disorder characterized by an inability to recognize and identify objects or persons. People with agnosia may have difficulty recognizing the geometric features of an object or face or may be able to perceive the geometric features but not know what the object is used for or whether a face is familiar or not. Agnosia can be limited to one sensory modality such as vision or hearing. For example, a person may have difficulty in recognizing an object as a cup or identifying a sound as a cough. Agnosia can result from strokes, dementia, developmental disorders, or other neurological conditions. It typically results from damage to specific brain areas in the occipital or parietal lobes of the brain. People with agnosia may retain their cognitive abilities in other areas.

Is there any treatment?

Treatment is generally symptomatic and supportive. The primary cause of the disorder should be determined in order to treat other problems that may contribute to or result in agnosia.

What is the prognosis?

Agnosia can compromise quality of life.

Section 31.2

Right Hemisphere Brain Damage

"Right Hemisphere Brain Damage," © 2013 American Speech-Language-Hearing Association (www.asha.org). Reproduced with permission of the American Speech-Language-Hearing Association via Copyright Clearance Center.

What is right hemisphere brain damage?

Right hemisphere brain damage is damage to the right side of the brain. The brain is made up of two sides, or hemispheres. Each hemisphere is responsible for different body functions and skills. In most people, the left side of the brain contains the person's language centers. The right side controls cognitive functioning (thinking skills).

Damage to the right hemisphere of the brain leads to cognitive-communication problems, such as impaired memory, attention problems, and poor reasoning. In many cases, the person with right brain damage is not aware of the problems that he or she is experiencing (anosognosia).

What are some signs or symptoms of right hemisphere brain damage?

Cognitive-communication problems that can occur from right hemisphere damage include difficulty with the following:

- Attention
- Left-side neglect
- Memory
- Organization
- Orientation
- Problem solving
- Reasoning
- Social communication (Pragmatics)

Attention: Difficulty concentrating on a task and paying attention for more than a few minutes at a time. Doing more than one thing at a time may be difficult or impossible.

Left-side neglect: A form of attention deficit. Essentially, the individual no longer acknowledges the left side of his/her body or space. These individuals will not brush the left side of their hair, for example, or eat food on the left side of their plate, as they do not see them or look for them. Reading is also affected as the individual does not read the words on the left side of the page, starting only from the middle.

Memory: Problems remembering information, such as street names or important dates, and learning new information easily.

Orientation: Difficulty recalling the date, time, or place. The individual may also be disoriented to self, meaning that he/she cannot correctly recall personal information, such as birth date, age, or family names.

Organization: Trouble telling a story in order, giving directions, or maintaining a topic during conversations.

Problem solving: Difficulty responding appropriately to common events, such as a car breakdown or overflowing sink. Leaving the individual unsupervised may be dangerous in such cases, as he or she could cause injury to himself or herself, or others.

Reasoning: Difficulty interpreting abstract language, such as metaphors, or responding to humor appropriately.

Social communication (pragmatics): Problems understanding nonverbal cues and following the rules of communication (e.g., saying inappropriate things, not using facial expressions, talking at the wrong time).

What treatment is available for individuals with right hemisphere brain damage?

A person with right hemisphere brain damage should see a speech-language pathologist (SLP), a professional trained to work with people with communication disorders, in addition to his or her doctor.

The SLP will work with the person and develop a treatment plan designed to improve his or her cognitive-communication abilities.

How can I communicate more effectively with a person with right hemisphere brain damage?

- Ask questions and use reminders to keep the individual on topic.

- Avoid sarcasm, metaphors, etc., when speaking to the individual.

- Provide a consistent routine every day.
- Break down instructions to small steps and repeat directions as needed.
- Decrease distractions when communicating.
- Provide appropriate supervision to ensure the person's safety.
- Stand to the person's right side and place objects to the person's right if he or she is experiencing left-side neglect.
- Use calendars, clocks, and notepads to remind the person of important information.

What causes right hemisphere brain damage?

The causes of right hemisphere brain damage include the following:

- Infection/illness
- Stroke
- Surgery
- Traumatic brain injury (TBI)
- Tumor

How effective are treatments for right hemisphere brain damage?

ASHA has developed a treatment efficacy summary on right hemisphere brain damage that describes evidence about how well treatment works. This summary is useful not only to individuals with right hemisphere brain damage and their caregivers but also to insurance companies considering payment for much needed services for right hemisphere brain damage.

Section 31.3

Vascular Dementia

Excerpted from "Dementia: Hope through Research," by the National Institute of Neurological Disorders and Stroke (NINDS, www.ninds.nih.gov), part of the National Institutes of Health, May 16, 2012.

What Is Dementia?

Dementia is not a specific disease. It is a descriptive term for a collection of symptoms that can be caused by a number of disorders that affect the brain. People with dementia have significantly impaired intellectual functioning that interferes with normal activities and relationships. They also lose their ability to solve problems and maintain emotional control, and they may experience personality changes and behavioral problems such as agitation, delusions, and hallucinations. While memory loss is a common symptom of dementia, memory loss by itself does not mean that a person has dementia. Doctors diagnose dementia only if two or more brain functions—such as memory, language skills, perception, or cognitive skills including reasoning and judgment—are significantly impaired without loss of consciousness.

There are many disorders that can cause dementia. Some, such as Alzheimer disease, or AD, lead to a progressive loss of mental functions. But other types of dementia can be halted or reversed with appropriate treatment.

With AD and many other types of dementia, disease processes cause many nerve cells to stop functioning, lose connections with other neurons, and die. In contrast, normal aging does not result in the loss of large numbers of neurons in the brain.

Vascular Dementia

Vascular dementia is the second most common cause of dementia, after AD. It accounts for up to 20 percent of all dementias and is caused by brain damage from cerebrovascular or cardiovascular problems—usually strokes. It also may result from genetic diseases, endocarditis (infection of a heart valve), or amyloid angiopathy (a process in which amyloid protein builds up in the brain's blood vessels, sometimes causing hemorrhagic or bleeding strokes). In many cases, it may coexist with AD. The incidence of vascular dementia increases with advancing age and is similar in men and women.

Symptoms of vascular dementia often begin suddenly, frequently after a stroke. Patients may have a history of high blood pressure, vascular disease, or previous strokes or heart attacks. Vascular dementia may or may not get worse with time, depending on whether the person has additional strokes. In some cases, symptoms may get better with time. When the disease does get worse, it often progresses in a stepwise manner, with sudden changes in ability. Vascular dementia with brain damage to the mid-brain regions, however, may cause a gradual, progressive cognitive impairment that may look much like AD. Unlike people with AD, people with vascular dementia often maintain their personality and normal levels of emotional responsiveness until the later stages of the disease.

People with vascular dementia frequently wander at night and often have other problems commonly found in people who have had a stroke, including depression and incontinence.

There are several types of vascular dementia, which vary slightly in their causes and symptoms. One type, called multi-infarct dementia (MID), is caused by numerous small strokes in the brain. MID typically includes multiple damaged areas, called infarcts, along with extensive lesions in the white matter, or nerve fibers, of the brain.

Because the infarcts in MID affect isolated areas of the brain, the symptoms are often limited to one side of the body or they may affect just one or a few specific functions, such as language. Neurologists call these local or focal symptoms, as opposed to the global symptoms seen in AD, which affect many functions and are not restricted to one side of the body.

Although not all strokes cause dementia, in some cases a single stroke can damage the brain enough to cause dementia. This condition is called single-infarct dementia. Dementia is more common when the stroke takes place on the left side (hemisphere) of the brain and/or when it involves the hippocampus, a brain structure important for memory.

Another type of vascular dementia is called Binswanger disease. This rare form of dementia is characterized by damage to small blood vessels in the white matter of the brain (white matter is found in the inner layers of the brain and contains many nerve fibers coated with a whitish, fatty substance called myelin). Binswanger disease leads to brain lesions, loss of memory, disordered cognition, and mood changes. Patients with this disease often show signs of abnormal blood pressure, stroke, blood abnormalities, disease of the large blood vessels in the neck, and/or disease of the heart valves. Other prominent features include urinary incontinence, difficulty walking, clumsiness, slowness, lack of facial expression, and speech difficulty. These symptoms, which usually begin after the age of 60, are not always present in all patients and may sometimes appear only temporarily. Treatment of Binswanger disease is symptomatic, and may include the use of medications to control high blood pressure, depression, heart arrhythmias, and low blood pressure. The disorder often includes episodes of partial recovery.

Another type of vascular dementia is linked to a rare hereditary disorder called CADASIL, which stands for cerebral autosomal dominant arteriopathy with subcortical infarct and leukoencephalopathy. CADASIL is linked to abnormalities of a specific gene, Notch3, which is located on chromosome 19. This condition causes multi-infarct dementia as well as stroke, migraine with aura, and mood disorders. The first symptoms usually appear in people who are in their twenties, thirties, or forties and affected individuals often die by age 65. Researchers believe most people with CADASIL go undiagnosed, and the actual prevalence of the disease is not yet known.

Other causes of vascular dementia include vasculitis, an inflammation of the blood vessel system; profound hypotension (low blood pressure); and lesions caused by brain hemorrhage. The autoimmune disease lupus erythematosus and the inflammatory disease temporal arteritis can also damage blood vessels in a way that leads to vascular dementia.

Treatment for Vascular Dementia

There is no standard drug treatment for vascular dementia, although some of the symptoms, such as depression, can be treated. Most other treatments aim to reduce the risk factors for further brain damage. However, some studies have found that cholinesterase inhibitors, such as galantamine and other AD drugs, can improve cognitive function and behavioral symptoms in patients with early vascular dementia.

The progression of vascular dementia can often be slowed significantly or halted if the underlying vascular risk factors for the disease are treated. To prevent strokes and TIAs (transient ischemic attacks), doctors may prescribe medicines to control high blood pressure, high cholesterol, heart disease, and diabetes. Doctors also sometimes prescribe aspirin, warfarin, or other drugs to prevent clots from forming in small blood vessels. When patients have blockages in blood vessels, doctors may recommend surgical procedures, such as carotid endarterectomy, stenting, or angioplasty, to restore the normal blood supply. Medications to relieve restlessness or depression or to help patients sleep better may also be prescribed.

Chapter 32

Communication Problems after Stroke

Many people have communication problems after a stroke. About a third of stroke survivors have some difficulty with speaking or understanding what others say, and this can be frightening and frustrating. This text is aimed at family members and carers who support people with these difficulties. It explains the types of problems that can arise, the help and support available, and offers some tips to aid communication.

What Is a Stroke?

A stroke is an injury to the brain. The brain controls everything we do including everything we interpret and understand.

A stroke can cause problems with communicating if there is damage to the parts of the brain responsible for language.

These functions are controlled by the left side of the brain in most people. As one side of the brain controls the opposite side of the body, many people who have communication problems after stroke also have weakness or paralysis on the right side of their body.

Stroke can also cause communication problems if muscles in the face, tongue, or throat are affected.

How Can Stroke Affect Communication?

The range of communication problems someone has will depend on where in the brain the stroke happened and how large an area was damaged.

A stroke can affect how you speak, understand speech, read, or write.

A stroke can affect communication in different ways. The main conditions that can happen after stroke are:

- aphasia;

- dysarthria;

- dyspraxia.

Aphasia

Aphasia (sometimes called dysphasia) is the name for the most common language disorder caused by stroke. Aphasia can affect how you speak, your ability to understand what is being said, and your reading or writing skills. It does not affect intelligence, although sometimes people think it does.

Aphasia can be very mild, and sometimes only affects one form of communication, such as reading. However, it is more common for several aspects of communication to be affected at the same time.

There are different types of aphasia:

- If your problems are mainly with understanding what is being said, this is called receptive aphasia.

- If you mostly understand others, but have difficulties expressing what you want to say, this is called expressive aphasia.

- A combination of problems that changes all or most of your communication may be referred to as mixed aphasia, or global aphasia if the effects are severe.

In the following text are some examples of the different ways aphasia can affect you.

People with receptive aphasia may:

- not understand much of what other people say and feel as though others are talking in an unknown foreign language;

- not understand when people speak in long, complex sentences and may forget the start of what they said;

- not understand others if there is background noise or if different people are talking in a group;
- be able to read newspaper headlines, but not understand the rest of the text;
- be able to write but unable to read back what they've written.

People with expressive aphasia may [experience the following]:

- Not be able to speak at all: They may communicate by making sounds but not be able to form words.
- Have difficulty speaking in normal sentences: They may say only single words or very short sentences, missing out crucial words. They may write in a similar way.
- Speak with frequent pauses and be unable to find the word they want to say—yet it may be on the tip of their tongue.
- Answer 'yes' or 'no,' but mean the opposite so their answers are not reliable.
- Think of the word they want to say, but another word comes out—for example, 'milk' instead of 'water.'
- Speak at a normal rate, but much of what they say is unrecognizable and has limited meaning: They may not realize this and others may wrongly think they are confused.
- Describe or refer to objects and places, but not be able to name them: They miss out the words they can't think of.
- Say only a few set words in answer to any question: They may be emotional words, such as swear words.
- Get stuck on a single word or sound and end up repeating it.

Dysarthria

Dysarthria happens when a stroke causes weakness of the muscles you use to speak.

This may affect the muscles you use to move your tongue, lips or mouth, control your breathing when you speak, or produce your voice.

Dysarthria does not affect your ability to find the words you want to say or to understand others, unless you have other communication problems at the same time. If you have dysarthria, your voice may sound different and you may have difficulty speaking clearly. You may find your voice sounds slurred, strained, quiet, or slow.

Other people may find your voice hard to understand. If breath control is affected, you may need to speak in short bursts rather than in complete sentences.

Dyspraxia

Dyspraxia is a condition that affects movement and coordination. Dyspraxia of speech happens when you cannot move muscles in the correct order and sequence to make the sounds needed for clear speech.

The individual muscles you use to produce clear speech may be working well and you may have no weakness or paralysis, but you cannot move them as and when you want to in the right order and in a consistent way.

If you have dyspraxia, you may not be able to pronounce words clearly, especially when someone asks you to say them. You may try several times to repeat them and may want to keep trying to correct yourself. At times, you may be unable to make any sound at all.

It can be frightening and distressing to have difficulty communicating after stroke. It can be difficult to join in conversations and this can be very frustrating. If the ability to read is affected, everyday activities such as choosing from a menu or reading signs or prescriptions can become problems.

What Other Effects of Stroke Affect Communication?

Stroke can cause other problems that affect a person's ability to communicate well. It may help to be aware of these during conversations.

Changes to the Emotional Content of Communication

A stroke can sometimes cause subtle changes to emotional aspects of speech.

For example, your tone of voice may sound flat or your facial expression may not vary. You may have difficulty understanding humor or when to take turns in conversation. You may be aware of these effects and frustrated by them, or you may be unaware. These types of changes can happen even if there are no other communication problems after stroke.

They are due to changes on the right side of the brain and can be misinterpreted as depression.

Changes to Perception

A stroke can alter your vision and sometimes your hearing. This can make reading and writing problems worse. Make sure the doctor is made aware of such problems so that they can be fully assessed.

Tiredness

Many people find that they feel very tired after a stroke, both physically and mentally.

Having a conversation may also take more effort than it used to, and other people may not realize this. The ability to communicate can vary significantly depending on how tired or stressed someone is feeling.

Memory and Concentration Problems

Stroke can affect your short-term memory and aspects of your thinking processes, such as the ability to focus and concentrate.

This can make communication slower and more difficult.

Physical problems

Physical weakness or paralysis after stroke may affect facial expressions and body language. Physical problems can also make writing difficulties worse if your dominant hand is affected. Physical pain or discomfort can be a distraction. Swallowing problems are also common after stroke and often associated with dysarthria.

Changes to Mood or Personality

It can be frightening and frustrating if a stroke has affected your ability to communicate. Changes in the brain caused by the stroke can also affect mood, emotions, and personality in other ways that can be difficult to control.

Tips for Helping Conversation

Helping someone with aphasia to understand you:

- Keep your own language clear and simple.

- Speak in a normal tone of voice.

- Don't rush the conversation. Give the person time to take in what you say and to respond.

- Assume the person can hear and understand well, in spite of any difficulties responding, unless you learn otherwise.

- Stick to one topic at a time using short sentences. For example, instead of saying, "Your wife called and she will be here at 4 pm to pick you up and take you home," say: "Your wife called."

(pause) "She will be here at 4 pm." (pause) "You can go home then."

- Use all forms of communication to help reinforce what you are saying, such as clear gestures, drawing, and communication aids.

- Use adult language and don't talk down to the person with aphasia. Even if someone understands little or nothing, remember they are not a child.

Helping Someone with Aphasia to Express Themselves

- Don't interrupt them. Watch out for when they are finished, or when they are looking for help. Ask if your help is needed before giving it.

- If it helps them to remember things, make use of a diary, calendar, or photos. Lists of words or options to select from can help.

- If they can't think of a word, ask how it is spelt. Write down the first letter or syllable as a prompt.

- Write down key words with a marker pen. Write clearly in lower case and don't underline. Keep the lists of words to refer back to.

- If they prefer, guess the word they can't find and ask if it's correct.

- If they are keen to find the right word, give them more time to respond, or guess their meaning and check if you're correct. Otherwise, if they prefer and you've understood the message, just carry on the conversation.

- If easier for them, establish the general topic of their message by asking careful questions that only require a 'Yes' or 'No' answer. Give them plenty of time to respond. Don't ask too many questions too quickly, as they may feel overwhelmed and become frustrated.

- Look as well as listen—you will get a lot of information from natural gestures, facial expressions, and body language. Check these are consistent with their message.

- Encourage them to give you extra help. Ask if there is anything they can point to, gesture, write, or draw to help you understand. If they write or draw for you, allow extra time if they are learning to do so with their non-dominant hand.

- If they are repeating a single sound or word, it may help to distract them by changing topic or activity. Allow time for their memory to clear before asking another question.

- Don't pretend to understand. If you're having difficulty, be honest and tell them: "I'm sorry, I don't understand—let's try again." Or arrange another time to come back to the topic—and don't forget!

Other Useful Tips

- Remember they may have difficulty with attention and concentration. So minimize distractions such as background noise. Focus on just one topic and one person at a time.

- At the start of conversation, check the person is comfortable and there are no problems. If they normally wear glasses, a hearing aid, or dentures, make sure these are available. This can make a big difference to communication.

- Check you have both understood before moving to another topic. Summarize what they said and ask if this is correct. If not, try asking a question in a different way.

- Try to keep conversation natural and meaningful to them. Talk about real hobbies and people.

- Look at a photo album together and talk about the places visited and the people in the photos.

- A personal file, with useful, meaningful information about the person, their life, and their interests, will be a way for them to talk about themselves. This can also take the pressure off speaking.

- Keep a diary of visits and what you talked about. Encourage family and friends to write in it when they come. Point out progress others have noticed and that they may have not.

- Tell them in advance if you want to discuss something important, so you can both prepare.

- Don't be afraid to acknowledge when you both feel frustrated or tired, or if you have a day when communication seems impossible. This happens. It may be no one's fault if conversation breaks down.

- If you're extra busy, it may help you both to agree regular times for communication practice. This might be short periods (around 30 minutes) and planned at times when you are both relaxed.

Chapter 33

Swallowing
Problems after Stroke

Swallowing is a complex activity that involves the coordination of many nerves and muscles. At least 40 percent of stroke survivors will initially experience some difficulty swallowing, although for many people it improves quite quickly. This text explains the signs of swallowing problems, the complications that can happen, the key ways to manage these difficulties, and some tips for safer swallowing.

How Can a Stroke Affect Swallowing?

Swallowing problems occur after stroke when the parts of your brain that control swallowing are affected. The medical term used to describe any difficulties or pain in eating, chewing, drinking, or swallowing is dysphagia.

Muscle weakness, problems with attention and concentration, balance difficulties, and poor coordination can also affect your ability to swallow food and drink safely.

Most people regain the ability to swallow safely within several weeks. How long it takes depends on the severity of your stroke and the parts of your brain which have been affected. Recovery is different for everyone.

What Are the Signs of Swallowing Problems?

Common signs include:

- not being able to swallow;
- difficulty chewing or swallowing;
- coughing or choking before, during, or after swallowing;
- difficulty controlling food or fluid in the mouth;
- bringing food back up, sometimes through the nose;
- drooling;
- a hoarse voice;
- a gargly or a wet sounding voice;
- the sensation of food or drink catching in your throat.

In the long term symptoms may include unexplained weight loss or frequent chest infections.

What Are the Hazards?

There are several reasons why swallowing problems need to be managed properly:

Aspiration: This is the medical term used to describe something going down the wrong way. The entrances to your airway and your stomach are very close together. Aspiration occurs when food, fluid, and/or saliva enters your airway and lungs. Usually if this happens you will cough. However, the effects of the stroke may mean you are not aware something has gone down the wrong way and the coughing reflex may not happen. Signs of aspiration can include coughing and a change in your voice. Sometimes people do not have any noticeable signs of aspiration and this is known as silent aspiration.

Aspiration pneumonia: This is a chest infection that occurs when food or fluid get into your lungs then irritate and damage them. Symptoms of aspiration pneumonia include a cough, high temperature, chest pain, and difficulty breathing. The condition will usually be treated with antibiotics.

Malnutrition: If you are not able to swallow properly, you may not be able to eat a balanced diet that includes all the nutrients you need and you may develop malnutrition.

Dehydration: It is important that your body gets enough water and remains hydrated. If you have difficulty swallowing, you may become dehydrated.

How Are Swallowing Problems Assessed?

Immediate screening: After you have been admitted to hospital, your swallowing should be screened by a trained healthcare professional, such as a nurse, doctor, or speech and language therapist. This should happen before you are given anything to eat or drink or any medication to swallow. Ideally this should take place within four hours of you being admitted. They will usually ask you to swallow a small amount of water and may ask you to swallow different consistencies in order to observe your swallowing ability.

Assessment: If the screen identifies problems you should then have a specialist assessment of your swallowing. This should take place no more than 72 hours after your admission to hospital and ideally within 24 hours. The assessment will usually be carried out by a speech and language therapist or another specially trained professional. It may include advice on how to manage your swallowing problems and may include a referral for further investigation.

Further investigation: The following two tests are common:

- A videofluoroscopy is a procedure that involves taking a series of x-ray images of the parts of your body involved in swallowing. You may be asked to swallow food and drink of different consistencies that are mixed with a non-toxic solution, which will show up on an x-ray. The images will show if the food or drink is going down the wrong way into your airway. These images may identify what is wrong with your swallowing and may help identify strategies that may help.

- A fiberoptic endoscopic evaluation of swallowing (FEES) involves a long thin, flexible tube that has a light and a camera on the end (endoscope). It is placed up one nostril and moved into position so that it can view images of the back of your throat and the structures involved in swallowing. The findings may show what happened to the food and drink before and after the swallow. It may also identify the nature and cause of aspiration and be helpful in deciding on treatment and rehabilitation. The advantages of this test are that it is easy and safe to do with relatively little discomfort and it can be completed at the bed side.

Hydration assessment: Your body's level of hydration should be assessed when you are admitted. This is done by taking a blood or urine test. This should then be monitored to make sure you do not become dehydrated.

Malnutrition screening: Different screening tools for malnutrition may be used, for example the MUST—the Malnutrition Universal Screening Tool. Screening involves measuring your height and weight to calculate your body mass index (BMI), noting any unplanned weight loss and any illnesses. Screening should be repeated weekly while you are in the hospital or when there is concern that you may be malnourished.

Nil by mouth: If the health care team feels that your swallow is unsafe, they may advise that you should not eat or drink anything until you have your swallow assessed. While you are nil by mouth you should be given fluids and foods by other means to keep you hydrated and maintain your nutrition levels.

How Are Swallowing Problems Treated and Managed?

A team of different healthcare professionals, usually including a doctor, speech and language therapist, dietitian, and nutrition nurse, will work closely with you, your family, and any carers to manage your swallowing difficulties. The aim of managing your swallowing problems will be to avoid aspiration, to help you swallow safely, to make sure your body remains hydrated, to make sure you get the nutrients you need to stay healthy and to maximize your quality of life. Swallowing problems can impact your overall recovery from stroke, so it is important you get the right help.

The health care team should involve you and your family in any decisions and provide you with information. Until you are able to swallow safely, written guidance should be provided to any staff or carers involved in giving you nutrition or fluids. Any methods you use to manage your swallowing problems should be reviewed regularly to ensure they continue to be suitable.

The methods listed in the following text may help you to manage your swallowing difficulties. These may be included in a program of swallowing therapy designed and monitored specifically for you.

Food and fluid alterations: The presentation of your food may need changing to ensure you can swallow it safely. This may involve altering the temperature, texture, taste, and thickness. For example, fruit and vegetables might be pureed or a thickener may be added to a drink.

Commercial thickeners can be used to vary the consistency of your food from solid to liquid and from thin to pudding-like. If you require food or fluid alterations, you should be referred to a dietitian or nutrition team so they can make sure you get the right balance of nutrients and this is monitored. As your swallowing improves, you may be able to progress to a normal diet.

Meal changes: The time, how often you eat, and the size of your portions may need to be changed, particularly if you are finding eating tiring, have difficulty concentrating, and are sometimes not hungry.

Postural/swallowing techniques: You may be advised to undertake different postures and swallowing techniques that change the way you swallow your food and drink. These can help you to swallow more easily and safely. You may also be provided with specialist seating equipment to help you sit in the best position. A physiotherapist and occupational therapist may assist with this.

Environmental changes: Your environment affects the way that you swallow. To make meal times as safe and pleasurable as possible, it is important to make the environment as suitable as possible. This may involve reducing distractions and noise, getting the right lighting levels and helping you to have some social interaction at mealtimes.

Exercises: You may be given a number of chewing and swallowing exercises to help maintain and improve the muscles you use for eating and drinking.

Practical help: You may find it takes you a long time to eat. You may be offered assistance at mealtimes or given equipment or utensils to help you eat independently and safely. For example, you may be provided with cutlery that is easier to grip, a non-slip mat to place items on, or a cup that is specially shaped so you don't have to tilt your head back when drinking.

Other Feeding Methods

If you are unable to get the nutrition and fluids you need by eating and drinking then you may be given food and drink by a tube (enteral feeding.) The medical professionals should discuss their expectations for the use of tube feeding with you, including what would happen without tube feeding, the quality of life you will have with or without tube feeding, and the impact on you and your carers. The most common types of tube feeding you may be given are:

Nasogastric (NG) tube: This is a thin tube that goes up your nose, down the back of your throat, and into your stomach to enable you to be fed a liquid containing all the nutrients your body needs. The tube is connected to a container of liquid feed and you are given doses of feed continuously or at regular intervals called bolus feeds. The tube may cause some irritation but, once in place, the tube is usually comfortable and you will soon forget it is there.

If you are going to have a nasogastric tube, it should be put in place within 24 hours of admission to the hospital. If you tolerate an NG tube well and don't need it for longer than six weeks then you shouldn't need to have a PEG tube.

Percutaneous endoscopic gastrostomy (PEG) tube: If you have longer-term swallowing problems, you may need to be fed through a PEG tube. This is a tube that is inserted directly through the wall of your abdomen into your stomach and can be easily hidden by your clothes. It is inserted while you are awake, but sedated.

There is a possibility of complications including the tube getting out of place, becoming blocked or leaking, and there is a risk of infection and internal bleeding. If you have not eaten for some time before the tube is fitted, it can also take time for your bowel to get used to the feeds.

You may experience diarrhea, bloating, constipation, and reflux or vomiting at first.

There are both advantages and disadvantages associated with nasogastric and percutaneous endoscopic gastrostomy tubes. These should be discussed with you before any decision is made. Both tubes offer an alternative to eating and drinking or they may be used to give you vital nutrition and fluids if you are only eating or drinking small amounts. Your health care team will advise you which approach they feel is appropriate for you. Both tubes may be removed on medical advice if your swallow improves.

Maintaining Good Health

Nutrition Support

If you are at risk of malnutrition, you may be given nutrition support. This could be nutritional supplements, special nutrient-rich foods, dietary advice, and/or tube feeding. The aim will be to ensure you get the right balance of nutrients. This is important as malnutrition is associated with a slower recovery and poorer outcome for stroke survivors. If you have not eaten anything for a while, food may need to be reintroduced gradually. Your nutrition support should be reviewed regularly.

Oral Care

It is important to look after your mouth, teeth, and gums to make sure your mouth does not become dry or sore. Some medication can also add to difficulties by giving you a dry mouth or affecting your ability to manage your saliva. If you are not able to swallow, you or your carer should regularly take steps to maintain good oral health (ideally every four hours). These include brushing your teeth, cleaning your gums, and cleaning any dentures. You may need to keep your mouth moist by using wet swabs and putting some petroleum jelly around your lips. Your health care team may be able to offer further advice about oral care to suit your needs.

Coping with Swallowing Problems in the Long Term

Eating and drinking are a large part of daily life. As well as ensuring your body gets the necessary fluids and nutrients to maintain good health, they are also pleasurable and social activities. If you have long-term swallowing difficulties you may feel you have lost the enjoyable experience of eating, both alone and in company. This can also have an impact on your family.

You may need to be fed through a tube in the long term or continue to have modified foods. Once you leave hospital, you and your carers should be provided with support and information to manage any ongoing swallowing problems. This should include details of your difficulties, the support you need, how to put into practice any eating and drinking plans, and when to ask for further support. Support may include the following:

Tube Feeding Support

If you need NG or PEG tube feeding on a long-term basis you should be supported in the community by a team of different health care professionals including a dietitian, nurses, your physician, pharmacist, and, if appropriate, a speech and language therapist. You should be given:

- an individual care plan covering the aims of your treatment and the plans for monitoring this;

- an opportunity to discuss your treatment options and the physical, psychological, and social issues your tube feeding brings;

- training for you and your carer and an instruction manual covering all aspects of your tube feeding such as how to overcome common problems;

- regular checkups at a specialist clinic;

- general and emergency contact numbers for a relevant professional you can contact if you have any questions and for relevant support organizations;

- information about your tube feeding equipment delivery arrangements.

Products

You should be provided with any products you need, such as a food thickener which is available from your GP. You may like to use molds to shape pureed food so it looks more attractive.

Training and Support from Others

You and/or your carer should be given training to manage your swallowing difficulties. For example, your carer may be shown a particular technique to help you swallow. Your carer should know how to create the best environment for safe, efficient and pleasurable eating and drinking.

They should be able to identify problems and know when to ask for a review of your swallowing difficulties. If you have difficulties with memory and attention, your carer may need to prompt you to eat meals or snacks and sit with you till you finish a meal. If you don't feel like eating, your family may be able to help by identifying foods you particularly like.

Support in a Care Home

If you move into a care home, any staff involved in your care should be trained in recognizing and managing swallowing difficulties and oral hygiene. The care home should make sure they have enough staff to assist you if you take longer to eat.

Tips for Safe Swallowing

Everyone is different but the following suggestions may help you swallow more safely. Always check with a medical professional if you are unsure of what will help you.

- Allow yourself time.

- Eat in a quiet environment, free from distractions and interruptions.

- Try to remain calm. Being tense makes swallowing more difficult.

- Take one mouthful at a time, ensuring that all the food has been swallowed before taking the next.

- Make sure the food is a temperature and consistency you can swallow safely.

- Do not mix food and drink in the same mouthful.

- Arrange comfortable and safe seating for you and anyone helping you to eat.

- Remain sitting upright for 30 minutes after eating or drinking.

- Make sure you get any medication prescribed in a suitable form, e.g., liquid.

- Make food look attractive so you feel more like eating it.

- Persist with thickeners and drink supplements, as prescribed, to ensure you swallow safely.

- Have meals at regular times and possibly try having smaller meals more frequently.

- Write yourself reminders to eat or ask family and carers to remind you.

- Make sure your carers and family understand your swallowing problems and how they can support and encourage you.

- Speak to your doctor, nurse, speech and language therapist, or another health care professional should you need more help and information.

Chapter 34

Muscle Spasticity and Weakness after Stroke

Chapter Contents

Section 34.1

Overview of Spasticity

"Spasticity Information Page," by the National Institute of Neurological Disorders and Stroke (NINDS, www.ninds.nih.gov), part of the National Institutes of Health, October 4, 2011.

Spasticity is a condition in which there is an abnormal increase in muscle tone or stiffness of muscle, which might interfere with movement, speech, or be associated with discomfort or pain. Spasticity is usually caused by damage to nerve pathways within the brain or spinal cord that control muscle movement. It may occur in association with spinal cord injury, multiple sclerosis, cerebral palsy, stroke, brain or head trauma, amyotrophic lateral sclerosis, hereditary spastic paraplegias, and metabolic diseases such as adrenoleukodystrophy, phenylketonuria, and Krabbe disease. Symptoms may include hypertonicity (increased muscle tone), clonus (a series of rapid muscle contractions), exaggerated deep tendon reflexes, muscle spasms, scissoring (involuntary crossing of the legs), and fixed joints (contractures). The degree of spasticity varies from mild muscle stiffness to severe, painful, and uncontrollable muscle spasms. Spasticity can interfere with rehabilitation in patients with certain disorders, and often interferes with daily activities.

Treatment may include such medications as baclofen, diazepam, tizanidine, or clonazepam. Physical therapy regimens may include muscle stretching and range of motion exercises to help prevent shrinkage or shortening of muscles and to reduce the severity of symptoms. Targeted injection of botulinum toxin into muscles with the most tone can help to selectively weaken these muscles to improve range of motion and function. Surgery may be recommended for tendon release or to sever the nerve-muscle pathway.

The prognosis for those with spasticity depends on the severity of the spasticity and the associated disorder(s).

Section 34.2

Foot Drop

Excerpted from "Foot Drop Information Page," by the National
Institute of Neurological Disorders and Stroke (NINDS, www.ninds.nih.gov),
part of the National Institutes of Health, January 29, 2009.

What is foot drop?

Foot drop describes the inability to raise the front part of the foot
due to weakness or paralysis of the muscles that lift the foot. As a
result, individuals with foot drop scuff their toes along the ground
or bend their knees to lift their foot higher than usual to avoid the
scuffing, which causes what is called a steppage gait. Foot drop can
be unilateral (affecting one foot) or bilateral (affecting both feet). Foot
drop is a symptom of an underlying problem and is either temporary
or permanent, depending on the cause. Causes include: neurodegenerative disorders of the brain that cause muscular problems, such as
multiple sclerosis, stroke, and cerebral palsy; motor neuron disorders
such as polio, some forms of spinal muscular atrophy and amyotrophic
lateral sclerosis (commonly known as Lou Gehrig disease); injury to
the nerve roots, such as in spinal stenosis; peripheral nerve disorders
such as Charcot-Marie-Tooth disease or acquired peripheral neuropa-
thy; local compression or damage to the peroneal nerve as it passes
across the fibular bone below the knee; and muscle disorders, such as
muscular dystrophy or myositis.

Is there any treatment?

Treatment depends on the specific cause of foot drop. The most common treatment is to support the foot with lightweight leg braces and
shoe inserts, called ankle-foot orthotics. Exercise therapy to strengthen
the muscles and maintain joint motion also helps to improve gait.
Devices that electrically stimulate the peroneal nerve during footfall
are appropriate for a small number of individuals with foot drop. In
cases with permanent loss of movement, surgery that fuses the foot
and ankle joint or that transfers tendons from stronger leg muscles is
occasionally performed.

What is the prognosis?

The prognosis for foot drop depends on the cause. Foot drop caused by trauma or nerve damage usually shows partial or even complete recovery. For progressive neurological disorders, foot drop will be a symptom that is likely to continue as a lifelong disability, but it will not shorten life expectancy.

Section 34.3

Hand Paralysis in Animals Restored after Brain-Activated Muscle Stimulation

"Brain-Activated Muscle Stimulation Restores Monkeys' Hand Movement after Paralysis," by the National Institute of Neurological Disorders and Stroke (NINDS, www.ninds.nih.gov), part of the National Institutes of Health, June 11, 2012.

An artificial connection between the brain and muscles can restore complex hand movements in monkeys following paralysis, according to a study funded by the National Institutes of Health.

In a report in the [April 18, 2012 issue of the] journal *Nature*, researchers describe how they combined two pieces of technology to create a neuroprosthesis—a device that replaces lost or impaired nervous system function. One piece is a multi-electrode array implanted directly into the brain which serves as a brain-computer interface (BCI). The array allows researchers to detect the activity of about 100 brain cells and decipher the signals that generate arm and hand movements. The second piece is a functional electrical stimulation (FES) device that delivers electrical current to the paralyzed muscles, causing them to contract. The brain array activates the FES device directly, bypassing the spinal cord to allow intentional, brain-controlled muscle contractions and restore movement.

The research team was led by Lee E. Miller, PhD, professor of physiology at Northwestern University's Feinberg School of Medicine in Chicago. Prior to testing the neuroprosthesis, Dr. Miller's group recorded the brain and muscle activity of two healthy monkeys as the animals performed a task requiring them to reach out, grasp a ball, and release it. The researchers then used the data from the brain-controlled FES device to determine the patterns of muscle activity predicted by the brain activity.

To test the device, the researchers gave monkeys an anesthetic to locally block nerve activity at the elbow, causing temporary paralysis of the hand. With the aid of the neuroprosthesis, both monkeys regained movement in the paralyzed hand, could pick up and move the ball in a nearly routine manner and complete the task as before.

Dr. Miller's research team also performed grip strength tests, and found that their system restored precision grasping ability. The device allowed voluntary and intentional adjustments in force and grip strength, which are keys to performing everyday tasks naturally and successfully.

This new research moves beyond earlier work from Dr. Miller's group showing that a similar neuroprosthesis restores monkeys' ability to flex or extend the wrist despite paralysis. "With these neural engineering methods, we can take some of the important basic physiology that we know about the brain, and use it to connect the brain directly to muscles," Dr. Miller said. "This connection from brain to muscles might someday be used to help patients paralyzed due to spinal cord injury perform activities of daily living and achieve greater independence."

In 2008, a team led by Eberhard Fetz, PhD at the University of Washington in Seattle coupled the activity of single neurons to an FES device similar to the one used for Miller's study. Monkeys learned to activate individual neurons to control the FES device and move a joystick, and could adapt neurons previously unassociated with wrist movement to complete the task. The investigators suggest that this process of learning and adaption plays an important role in how the BCI translates the brain's activity patterns into adaptive control of the FES device.

The unique design of the ball grasp-and-release task used with the animals in this study is a further contribution to advanced neuroprosthetic testing and development. Daofen Chen, PhD, a program director at NIH's National Institute of Neurological Disorders and Stroke (NINDS), described how researchers in the field are striving toward devices that will go beyond simple arm movements and allow fine hand and finger movements. "We've learned a lot from non-human primate studies focused on understanding neural control of arm and wrist movements," said Dr. Chen. "Dr. Miller's study builds on those efforts and focuses on the complex hand and finger movements needed to grasp an object."

FES devices are currently used for foot drop, a clinical condition seen in patients with stroke or partial spinal cord injury where weak or paralyzed muscles cause the toes to catch on the ground while walking, leading to trips and falls. FES can be activated with shoe sensors, or coordinated with walking movements, to stimulate muscles and lift the toes at the appropriate time during a step.

Other FES devices in current clinical use take advantage of the patient's residual muscle activity. For example, a prosthetic arm can use sensors built into the shoulder, sensing a shrugging motion that is used to stimulate muscles to open or close the hand. However, this is a less precise and less natural method of control, and it is not an option for patients with higher level spinal cord injuries and little or no shoulder and arm movement. For these patients, the creation of a brain-controlled FES device that connects brain activity directly to muscle stimulation would provide an opportunity to restore hand function.

The temporary nerve block used in the current study is a useful model of paralysis, but it does not replicate the chronic changes that occur after prolonged brain and spinal cord injuries, Dr. Miller cautioned. He said the next steps include testing this system in primate models of long-term paralysis, and studying how the brain changes as it continues to use this neuroprosthesis.

Reference: Ethier C et al. "Restoration of grasp following paralysis through brain-controlled stimulation of muscles." *Nature*, published online April 18, 2012.

Section 34.4

Robot Therapy Helps Stroke Patients Regain Motor Function

Excerpted from "Robot Therapy Helps Stroke Patients Regain Motor Function," by Charlene Laino, *Neurology Today*, March 2009. © 2009 American Academy of Neurology. Reprinted with permission.

In a small study, 15 chronic stroke patients with weakness of the distal right arm and hand were all able to grasp and release objects more easily after treatment with a robotic device that cradled the lower arms and hands.

Robotic therapy helped patients with chronic moderate-to-severe motor deficits after stroke to regain modest motor function, a small study shows.

Fifteen chronic stroke patients with weakness of the distal right arm and hand were all able to grasp and release objects more easily after treatment with a robotic device that cradled the lower arms and hands, Steven C. Cramer, MD, director of the Stroke Center at the University of California-Irvine, reported in February 2009 at the American Stroke Association International Stroke Conference. The patients had had strokes four months to 10 years before starting the two-week course of therapy.

The better the baseline motor skills, the greater the recovery, Dr. Cramer said.

The study expands previous work in which the hand-wrist robot had favorable effects on hand and arm function in 13 patients with chronic stroke, reported in 2008 in *Brain*.

The Hand-Wrist Assisting Robotic Device—nicknamed HOWARD—wraps around the hand and, in concert with a computer program, directs the thumb and fingers through a physical therapy session, said Dr. Cramer, who was also a co-investigator on the 2008 study.

Users initiate hand movements on their own; HOWARD monitors the movement, helps train the hands into the positions it needs to be in to perform various tasks, and provides assistance to complete each activity, he said.

The therapy was built upon principles of motor learning including use of intense, active repetitive movement and sensorimotor integration, he said.

Section 34.5

Constraint-Induced Movement Therapy

"In Most Comprehensive Study Yet, Two-Week Regimen Helps Stroke Survivors Regain Arm Control," by the National Institute of Child Health and Human Development (NICHD, www.nichd.nih.gov), part of the National Institutes of Health, October 31, 2006. Reviewed by David A. Cooke, MD, FACP, January 24, 2013.

In the largest, most comprehensive study of its kind to date, researchers supported by the National Institutes of Health (NIH) showed clinical improvements out to one year when stroke survivors who had lost function in one arm were given a unique, two-week rehabilitation regimen.

Steven Wolf, PhD, professor of rehabilitation medicine at Emory University, led a multi-center team that tested the effects of constraint-induced movement therapy (CIMT) in 222 patients. The study, which is featured in the November 1, 2006, issue of the *Journal of the American Medical Association*, was funded by the National Institute of Child Health and Human Development (NICHD) and the National Institute of Neurological Disorders and Stroke (NINDS).

"This study provides the strongest evidence to date that constraint induced movement therapy can help stroke patients regain lost arm function," said NIH Director Elias A. Zerhouni, MD. "This is welcome news for stroke patients and those who care about them."

Each year, more than 700,000 Americans are hospitalized for stroke, an interruption of blood flow in the brain. Up to 85 percent of survivors have weakness on one side of their body.

CIMT involves training the weakened hand and arm through repetitive exercises, while restraining the unaffected hand and arm with a mitt like a boxing glove. The theory behind the hand restraint is that it forces the wearer to use the affected hand and arm.

"We now have an intervention that is beneficial for between 5 and 30 percent of the stroke population. CIMT should be considered as a valuable form of rehabilitation, and opens the door to further explorations," said Dr. Wolf.

Known as the EXCITE trial, for Extremity Constraint Induced Therapy Evaluation, Dr. Wolf's study involved people who had weakness in one arm caused by a stroke within the prior three to nine months. About half of the trial participants received customary care, ranging from no treatment to standard physical therapy, while the other half received CIMT.

Study participants were asked to wear the restraint every day, and come in for training every weekday for several hours, for a period of two weeks. They were evaluated immediately after treatment, and again 4, 8, and 12 months later, through a series of tasks designed to measure arm dexterity, and a set of questions about how well and how often they used the impaired arm in daily activities.

Compared to the group that received only customary care, the group that received CIMT showed improved function of the stroke-affected arm in timed tasks and in self-reported daily use at all-time points. At the earliest time points, some participants were unable to perform certain tasks at all, but those who received CIMT were more likely to regain the ability to perform those tasks by the end of the year-long study period.

Previous neuroimaging studies have revealed that CIMT stimulates increased activity in the part of the brain that controls the rehabilitated arm. "The work of Dr. Wolf and his colleagues shows that it's possible to harness this remarkable plasticity in the brain to significantly improve the lives of patients," said John Marler, MD, associate director of clinical trials at NINDS.

Beth Ansel, PhD, a project director of the National Center for Medical Rehabilitation Research, the NICHD division that funded the study, said its results represent an important milestone after many years of research. "These studies began as basic research with laboratory animals, progressed to studies with patients, and now are poised to change patient care," she said.

Reference: Wolf SL, et al. Effect of Constraint-Induced Movement Therapy on Upper Extremity Function 3 to 9 Months After Stroke. The EXCITE Randomized Clinical Trial. *JAMA*, November 1, 2006, Vol. 296, No. 17, pp. 2095–2104.

Chapter 35

Balance Problems after Stroke

Problems with balance are common after stroke. If your balance has been affected, you may feel dizzy or unsteady which could lead to a fall or loss of confidence when walking and moving around. This text explains how stroke can affect your balance, what can help, and how you can look after yourself.

Balance involves the coordination and stability of our bodies in our surroundings. It affects most day-to-day activities, such as moving around and reaching for objects.

If your balance is impaired, you may feel dizzy or unsteady. This can reduce your confidence and increase your risk of having a fall. If your balance problems have lasted for a long time, you might find that they affect your quality of life.

Balance is very complex and it involves many different parts of the body such as your ears, eyes, and sensors in your muscles and joints.

These work together automatically and subconsciously so you are usually unaware of them unless something goes wrong.

You are more likely to have problems with your balance if your stroke has affected the left side of your body.

How Can Your Balance Be Affected by Stroke?

A stroke can affect any, or all, parts of your balance system, and the way in which they work together. Usually your body can overcome mild problems, but if they are more severe, your system will be unable to work effectively and you will probably feel unsteady.

Weakness on One Side of Your Body

When your balance is affected after a stroke, it is usually because of weakness on one side of your body. At worst, you may find it difficult to sit up safely, or you may have difficulty standing if you cannot keep your leg straight when you stand on it. On the other hand, you may be able to walk but find that you cannot lift your toes quickly enough to stop them catching when you step. This is a condition called drop foot.

Another common problem is having difficulty adapting to unpredictable situations (such as crowds or uneven surfaces). Or you may find that you have less energy so that you tire easily and then become unsteady.

Loss of Sensation

The second main factor affecting balance is loss of sensation in your affected side, particularly your leg. If you cannot feel where your leg and foot are, especially when your foot is safely on the ground, it is very difficult to know how to move. You will automatically use your vision to compensate for the lack of feeling, which takes a lot of concentration and is tiring. It also means that you may be less aware of your surroundings. All of this increases your risk of having slips, trips, and falls.

Injury to Your Brain

Sometimes if a stroke happens in your cerebellum or brainstem—the areas that control balance in the brain—you may be left with a sensation that you are moving when you are not.

Lack of Concentration

After a stroke, moving around and keeping your balance is no longer automatic. It takes a lot of concentration, which is hard work.

If your attention is distracted, it might be harder to concentrate on your balance.

Many people who fall report that they were not paying attention, were thinking of other things, or doing several things at the same time when they fell. One example is walking and talking at the same time—some stroke survivors often stop walking if you speak to them, or keep walking and do not answer. Other examples include coping with unpredictable situations such as crowds and uneven surfaces, turning, or changing direction when walking or carrying things.

Less Common Problems That Can Affect Your Balance

Perceptual problems: Some strokes can affect your ability to interpret your surroundings. This is often associated with strokes that occur in the right side of the brain. It can be difficult to maintain your balance and plan how to move if the world around you does not make sense. You may feel unsure of your position and think that you are upright even when you are leaning heavily to your weak side, sometimes to the extent that you cannot sit up safely. This is called pusher syndrome and can happen (usually just in the early days) after a severe stroke.

A related problem is neglect. This occurs when you are not aware of one side of your body (usually the left side). Again, it is difficult to move if you are not aware of one of your legs. People with neglect may try to move but forget to move their weak leg causing loss of balance.

Vision is an important aspect of balance. Visual problems are quite common after stroke. They vary and include difficulty focusing, double vision, eye movement problems, and blind patches. Again it is difficult to make the subtle and rapid changes to your posture and movements necessary to keep your balance if you cannot see clearly around you.

Dizziness or vertigo (a feeling that the world is spinning) is quite common after stroke, but for most people this does not usually last long.

Ataxia is the name for clumsy, uncoordinated movements. It is associated with strokes that happen in the back of the brain (the cerebellum or posterior circulation).

People with ataxia have difficulty producing movements quickly enough and in the right order to prevent losing their balance or to recover from a trip or slip.

Side Effects of Medication

Some medicines commonly prescribed after stroke can cause dizziness and/or weakness.

These include some drugs for high blood pressure, diabetes, and depression. In rare cases, clopidogrel, a commonly used blood thinning medicine, can cause dizziness.

Interactions between different medicines can also cause problems with balance. Talk to your doctor if you have any concerns about the medicine you are taking. Never stop taking any medication without speaking to your doctor first.

Other causes of balance problems: A range of other conditions not directly related to stroke, such as inner ear infections and migraines, can also cause dizziness and loss of balance.

Tips to Avoid a Fall

The following tips may help to prevent you from having a fall.

- Keep all floors clear of trailing wires, frayed carpet, or anything else you might trip on.

- Mop up any spills straightaway.

- Organize your home so that you are less likely to bump into things. Remove clutter and arrange your furniture so that you do not have to walk around it.

- Most falls happen when people are not paying attention, are thinking of other things or doing several things at once. Try to avoid doing two things at once such as walking and carrying something. Use a trolley to move things around (for example, to take your plate or a cup from the kitchen to dining table) rather than carrying it.

- Try to avoid walking and talking. Stop if you want to talk to someone.

- Focus on your movements when you are doing something that is tricky—such as turning, going up and down stairs, or getting in and out of the bath or bed. These are all common times when falls happen. Step around carefully when you are turning (rather than twisting), hold on to whatever solid objects are around and take your time. Use aids if you have them and ask someone to help you if they are available.

- Move at a pace that is comfortable for you. Do not be persuaded by the pressures of everyday life to do things more quickly.

- Talk to an occupational therapist about getting handrails for the stairs and/or bathroom. Your doctor can refer you to see one.

- Use high wattage light bulbs so you can see clearly, particularly around stairs. If you get up in the night, make sure you turn the light on.

- Keep your home warm—cold muscles work less well and this can lead to accidents.

- Remember to use any walking aids, such as sticks or frames that your therapist has recommended.

- In case you do have a fall, you may want to consider getting a personal alarm.

- Wear well-fitting shoes with thin soles, high sides, and a good grip. Never walk on slippery floors in socks or tights.

- Talk to a podiatrist (also called a chiropodist) about any foot problems—these can increase the risk of falls if left untreated. Your physician may be able to refer you to one, or details will be in your local phone book.

- Have regular eye tests. Wear any glasses that have been prescribed for you.

Chapter 36

Pain and Fatigue after Stroke

Chapter Contents

Section 36.1

Pain after Stroke

After a stroke you might experience various physical effects, such as weakness, paralysis, or changes in sensation. Unfortunately you may also experience pain. This text will help you to understand some of the causes of pain after stroke and the treatments that may be available.

There are many different types of pain you may experience after having a stroke.

Weakness on one side of your body is one of the most common effects of stroke. This can lead to painful conditions such as muscle stiffness (spasticity) and shoulder problems. Some people also experience central poststroke pain, headaches, and sore swollen hands after stroke.

As with many effects of stroke, pain may persist for some time, but treatments such as medication and physiotherapy are often successful in relieving pain.

Many people also benefit from attending pain management clinics and learn coping techniques to help them to manage any long-term pain.

Spasticity and Contractures

After a stroke you may find that you have muscle tightness or stiffness—this is called spasticity. It is a common problem and affects over a third of stroke survivors. Usually it occurs on the weaker side of your body.

Spasticity happens when there is damage to the area of your brain that controls your muscles. If you have spasticity you will have increased muscle tone. Muscle tone is the amount of resistance or tension in your muscles, and it is what enables us to hold our bodies in a particular position. This increased muscle tone can make it difficult to move your limbs. Spasticity may also cause your muscles to tense and contract abnormally, causing spasms, which can be very painful.

Spasticity can also damage your tissues and joints and can sometimes cause painful night cramps.

It is important to treat spasticity as soon as possible because your joints and muscles may become so stiff that it is impossible to move them (this is called a contracture).

How Is Spasticity Treated?

If you have weakness after your stroke you should be assessed for spasticity. A team of specialists will decide on the best treatment for you. This may include a combination of physiotherapy, medication, and Botox.

Physiotherapy

If you have spasticity you should have physiotherapy every day to move your joints. This will help to stretch your muscles, keeping them flexible and reducing the possibility of contractures.

Your physiotherapist will gently place your affected limb into as many different positions as possible. This is called passive stretching and should be taught to your family and carers so that they can help you to practice your exercises.

Botox

If spasticity affects only one or two specific parts of your body, you may be given botulinum toxin A (Botox) as an injection directly into your muscle. Botox works by blocking the action of the nerves on the muscle, reducing your muscle's ability to contract. It reduces muscle tone, which can help you to straighten out your limbs.

Botox is only useful for small muscles, such as those in the hands. The muscle-relaxing effects of Botox usually last for about three months and you should not notice any changes in sensation in your muscles.

Botox treatment should be given with further rehabilitation such as physiotherapy, or other treatments like splinting or casting.

You should also have an assessment three to four months after the treatment, and be offered further Botox treatments if helpful.

Medication

If you find that you are still experiencing muscle stiffness, you may be prescribed medication to help reduce this stiffness and the pain that often accompanies muscle spasms. There are different types of drugs that you could be given. They all work in slightly different ways, but they all help to relax your muscles. When your muscles are relaxed they can move more easily and you can stretch them further. You may also find that it becomes easier to straighten or bend your affected limbs, and you may notice fewer muscle spasms.

You will usually be prescribed baclofen or tizanidine first. If these drugs do not work, there are other drugs that may help, but they should only be prescribed by someone who specializes in managing spasticity.

How Are Contractures Treated?

Splinting and Casting

If your spasticity is not fully controlled and you develop contractures, your physiotherapist may use a splint or a cast that molds to or lies along your affected limb and holds it in place. This treatment helps to stretch out the muscles in your tight limbs and is usually combined with physiotherapy. Sometimes this treatment is used to try to prevent contractures from forming by making sure that your body is not in an abnormal position. Unfortunately sometimes splints and casts can be uncomfortable. Talk to your physiotherapist about what would be best for you.

Surgery

If you have severe contractures, you may need surgery to lengthen your tendons.

Tendons are the bands that connect your muscle to the bone, and lengthening your tendons allows the joint to be stretched out. This procedure is performed under anaesthetic. Surgery is always a last resort.

Shoulder Pain

Shoulder pain is common after a stroke, and usually affects the side of your body that is affected by the stroke. There are different types of shoulder pain that you might experience and experts do not yet fully understand the exact causes.

Frozen Shoulder

After a stroke you may find that your shoulder is very stiff and that it hurts when you move it. This is called frozen shoulder or capsulitis. Muscles and ligaments around our shoulder joints hold the bone in our upper arms in place. There is a layer of tissue that surrounds this joint which is called a capsule. If your arm muscles are very weak, stiff, or paralyzed, the effect of gravity puts a strain on your ligaments and your capsule. This can cause these parts of your shoulder joint to become inflamed, stretched, and damaged. Having weakness in your arm muscles may contribute to this pain in your shoulder.

Subluxation

Another cause of shoulder pain is shoulder subluxation. This means partial dislocation—where the bone of the upper arm and the shoulder blade have moved apart. This might be because the muscles that normally hold this joint in place are too weak to do this properly.

How Is Shoulder Pain Treated?

Prevention

If you have weakness in your arm following your stroke, your medical team will try to prevent shoulder pain developing. They will make sure that anyone who handles your arm knows how to do so with care and without causing strain on your shoulder joint.

They should also ensure that your arm and shoulder are positioned correctly. Correct positioning is vital because it can help to reduce the strain on your ligaments and capsule, helping to prevent frozen shoulder from developing. It may also help to prevent your shoulder blade and upper arm bone from moving apart (subluxation). Your medical team may use foam supports to make sure that your shoulder is supported in the correct position. Your arm can also be supported using a pillow. Overhead arm slings should not be used because there is not enough evidence that they work and they may increase your risk of developing shoulder pain or contractures.

Your physiotherapist may use cuffs or straps to keep your arm and shoulder in the correct position, but for some people this may lead to spasticity.

Your physiotherapist may also use electrical stimulation on the muscles around your shoulder to help prevent or treat subluxation.

Reducing Pain

You may be given painkillers such as paracetamol or codeine to help relieve the pain in your shoulder. For more severe pain you may be given a non-steroidal anti-inflammatory drug (NSAID) such as diclofenac or ibuprofen. These types of drug help to relieve pain and can also help to reduce swelling in your shoulder capsule.

If you have an inflamed shoulder a steroid, such as triamcinolone, may be injected into your joint to help reduce the pain. Botox can sometimes be injected into specific muscles around your shoulder to help reduce pain and increase flexibility, particularly where the pain is associated with spasticity.

Moving Your Shoulder

It is important to keep the muscles in your shoulder and arm active so that any stiffness does not get worse. Your physiotherapist may use stretching exercises to move your shoulder joint in all directions. They can also provide you with advice about how to protect your shoulder during everyday movements such as reaching for something or getting dressed.

Central Post-Stroke Pain (CPSP)

Up to 12 percent of people who have a stroke will develop a particular type of pain called central post-stroke pain (CPSP). This is also known as Dejerine Roussy Syndrome, or central pain syndrome.

There are different types of pain you might experience if you have CPSP. Many people describe it as an icy burning sensation, or a throbbing or shooting pain. Some people also experience pins and needles or numbness in the areas affected by the pain.

For most stroke survivors with CPSP, the pain occurs in the side of their body that has been affected by the stroke. The pain may begin immediately after your stroke but more often it begins several months later.

Some people find this pain becomes worse because of other factors such as movement or a change in temperature.

The exact cause of CPSP is unknown, but it is thought to be due to damage to certain parts of the brain and body. CPSP is a form of neuropathic pain, which means that the painful sensation does not occur because your body is injured or because something is making it hurt.

The pain may be caused by damage to the brain, brainstem, or spinal cord (together, these are called the central nervous system) or be due to damage to the sensory pathways. These are pathways between the brain and the body which carry messages about pain. In some cases, CPSP is due to damage to the thalamus, which is the brain's pain center. When this part of the brain is damaged it can sometimes cause feelings of pain when you are feeling a sensation that is not normally painful.

How Is CPSP Treated?

Unfortunately there is no cure for CPSP, but around 70 percent of stroke survivors with CPSP find that medication helps to relieve their pain. Ordinary painkillers are not usually helpful in relieving CPSP, but some drugs which were originally created for treating other conditions are helpful for some people. They include amitriptyline, which is a drug used to treat depression, and gabapentin and pregabalin, which are used to treat epilepsy.

You will usually be started on a low dose, which is then gradually increased. If the first medication you try does not work, you should be offered another drug to try either with, or instead of, the first one.

In rare cases, if your pain is severe and other treatments have been unsuccessful, your medical team may offer you deep brain stimulation. This is a procedure where small electrical leads are placed deep within your brain and are connected to a battery-powered machine, which sits under your skin. This procedure can only be carried out in specialist centers and it is not suitable for everyone. Research shows that deep brain stimulation is effective in reducing pain for some people, though only a small number of people have taken part in the studies.

Other Painful Conditions

Swollen Hand

You might find that after your stroke your hand swells up and becomes painful. This usually happens if you are not moving your hand very much, for example, if it is paralyzed. The swelling happens because the fluid in the tissue in your hand cannot circulate properly because the muscles are not moving. When your muscles are not moving regularly, this fluid can collect, causing swelling and discomfort. This can get worse if your hand is often hanging downward. This painful swelling can make it even more difficult to move your hand and arm, which can make spasticity worse.

To overcome this problem it is best to raise your hand and place it on a pillow or a cushion, and to get your hand moving again gently with the help of your physiotherapist.

Wearing a tight-fitting glove can sometimes help to push the fluid out of your hand—this is called an edema glove. This will need to be fitted correctly to avoid causing too much pressure. Your physiotherapist should be able to make a referral for you to have this done. You might find that painkillers such as paracetamol help to relieve the pain caused by this swelling in your hand.

Headache

There are many reasons why you might experience headaches following your stroke. Some reasons might be the same as before your stroke, such as stress, depression, or lack of sleep.

If you are having headaches after your stroke, they could be a side effect of medication that you have started taking. Common examples include nifedipine (Adalat), which is given for high blood pressure, dipyridamole (Persantine), a blood-thinning medication, and glyceryl trinitrate, which is given for angina and to lower blood pressure. Talk to your doctor, because if you are experiencing headaches or any other side effects from medication, there may be an alternative drug you can try instead.

Occasionally, headaches may be a direct after-effect of your stroke if there is swelling of the brain. This swelling, which can be caused by a stroke, can irritate the membrane that covers the brain, resulting in a headache. This is more common if you have had a stroke caused by a bleed in the brain.

Headaches can also occur because of a change to the levels of cerebrospinal fluid (CSF). This is the fluid that fills the space between our brain and our skull. If there is an increased or reduced amount of CSF, this can cause headaches.

The pain from the headaches you are experiencing should lessen over time and can usually be controlled by painkillers such as paracetamol. You should not take aspirin if your stroke was caused by a bleed.

Drinking plenty of water (two to three liters per day) and avoiding caffeine and alcohol (which cause dehydration) may help to reduce these headaches. Increasing the amount of fluid in your body will improve the blood circulation to your brain.

Sometimes taking painkillers for headaches too often (for more than about 10 days a month) can cause headaches. Treatment usually involves stopping all pain relief medication for one month, but talk to your doctor first if you think this is the cause of your headaches. Do not stop taking any medication without getting medical advice.

If you ever experience a sudden, severe headache or a persistent headache, you should seek medical attention urgently to find out what is causing it. One of the symptoms of a stroke caused by bleeding on the surface of the brain (subarachnoid hemorrhage) is a very sudden and severe headache, as if you have been hit on the back of the head.

Section 36.2

Fatigue after Stroke

Reprinted with permission from *Stroke Connection Magazine*, November/
December 2010–p. 16. © 2010 American Heart Association, Inc.

A stroke leaves physical and emotional damage—it can also zap energy and cause fatigue. Researchers report that up to 70 percent of survivors experience fatigue that includes overwhelming physical and/ or mental tiredness or exhaustion.

Symptoms include difficulty with self-control, emotions, and memory. How severe and long-lasting fatigue is ranges from mild and seldom to overwhelming and constant. Some report feeling tired even after a good night's sleep and that symptoms never seem to get better. Others say they feel tired when they perform a task requiring physical or mental focus. Most report that fatigue occurs without warning and makes it harder to do daily, routine activities as well as social or work activities.

Causes

Because research in this area is limited, we aren't certain what causes fatigue, but there are several possible causes.

Medical conditions a survivor has, such as heart disease, diabetes, respiratory disease, anemia, pre-stroke fatigue, or migraines, can contribute to fatigue. That's because the stroke or medication side effects may worsen fatigue or even mask it. Sleep apnea is also common among survivors. It is reported at high rates among those who report post-stroke fatigue, although no solid relationship has been proven.

Poor heart health may also play a part due to higher levels of exertion. Survivors expend twice as much energy just standing upright and keeping their balance.

Survivors are often concerned about falling and may feel unsure about doing some tasks. This stress can increase physical and mental demands and lead to fatigue. Lack of control in movement and walking appear to increase when a person is tired. Anxiety, stress, and depression, which are common after stroke, are associated with lack of energy, although research has not determined their specific relationships to post-stroke fatigue.

Fighting Post-Stroke Fatigue

Talk to your family and work with your healthcare team to determine the best plan of care for you. Here are some other tips:

1. Check your prescriptions for potential side effects, including fatigue.

2. Ask for treatment options if you are experiencing anxiety, depression, or difficulty sleeping. Family support and understanding can also help. Let your family know that post-stroke fatigue is different from fatigue they've experienced.

3. Maintain good health to prevent or control other medical conditions, such as heart disease or diabetes, which can affect your energy level. Currently there is no prescription specifically for tiredness, although many related symptoms can be treated.

4. Talk to your physical therapist to understand fitness, balance disorders, uncoordinated movement, and walking related to fatigue. He or she can create an exercise program to increase your endurance. Balance and coordination exercises will help you perform tasks with less energy, increase your confidence, and decrease your anxiety.

5. Try to schedule demanding physical or mental activities throughout the day or week. That way you'll plan to take rest breaks before you feel tired and break up the concentrated periods of time that you're exerting yourself.

6. Consider modifying your home and work environment to make them more efficient. Use assistive technology when possible.

Physical therapists can help patients reduce post-stroke fatigue. In most states, patients can make an appointment directly with a physical therapist, without a physician referral. Learn more about conditions physical therapists can treat and find a physical therapist in your area at moveforwardpt.com.

Chapter 37

Bowel System Problems and Their Management

Bowel System: Common Problems

Listed in the following text are common bowel problems, symptoms, and management techniques.

Constipation: The inability to have a bowel movement for three or more days

Symptoms:

- Hard stools
- Inability to have a bowel movement in many days
- Feeling bloated in the stomach area

This chapter contains text from "Bowel System: Common Problems," May 2011, Copyright © Rehabilitation Institute of Chicago. All rights reserved. Reprinted with permission. For additional information, visit the website of the LIFE Center at the Rehabilitation Institute of Chicago, http://lifecenter .ric.org. It also contains text from "Bowel System: Creating and Managing a Bowel Program," August 2012, Copyright © Rehabilitation Institute of Chicago. All rights reserved. Reprinted with permission. For additional information, visit the website of the LIFE Center at the Rehabilitation Institute of Chicago, http://lifecenter.ric.org.

Causes:

- Insufficient fluid intake (less than one liter per day)
- Inactivity
- Poor diet—low in fiber-containing foods such as fruit, vegetables, and whole grains
- Side effects of medicines—especially iron, codeine, and pain medication
- Repeatedly ignoring urge to move bowels

Treatment:

- Drink at least six to eight glasses of fluid each day.
- Eat a diet high in fiber.
- Ask the doctor about using a stool softener or laxative.
- If constipation persists, ask your doctor about using suppositories or an enema.

Any person with a spinal cord injury who experiences the above symptoms along with abdominal pain that does not go away after removal of the stool should contact their physician immediately. This may be a sign of autonomic dysreflexia, a serious condition of over activity of the nervous system. Autonomic dysreflexia can happen to people who have injuries at or above T6.

Impaction: Hard stool plugging the rectum

Symptoms:

- Hard stools
- Bloated feeling in the stomach
- Leaking of loose or liquid stool

Causes:

- Insufficient fluid intake
- Inactivity
- Poor diet
- Side effect of medications
- Chronic constipation

Treatment:

Many people who experience impactions are able to remove the stool by hand. Check with your physician or health care provider to find out if this is appropriate.

Diarrhea: Loose or liquid stool, usually three or more times a day

Symptom:

- Large amounts of loose or watery stool

Causes:

- Illness, such as a cold or flu
- Poor diet, including too much spicy or greasy food
- Excessive use of laxatives or stool softeners

Treatment:

- Do a rectal check looking for impaction.
- Check with your health care provider regarding the use of specific fiber supplements.
- Stop all laxatives and stool softeners.
- Drink plenty of fluids.

Hemorrhoids: Swelling or bleeding of tissue around the rectum

Symptoms:

- Red, bulging areas inside or outside the rectum
- Pain or rectal bleeding after a bowel movement

Causes:

- Long history of hard stools or constipation
- Removal of stool by hand

Treatment:

- Use medications ordered by doctor such as Anusol or Preparation H.

- If stool is hard, follow guidelines for constipation.
- Drink plenty of liquids.

Incontinence: Problems controlling bowel movements

Symptoms:

- Inability to start or stop bowel movements
- Lack of awareness of bowel movements

Causes:

- Decreased mobility
- Inability to communicate the need to use the toilet
- Side effects of medication
- Uncontrolled diarrhea

Treatment:

- Assess bowel habits to find a pattern. Some people have bowel movements every day; others have bowel movements every two or three days. Try to anticipate when a bowel movement might occur and sit on the toilet at that time.
- Sit on the toilet after eating for 30 minutes up to an hour.
- Avoid using a bed pan as much as possible; use the toilet or a commode.
- Check with your health care provider about using suppositories to regulate bowel movements.

Bowel System: Creating and Managing a Bowel Program

Following an injury or medical condition, bowel habits often change. A daily bowel program routine will help in managing bowels and preventing accidents.

The bowel program may take a while to develop. It generally starts with trying to identify a regular pattern of bowel activity. You and your nurse will work together to create the right program for you.

At first, the program may mean consistent toileting and/or using a suppository every day, which allows the rectum to empty. After a while, you may not need a suppository at all.

Some people use other medications as part of the bowel program. Medicines are used to soften the stool, firm up the stool, or stimulate bowel activity.

A bowel program works best after a meal or at the time of day you usually have a bowel movement. For example, some people have a bowel movement in the morning after breakfast or a cup of coffee.

Following instructions for diet and fluids is an important part of a bowel program.

Diet

- Choose foods that are high in fiber such as fruits, vegetables, and whole grains. These foods add bulk to the stool. The right amount of fiber promotes solid, soft stool that is easier to pass.

- Certain foods can cause diarrhea. Foods that cause diarrhea vary from person to person. Often spicy or greasy food or sometimes caffeine-containing beverages can lead to diarrhea.

Liquids

- Drink at least 8 to 10 eight-ounce glasses of fluid a day. Liquids are very important for any bowel program. Examples: water, milk, juice, soup, and tea.

- Prune juice can be helpful when coping with constipation. Try four to six ounces per day.

- More fluid may be necessary if using a fiber supplement or with certain medications.

Activity

- Activity increases muscle movement in the bowel (peristalsis).

- People who are more active are less likely to be constipated.

Medications

Medications may be needed short-term or long term, depending on a number of factors. There are several types of medications related to bowel management.

- Bulk formers: Fiber supplements that help keep the stool formed; must be taken with adequate fluids. Examples: Metamucil, Citrucel, Benefiber

- Stool softeners: Add fluid to the stool so it is easier to pass; also must be taken with adequate fluids. Example: Colace

- Peristaltic stimulators: Increase bowel activity, causing the stool to move through more quickly and may be helpful with constipation caused by narcotic analgesics. Example: Senokot

- Laxatives: Promote bowel movements, but can also be too strong and can cause accidents; should not be used routinely as they may lead to further bowel problems. Example: Milk of Magnesia

- Suppositories: Start a bowel movement. Examples: glycerin, Dulcolax. Glycerin is less expensive. Dulcolax can cause cramping. If you find that you are not having a bowel movement after an everyday suppository program, call your doctor.

Some medications can interfere and make a bowel program more difficult.

- Magnesium hydroxide or aluminum hydroxide, when used together, can cause constipation. Examples: Maalox, Mylanta, Gaviscon

- Anti-ulcer drugs cause constipation. Examples: Cimetidine, Zantac, Ranitidine, protein pump inhibitors

- Narcotics can cause constipation and sometimes bowel obstructions. Examples: Tylenol with codeine, codeine, Vicodin, Norco

Long-term use of calcium, aspirin, antidepressants, iron supplements, and antihistamines can also cause constipation

Once a program is established, you will begin having bowel movements at regular times. Maintain your routine at those regular times. Skipping your program can cause constipation, impaction, and accidents. Consult with your physician or nurse to see whether you can remove any medications from your long-term program.

Additional Instructions

Rectal Check

A rectal check makes sure the rectal cavity is empty and is usually done at the beginning and end of a bowel program.

Supplies:

- Bed pads

- Glove

- Water-soluble lubricant (such as K-Y)
- Soap, water, washcloth, and towel

Procedure:

- Lie on left side if possible and place bed pads under buttocks.
- Put on glove. Lubricate gloved index finger with water-soluble lubricant. A dry glove can hurt tissue.
- Insert finger one to two inches into the rectum.
- If stool is present, gently remove and discard.
- Wash buttocks and dry skin very well.

Rectal Suppository

Insertion of a rectal suppository helps the bowel to empty.

Supplies:

- Bed pads
- Glove
- Water-soluble lubricant
- Suppository (as recommended by your physician/nurse)
- Toilet paper
- Soap, water, washcloth, and towel

Procedure:

- Lie on left side and place bed pads under buttocks.
- Put on glove. Lubricate gloved index finger. A dry glove can hurt tissue.
- Insert finger slowly into rectum, remove any stool and discard.
- Insert suppository into rectum, next to the rectal wall, not directly into stool.
- Transfer to a toilet after 20 minutes.
- If no bowel movement within 30–60 minutes, insert a second suppository.
- Wash buttocks and dry the skin very well.

Manual Removal of Impaction

Manual removal of an impaction rids the body of hard stool. This must be done very gently or the wall of the bowel may be hurt. This is not recommended for anyone with heart disease.

Supplies:

- Bed pads
- Glove
- Water-soluble lubricant
- Soap, water, washcloth, and towel

Procedure:

- Lie on side and place bed pads under buttocks.
- Lubricate gloved index finger. A dry glove can hurt tissue.
- Insert finger slowly into rectum, gently remove hard stool, and discard.
- Wash buttocks and dry skin very well.

If the stool is higher up in the rectum, call your doctor.

Digital Stimulation

This relaxes the sphincter muscle but is not recommended for anyone with heart disease or rectal feeling.

Supplies:

- Bed pads
- Glove
- Water soluble lubricant
- Toilet paper
- Washbasin, washcloths, and towel

Procedure:

- Place bed pad under buttocks if in bed.
- Lie on left side or sit on a toilet.
- Lubricate gloved index finger. A dry glove can hurt issue.

- Insert finger one inch into the rectum. Do not insert past the first joint (bend) on your finger.

- Gently move the finger in a circle. This will cause peristalsis and relax the sphincter. Perform for 30 seconds. Repeat three times.

- Use wash cloths or towels to clean and dry buttocks when finished.

Enema

Enemas help bowels to empty but are used only if other medications do not work. They should not be used regularly as they can disturb bowel function over time.

Supplies:

- Enema (30ml Bisacodyl or Fleets)

- Glove

- Bed pad

Procedure:

- Lie on left side and place pad under buttocks.

- Put on glove

- Remove cap and gently insert the lubricated tip of the enema into the rectum.

- If resistance is met do not force the tip, instead remove and do a rectal check. If stool is present, gently remove manually. If resistance is met with rectal check, stop and call your doctor.

- Gently squeeze contents from bottle into rectum and hold fluid in rectum.

- Transfer to toilet if able.

Bowel Record

If you are having trouble with bowels or bowel program, it may be helpful to write down what is happening and bring the record to doctor's appointment.

Chapter 38

Continence Problems after Stroke

It is common for people to have problems controlling their bladder and/or bowels after a stroke. Though initially very distressing, these problems are often resolved with time. This text explains some of the continence problems that may happen after stroke.

About half of people admitted to a hospital with a stroke will have lost control of their bladder, and a third will experience loss of bowel control. This is called incontinence.

It is quite normal for incontinence to be a source of concern after a stroke. For many people loss of toilet control is a very sensitive and personal issue and some people may feel like they have lost their dignity.

However, there is a lot that can be done to help, and just 15 percent of stroke survivors will continue to have continence problems a year after their stroke. It is generally easier to regain bowel control than bladder control.

Regaining control can improve both your morale and overall recovery.

Why Do Continence Problems Develop?

There are different reasons why you may develop continence problems after a stroke. For example, as with any serious illness or accident,

---

if you are not fully conscious or aware of your surroundings, you may wet or soil yourself without realizing it.

Your stroke may have damaged the part of the brain that controls your bladder and/or the bowel. As with other after-effects, it may take time to recover.

If you have difficulty walking or moving around (or you need help getting to the toilet) you may not always be able to get there in time. The same may be true if you have communication difficulties and cannot make yourself understood in time.

Any extra exertion involved in moving may itself make it more difficult to maintain control.

Being less mobile than usual can make you more prone to constipation (difficulty emptying your bowels), which in turn may cause continence problems. You may not be able to eat or drink as much as usual because of the stroke and may be undernourished or dehydrated. This may also lead to constipation.

Some medicines, including ones commonly prescribed after a stroke, may affect bladder or bowel control. For instance medicines called diuretics, which may be taken to help lower your blood pressure, may initially affect bladder control.

You may already have had mild continence problems before your stroke, which are likely to be made worse by any lengthy period in bed. Urine retention (being unable to empty your bladder completely) may cause your bladder to swell painfully. It is also more likely that you will suffer bladder infections during any period of inactivity, and these can cause temporary incontinence.

Which Continence Problems Can Occur after Stroke?

There are many different types of continence problems that can occur (sometimes in combination) as a result of stroke. These include [the following]:

- Frequency: Needing to pass urine more often

- Urgency: Feeling a sudden, urgent, and uncontrollable need to pass urine. This is due to bladder spasm or contractions. Often there is no time to get to the toilet, so you may have an accident.

- Nocturnal incontinence: Wetting the bed while asleep

- Functional incontinence: Caused when the physical effects of a stroke impede mobility or make it difficult to unfasten clothes in time to use the toilet

- Stress incontinence: Small amounts of urinary leakage on coughing, sneezing, or laughing. This usually happens because the muscles in the pelvic floor or urethral sphincter are weak or damaged.

- Reflex incontinence: Passing urine without realizing it. This happens when a stroke has affected the part of the brain that senses and controls bladder movement.

- Overflow incontinence: Where the bladder leaks due to being too full. This can be due to a loss of feeling in your bladder, or difficulty in emptying your bladder effectively (urine retention).

Bowel Problems

- Fecal incontinence: Uncontrolled bowel movement. This can be caused by damage to the part of the brain controlling the bowel, not being able to get to the toilet in time, diarrhea, or constipation.

- Constipation with overflow: Large stools can get stuck and block the bowel. Liquid stools above the blockage can flow around it causing watery stools to leak.

- Fecal impaction: Dry and hardened stools collect in the rectum, they can press on your bladder, and make any problems you have with emptying your bladder worse.

Initial Care after Stroke

Until you are well enough to start actively regaining control of your bladder or bowel, you may need to wear incontinence pads.

These should be changed rapidly by the nursing staff if they become soiled.

If you have good bladder and bowel function but are unable to indicate when you need the toilet, the nurses may offer you the toilet or commode every two hours or so.

While you are in bed, you may be transferred to the commode using a hoist, or offered a bottle or sheath urinal (designed for men) or a bedpan (for women). If your bladder is not emptying completely, then a catheter may be used to empty it. This involves gently inserting a fine tube to drain urine from the bladder into a bag. This may need to be done several times a day (intermittent catheterization) to keep you comfortable and reduce the risk of developing a urinary tract infection (UTI).

If you develop soreness through skin contact with your urine, or the catheterization causes discomfort, an indwelling (or semi-permanent) catheter may be used.

Fecal containment bags are used in intensive care, but you are more likely to wear pads if you are on a stroke unit.

Good hygiene and skin care are therefore important to protect your skin from damage.

Assessment

If you stay in a hospital after your stroke, in the second week or so, your medical team will carry out an assessment to establish the nature and cause of your difficulties and devise an effective treatment programme.

The continence assessment may include:

- a medical history of any problems you had before the stroke and your current medication that could be affecting control;

- a simple chart recording your fluid intake and output (by volume and frequency) over at least two days;

- a urine sample analysis to rule out infections;

- a chart recording bowel movements and consistency;

- further tests ranging from a simple physical examination to bladder ultrasound scan, abdominal X-ray, or specialist investigations to determine exactly how your bladder and bowel are working.

What Are the Treatments for Bladder Incontinence?

Once the underlying cause of incontinence has been determined, suitable treatment will be offered. This may include [the following]:

- Bladder training which reduces urgency and frequency by gradually retraining your bladder to be less active and to hold more urine. This is done by making regular visits to the toilet, and gradually extending the time between visits until your bladder learns how to hold on.

- Pelvic floor exercises help strengthen muscles so that they provide support. This will help improve bladder control and improve or stop leakage of urine.

- Bladder stimulation vibrating devices are sometimes effective where there is difficulty in emptying the bladder.

- Medication may help to reduce urine production, urgency, and frequency.

- Weight loss (if you are overweight) will often improve bladder control in the longer term.

What Are the Treatments for Bowel Incontinence?

Treatment for bowel (fecal) incontinence may include [the following]:

- Bowel training through regular visits to the toilet (usually after meals, when the bowels are stimulated to move by a natural reflex). You also learn to delay bowel movements once on the toilet to improve your ability to hold on.

- Medication to help reduce movement in the bowel or make the sphincter muscle tighter to avoid leakage

- Treatment for constipation using laxatives

- A bowel regimen which uses medicine to make you constipated followed by an enema (putting liquid into your anus) to clear the bowel in a controlled way

- Dietary changes such as eating more fiber if you have constipation and eating less fiber if you have diarrhea

Chapter 39

Vision Problems after Stroke

Following a stroke, you might experience problems with your vision, but you are not alone. Up to two thirds of people experience some changes to their vision after stroke. This text explains the different types of problems you might experience and how they can be treated.

Having trouble with your vision can be distressing and it can affect the rest of your recovery. For example, you may not be able to walk confidently if you cannot fully see where you are going. Like other effects of stroke, visual problems do often improve in time as the brain recovers. When this isn't possible, they can be quite difficult to adjust to.

Problems with vision can sometimes be missed, so if you think you or someone you know has visual problems after a stroke, talk to your doctor.

You may have had some visual problems before your stroke such as cataracts, age-related macular degeneration, diabetic retinopathy, or glaucoma. Also, you may have poor eyesight and need glasses to help you read, or to see long distance.

If you think your vision has become worse, it is important to have an eye examination to detect problems that are not related to your stroke so they can be treated. Correcting short sight with glasses or continuing to take eye drops for glaucoma can make a considerable difference to your eyesight.

How Can a Stroke Affect My Vision?

How you are affected depends on exactly where the stroke occurred in your brain.

There are four main types of visual problems and you may experience one or more:

- Central vision loss
- Visual field loss
- Eye movement problems
- Visual processing problems

Central Vision Loss

Central vision loss is the partial or complete loss of vision in one or both of your eyes.

Occasionally visual problems are due to a stroke affecting the eye only. This is called a retinal stroke and happens when there is a blockage in one of the blood vessels to your eye. If you have had a retinal stroke, you may have been aware of some blurring or blackouts of vision in one eye before your stroke.

However, usually visual problems after a stroke happen because of damage to your brain and not your eye. Central vision loss due to a stroke in the brain usually affects both eyes.

How Do I Know If I Have Central Vision Loss?

You may not be able to see anything at all, or you may only be able to see things around the edge of your vision, but not in the center.

How Is It Treated?

You may be given magnifiers (to increase the size of what you are looking at), minifiers (to help you concentrate on the remaining area of your vision), or anti-glare glasses or overlays (to reduce excessive contrast of images and glare).

Visual Field Loss

Your visual field is everything you can see—from straight ahead to outwards to the side (periphery).

Visual field loss after a stroke usually affects both eyes. It means that you are unable to see properly either to the left or to the right of the center of your field of vision.

Where you experience difficulties is directly related to where the stroke occurred in your brain.

Types of Visual Field Problems

There are many types of visual field loss, but the most common is a condition where you can see only the right half or the left half of the world out of each eye. It is called homonymous hemianopia and affects two thirds of people with visual field loss following stroke. This happens when a stroke occurs at the back of your brain.

Other types of visual field loss include:

- loss of a quarter of the visual field;

- loss of the entire upper or lower field of vision;

- patches (scotomas) missing in the field of vision.

How Do I Know If I Have Visual Field Loss?

You will usually experience loss of your visual field to one side. As a result, it is very common to have problems reading. It can be difficult to locate the start of sentences if you have left-sided field loss, and it's harder to see ahead along the line of text if you have right-sided field loss.

Chapter 40

Overview of Post-Stroke Rehabilitation and Types of Post-Stroke Therapies

In the United States more than 700,000 people suffer a stroke each year, and approximately two-thirds of these individuals survive and require rehabilitation. The goals of rehabilitation are to help survivors become as independent as possible and to attain the best possible quality of life. Even though rehabilitation does not cure the effects of stroke in that it does not reverse brain damage, rehabilitation can substantially help people achieve the best possible long-term outcome.

What is post-stroke rehabilitation?

Rehabilitation helps stroke survivors relearn skills that are lost when part of the brain is damaged. For example, these skills can include coordinating leg movements in order to walk or carrying out the steps involved in any complex activity. Rehabilitation also teaches survivors new ways of performing tasks to circumvent or compensate for any residual disabilities. Individuals may need to learn how to bathe and dress using only one hand, or how to communicate effectively when their ability to use language has been compromised. There is a strong consensus among rehabilitation experts that the most important element in any rehabilitation program is carefully directed, well-focused, repetitive practice—the same kind of practice used by all people when they learn a new skill, such as playing the piano or pitching a baseball.

From "Post-Stroke Rehabilitation Fact Sheet," by the National Institute of Neurological Disorders and Stroke (NINDS, www.ninds.nih.gov), part of the National Institutes of Health, July 26, 2011.

Rehabilitative therapy begins in the acute-care hospital after the person's overall condition has been stabilized, often within 24 to 48 hours after the stroke. The first steps involve promoting independent movement because many individuals are paralyzed or seriously weakened. Patients are prompted to change positions frequently while lying in bed and to engage in passive or active range of motion exercises to strengthen their stroke-impaired limbs. (Passive range-of-motion exercises are those in which the therapist actively helps the patient move a limb repeatedly, whereas active exercises are performed by the patient with no physical assistance from the therapist.) Depending on many factors—including the extent of the initial injury—patients may progress from sitting up and being moved between the bed and a chair to standing, bearing their own weight, and walking, with or without assistance. Rehabilitation nurses and therapists help patients who are able to perform progressively more complex and demanding tasks, such as bathing, dressing, and using a toilet, and they encourage patients to begin using their stroke-impaired limbs while engaging in those tasks. Beginning to reacquire the ability to carry out these basic activities of daily living represents the first stage in a stroke survivor's return to independence.

For some stroke survivors, rehabilitation will be an ongoing process to maintain and refine skills and could involve working with specialists for months or years after the stroke.

What disabilities can result from a stroke?

The types and degrees of disability that follow a stroke depend upon which area of the brain is damaged and how much is damaged. It is difficult to compare one individual's disability to another, since every stroke can damage slightly different parts and amounts of the brain. Generally, stroke can cause five types of disabilities: Paralysis or problems controlling movement; sensory disturbances including pain; problems using or understanding language; problems with thinking and memory; and emotional disturbances.

Paralysis or problems controlling movement (motor control): Paralysis is one of the most common disabilities resulting from stroke. The paralysis is usually on the side of the body opposite the side of the brain damaged by stroke, and may affect the face, an arm, a leg, or the entire side of the body. This one-sided paralysis is called hemiplegia if it involves complete inability to move or hemiparesis if it is less than total weakness. Stroke patients with hemiparesis or hemiplegia may have difficulty with everyday activities such as walking or grasping objects. Some stroke patients have problems with swallowing, called dysphagia, due to damage to the part of the brain that controls the muscles for swallowing. Damage to a lower part of the brain, the cerebellum, can affect the body's ability to coordinate movement, a disability called ataxia, leading to problems with body posture, walking, and balance.

Sensory disturbances including pain: Stroke patients may lose the ability to feel touch, pain, temperature, or position. Sensory deficits also may hinder the ability to recognize objects that patients are holding and can even be severe enough to cause loss of recognition of one's own limb. Some stroke patients experience pain, numbness, or odd sensations of tingling or prickling in paralyzed or weakened limbs, a symptom known as paresthesias.

The loss of urinary continence is fairly common immediately after a stroke and often results from a combination of sensory and motor deficits. Stroke survivors may lose the ability to sense the need to urinate or the ability to control bladder muscles. Some may lack enough mobility to reach a toilet in time. Loss of bowel control or constipation also may occur. Permanent incontinence after a stroke is uncommon, but even a temporary loss of bowel or bladder control can be emotionally difficult for stroke survivors.

Stroke survivors frequently have a variety of chronic pain syndromes resulting from stroke-induced damage to the nervous system (neuropathic pain). In some stroke patients, pathways for sensation in the brain are damaged, causing the transmission of false signals that result in the sensation of pain in a limb or side of the body that has the sensory deficit. The most common of these pain syndromes is called thalamic pain syndrome (caused by a stroke to the thalamus, which processes sensory information from the body to the brain), which can be difficult to treat even with medications. Finally, some pain that occurs after stroke is not due to nervous system damage, but rather to mechanical problems caused by the weakness from the stroke. Patients who have a seriously weakened or paralyzed arm commonly experience moderate to severe pain that radiates outward from the shoulder. Most often, the pain results from lack of movement in a joint that has been immobilized for a prolonged period of time (such as having your arm or shoulder in a cast for weeks) and the tendons and ligaments around the joint become fixed in one position. This is commonly called a frozen joint; passive movement (the joint is gently moved or flexed by a therapist or caregiver rather than by the individual) at the joint in a paralyzed limb is essential to prevent painful freezing and to allow easy movement if and when voluntary motor strength returns.

Problems using or understanding language (aphasia): At least one-fourth of all stroke survivors experience language impairments, involving the ability to speak, write, and understand spoken and written language. A stroke-induced injury to any of the brain's language-control centers can severely impair verbal communication. The dominant centers for language are in the left side of the brain for right-handed individuals and many left-handers as well. Damage to a language center located on the dominant side of the brain, known as Broca's area, causes expressive aphasia. People with this type of aphasia have difficulty conveying their thoughts through words or writing. They lose the ability to speak the words they are thinking and to put words together in coherent, grammatically correct sentences. In contrast, damage to a language center located in a rear portion of the brain, called Wernicke's area, results in receptive aphasia. People with this condition have difficulty understanding spoken or written language and often have incoherent speech. Although they can form grammatically correct sentences, their utterances are often devoid of meaning. The most severe form of aphasia, global aphasia, is caused by extensive damage to several areas of the brain involved in language function. People with global aphasia lose nearly all their linguistic abilities; they cannot understand language or use it to convey thought.

Problems with thinking and memory: Stroke can cause damage to parts of the brain responsible for memory, learning, and awareness. Stroke survivors may have dramatically shortened attention spans or may experience deficits in short-term memory. Individuals also may lose their ability to make plans, comprehend meaning, learn new tasks, or engage in other complex mental activities. Two fairly common deficits resulting from stroke are anosognosia, an inability to acknowledge the reality of the physical impairments resulting from stroke, and neglect, the loss of the ability to respond to objects or sensory stimuli located on the stroke-impaired side. Stroke survivors who develop apraxia (loss of ability to carry out a learned purposeful movement) cannot plan the steps involved in a complex task and act on them in the proper sequence. Stroke survivors with apraxia also may have problems following a set of instructions. Apraxia appears to be caused by a disruption of the subtle connections that exist between thought and action.

Emotional disturbances: Many people who survive a stroke feel fear, anxiety, frustration, anger, sadness, and a sense of grief for their physical and mental losses. These feelings are a natural response to the psychological trauma of stroke. Some emotional disturbances and personality changes are caused by the physical effects of brain damage. Clinical depression, which is a sense of hopelessness that disrupts an individual's ability to function, appears to be the emotional disorder most commonly experienced by stroke survivors. Signs of clinical depression include sleep disturbances, a radical change in eating patterns that may lead to sudden weight loss or gain, lethargy, social withdrawal, irritability, fatigue, self-loathing, and suicidal thoughts. Post-stroke depression can be treated with antidepressant medications and psychological counseling.

What medical professionals specialize in post-stroke rehabilitation?

Post-stroke rehabilitation involves physicians; rehabilitation nurses; physical, occupational, recreational, speech-language, and vocational therapists; and mental health professionals.

Physicians: Physicians have the primary responsibility for managing and coordinating the long-term care of stroke survivors, including recommending which rehabilitation programs will best address individual needs. Physicians also are responsible for caring for the stroke survivor's general health and providing guidance aimed at preventing a second stroke, such as controlling high blood pressure or diabetes and eliminating risk factors such as cigarette smoking, excessive weight, a high-cholesterol diet, and high alcohol consumption.

Neurologists usually lead acute-care stroke teams and direct patient care during hospitalization. They sometimes participate on the long-term rehabilitation team. Other subspecialists often lead the rehabilitation stage of care, especially physiatrists, who specialize in physical medicine and rehabilitation.

Rehabilitation nurses: Nurses specializing in rehabilitation help survivors relearn how to carry out the basic activities of daily living. They also educate survivors about routine health care, such as how to follow a medication schedule, how to care for the skin, how to move out of a bed and into a wheelchair, and special needs for people with diabetes. Rehabilitation nurses also work with survivors to reduce risk factors that may lead to a second stroke, and provide training for caregivers.

Nurses are closely involved in helping stroke survivors manage personal care issues, such as bathing and controlling incontinence. Most stroke survivors regain their ability to maintain continence, often with the help of strategies learned during rehabilitation. These strategies include strengthening pelvic muscles through special exercises and following a timed voiding schedule. If problems with incontinence continue, nurses can help caregivers learn to insert and manage catheters and to take special hygienic measures to prevent other incontinence-related health problems from developing.

Physical therapists: Physical therapists specialize in treating disabilities related to motor and sensory impairments. They are trained in all aspects of anatomy and physiology related to normal function, with an emphasis on movement. They assess the stroke survivor's strength, endurance, range of motion, gait abnormalities, and sensory deficits to design individualized rehabilitation programs aimed at regaining control over motor functions.

Physical therapists help survivors regain the use of stroke-impaired limbs, teach compensatory strategies to reduce the effect of remaining deficits, and establish ongoing exercise programs to help people retain their newly learned skills. Disabled people tend to avoid using impaired limbs, a behavior called learned non-use. However, the repetitive use of impaired limbs encourages brain plasticity and helps reduce disabilities.

Strategies used by physical therapists to encourage the use of impaired limbs include selective sensory stimulation such as tapping or stroking, active and passive range-of-motion exercises, and temporary restraint of healthy limbs while practicing motor tasks.

In general, physical therapy emphasizes practicing isolated movements, repeatedly changing from one kind of movement to another, and rehearsing complex movements that require a great deal of coordination and balance, such as walking up or down stairs or moving safely between obstacles. People too weak to bear their own weight can still practice repetitive movements during hydrotherapy (in which water provides sensory stimulation as well as weight support) or while being partially supported by a harness. A recent trend in physical therapy emphasizes the effectiveness of engaging in goal-directed activities, such as playing games, to promote coordination. Physical therapists frequently employ selective sensory stimulation to encourage use of impaired limbs and to help survivors with neglect regain awareness of stimuli on the neglected side of the body.

Occupational and recreational therapists: Like physical therapists, occupational therapists are concerned with improving motor and sensory abilities, and ensuring patient safety in the post-stroke period. They help survivors relearn skills needed for performing self-directed activities (also called occupations) such as personal grooming, preparing meals, and housecleaning. Therapists can teach some survivors how to adapt to driving and provide on-road training. They often teach people to divide a complex activity into its component parts, practice each part, and then perform the whole sequence of actions. This strategy can improve coordination and may help people with apraxia relearn how to carry out planned actions.

Occupational therapists also teach people how to develop compensatory strategies and change elements of their environment that limit activities of daily living. For example, people with the use of only one hand can substitute hook and loop fasteners (such as Velcro) for buttons on clothing. Occupational therapists also help people make changes in their homes to increase safety, remove barriers, and facilitate physical functioning, such as installing grab bars in bathrooms.

Recreational therapists help people with a variety of disabilities to develop and use their leisure time to enhance their health, independence, and quality of life.

Speech-language pathologists: Speech-language pathologists help stroke survivors with aphasia relearn how to use language or develop alternative means of communication. They also help people improve their ability to swallow, and they work with patients to develop problem-solving and social skills needed to cope with the after-effects of a stroke.

Many specialized therapeutic techniques have been developed to assist people with aphasia. Some forms of short-term therapy can improve comprehension rapidly. Intensive exercises such as repeating the therapist's words, practicing following directions, and doing reading or writing exercises form the cornerstone of language rehabilitation. Conversational coaching and rehearsal, as well as the development of prompts or cues to help people remember specific words, are sometimes beneficial. Speech-language pathologists also help stroke survivors develop strategies for circumventing language disabilities. These strategies can include the use of symbol boards or sign language. Recent advances in computer technology have spurred the development of new types of equipment to enhance communication.

Speech-language pathologists use special types of imaging techniques to study swallowing patterns of stroke survivors and identify the exact source of their impairment. Difficulties with swallowing have many possible causes, including a delayed swallowing reflex, an inability to manipulate food with the tongue, or an inability to detect food remaining lodged in the cheeks after swallowing. When the cause has been pinpointed, speech-language pathologists work with the individual to devise strategies to overcome or minimize the deficit. Sometimes, simply changing body position and improving posture during eating can bring about improvement. The texture of foods can be modified to make swallowing easier; for example, thin liquids, which often cause choking, can be thickened. Changing eating habits by taking small bites and chewing slowly can also help alleviate dysphagia.

Vocational therapists: Approximately one-fourth of all strokes occur in people between the ages of 45 and 65. For most people in this age group, returning to work is a major concern. Vocational therapists perform many of the same functions that ordinary career counselors do. They can help people with residual disabilities identify vocational strengths and develop résumés that highlight those strengths. They also can help identify potential employers, assist in specific job searches, and provide referrals to stroke vocational rehabilitation agencies.

Most important, vocational therapists educate disabled individuals about their rights and protections as defined by the Americans with Disabilities Act of 1990. This law requires employers to make reasonable accommodations for disabled employees. Vocational therapists frequently act as mediators between employers and employees to negotiate the provision of reasonable accommodations in the workplace.

When can a stroke patient get rehabilitation?

Rehabilitation should begin as soon as a stroke patient is stable, sometimes within 24 to 48 hours after a stroke. This first stage of rehabilitation can occur within an acute-care hospital; however, it is very dependent on the unique circumstances of the individual patient.

Recently, in the largest stroke rehabilitation study in the United States, researchers compared two common techniques to help stroke patients improve their walking. Both methods—training on a body-weight supported treadmill or working on strength and balance exercises at home with a physical therapist—resulted in equal improvements in the individual's ability to walk by the end of one year. Researchers found that functional improvements could be seen as late as one year after the stroke, which goes against the conventional wisdom that most recovery is complete by 6 months. The trial showed that 52 percent of the participants made significant improvements in walking, everyday function, and quality of life, regardless of how severe their impairment was, or whether they started the training at 2 or 6 months after the stroke.

Where can a stroke patient get rehabilitation?

At the time of discharge from the hospital, the stroke patient and family coordinate with hospital social workers to locate a suitable living arrangement. Many stroke survivors return home, but some move into some type of medical facility.

Inpatient rehabilitation units: Inpatient facilities may be free-standing or part of larger hospital complexes. Patients stay in the facility, usually for two to three weeks, and engage in a coordinated, intensive program of rehabilitation. Such programs often involve at least three hours of active therapy a day, five or six days a week. Inpatient facilities offer a comprehensive range of medical services, including full-time physician supervision and access to the full range of therapists specializing in post-stroke rehabilitation.

Outpatient units: Outpatient facilities are often part of a larger hospital complex and provide access to physicians and the full range of therapists specializing in stroke rehabilitation. Patients typically spend several hours, often three days each week, at the facility taking part in coordinated therapy sessions and return home at night. Comprehensive outpatient facilities frequently offer treatment programs as intense as those of inpatient facilities, but they also can offer less demanding regimens, depending on the patient's physical capacity.

Nursing facilities: Rehabilitative services available at nursing facilities are more variable than are those at inpatient and outpatient units. Skilled nursing facilities usually place a greater emphasis on rehabilitation, whereas traditional nursing homes emphasize residential care. In addition, fewer hours of therapy are offered compared to outpatient and inpatient rehabilitation units.

Home-based rehabilitation programs: Home rehabilitation allows for great flexibility so that patients can tailor their program of rehabilitation and follow individual schedules. Stroke survivors may participate in an intensive level of therapy several hours per week or follow a less demanding regimen. These arrangements are often best suited for people who require treatment by only one type of rehabilitation therapist. Patients dependent on Medicare coverage for their rehabilitation must meet Medicare's homebound requirements to qualify for such services; at this time lack of transportation is not a valid reason for home therapy. The major disadvantage of home-based rehabilitation programs is the lack of specialized equipment. However, undergoing treatment at home gives people the advantage of practicing skills and developing compensatory strategies in the context of their own living environment. In the recent stroke rehabilitation trial, intensive balance and strength rehabilitation in the home was equivalent to treadmill training at a rehabilitation facility in improving walking.

Chapter 41

Post-Stroke Rehabilitation Facilities

Chapter Contents

Section 41.1

How to Choose a Rehabilitation Facility

"Choosing a rehabilitation facility, especially after a serious event, can be a stressful process. That's why it's so important to learn what resources are available and to have the courage to ask questions. Getting answers to key questions will help patients and caregivers find the best resource to achieve optimal outcomes for recovery and to cope with their new situation," according to a brain aneurysm survivor who received rehabilitation therapy at the Rehabilitation Hospital of the Cape and Islands. Choosing the right rehabilitation facility can make a difference in how fully—and how quickly—the patient is able to resume his or her activities. It is highly recommend that you tour each facility you are considering. Talking with the admissions director and other staff will give you a better sense of the environment of care—and it will allow you to ask about specific areas of expertise. The facility's website often provides extensive information about programs, services, physicians, and other specialized resources as well. In a time of stress, it will be much easier for the primary caretaker to find an appropriate facility as close to the caretaker's home as possible to minimize drive time as much as possible.

How to Choose a Rehabilitation Facility: 20 Questions to Ask

The following questions can help you compare the services offered by different rehabilitation facilities.

Accreditations, Quality

1. Is the facility affiliated with any major hospitals?
2. Is the facility accredited?

3. Does the facility have a formal way to monitor quality of care?

4. Is the facility clean and well maintained?

Specialized Programs

5. Does the facility specialize in rehabilitation care?

6. Does the facility offer specialized programs?

7. Does the facility have the specialized resources to enhance its medical, nursing, and rehabilitation care?

Physicians and Nurses

8. Does the facility have a medical staff that is trained in rehabilitation?

9. Does the facility have a physician present at all times?

10. Are the nurses qualified to care for patients who need rehabilitation?

11. Are there enough nurses to provide high quality care to every patient?

Therapy Services

12. Does the facility offer specialized therapies?

13. Does the facility also offer outpatient physician and therapy services?

14. How much therapy do patients receive?

Team Approach to Care

15. Does the staff work as a team?

16. Are other specialists available if needed?

17. How is the treatment plan developed?

18. Who plans for the patient's discharge and handles insurance questions?

19. What happens if the family needs instruction about how to care for the patient after discharge?

20. How would you describe the staff?

Section 41.2

Inpatient Care for Stroke

Stroke rehabilitation focuses on restoration, compensation, and prevention. This means regaining skills, learning new skills to replace lost ones, and preventing future complications due to an injury or illness. Undergoing inpatient rehabilitation therapy is actually a milestone in recovery because it requires that a stroke survivor be medically stable and strong enough to participate daily in three hours of therapy. Further recovery is usually expected after discharge with continued outpatient therapy.

Therapeutic Goals

The goals of a rehabilitation program are to increase strength, endurance, and mobility and improve ability to perform activities of daily living. A wide variety of functional areas, such as cognitive, communication, and swallowing problems are also addressed as needed.

There are two types of recovery following an injury to the brain: Spontaneous and activity dependent (plasticity). Spontaneous recovery is based on the natural ability of the brain to clean up dead cells and to decrease swelling. Plasticity is the ability of certain areas of the brain to take over functions that the injured areas are no longer able to perform. Plasticity requires practice of tasks to be successful. Rehabilitation treatment maximizes all aspects of recovery.

Inpatient rehabilitation often addresses:

- basic daily skills—dressing, moving, and bowel and bladder control;
- communication;
- swallowing and eating.

Individual goals differ depending upon each patient's life situation, personality, and interests. Therapists work with patients and family to determine the best treatment. Be sure to discuss goals with therapists throughout the hospital stay.

Getting the Most out of a Rehabilitation Stay

Rehabilitation is a very active process and patient participation is key to success. As the saying goes, "you get out of it what you put into it."

- Start by talking with the case manager about plans for discharge and any concerns that may affect the rehabilitation process.

- Learn the names of the therapy team and communicate with them regularly.

- Arrive for therapies on time and give the best possible effort.

Rehabilitation Team

An interdisciplinary team approach is used to design a program for each patient. Your team meets daily to discuss medical status and progress. You and your family are an important part of this team effort. We want you to identify specific goals so they can be incorporated into the individualized treatment program.

Physician

You will have daily contact with an attending physician. The name of the attending doctor is always listed on the patient identification wrist band. All physicians at the Rehabilitation Institute of Chicago are physiatrists— specialists in Physical Medicine and Rehabilitation. They monitor your medical needs closely, and alter the rehabilitation program as needed. Ask questions and express any concerns to your physician. Each physician works with a resident who is training to be a physiatrist and will also be available for questions and information. The rehabilitation physician does not replace your family doctor after you leave. You will need to make an appointment with your family doctor one month after discharge. If you do not have a family doctor, please notify your care manager.

Nurse Practitioner

Nurse practitioners are also experienced in rehabilitation and are part of the medical team. They can be relied upon for medical care and information.

Nursing

The nursing team is trained in stroke and brain injury rehabilitation. Registered nurses (RN) and Patient Care Technicians (PCT) provide physical care and answer questions. Nurses give medications, care for wounds, and assist with pain management. They also determine bowel and bladder management, skin care, and safety. At the direction of, or with the assistance of the RN, PCTs help with bathing, showering, dressing, eating, transfers, turning, positioning, and toileting.

Nursing staff work with the team to plan for a safe discharge. Patients may be asked to identify a main caregiver who is responsible for learning home care; however, any family member or friend can learn and participate in your care. The RN provides discharge teaching on medications, skin, bladder and bowel care, and safety. Discharge teaching, actively involving you and your family member with hands-on care, may begin early in your stay so that you will feel well prepared at discharge.

Occupational (OT) and Physical Therapy (PT)

Our brain can actually reorganize based on the experiences it receives. For example, individuals who play a musical instrument have larger areas of their brains dedicated to controlling the small finger muscles used to play that instrument. The brain is able to adapt to our experiences, and if one area is damaged, it is possible that other areas can take over control. It is the therapists' job to choose activities that will encourage this type of reorganization such as [the following]:

- **Strengthening:** Arms and legs can become weak from lying in a hospital bed and because the stroke may have affected the area of the brain that controls these muscles. Both PTs and OTs work on strengthening arms, legs, trunk, and neck.

- **Range of motion:** Limited motion in a limb is common after stroke because of pain, decreased strength, stiffness, or spasticity (an uncontrolled muscle tightness caused by a constant reflex with no relaxation). It is important that muscles are stretched out so they don't get "stuck" in a certain position.

- **Balance and coordination:** Can also be affected by decreased strength, sensation, or the inability to feel where one's body is in space. Therapists work on sitting and standing balance. OTs can help improve fine motor coordination and strength in the hands and fingers.

- **Weight bearing activities:** To support body weight, strengthen weak muscles, and stretch tight muscles.

Physical therapy also addresses mobility tasks such as rolling in bed, getting from a chair to bed, and walking. Physical therapists determine if any devices or medical equipment are required at home (wheelchair, bedside commode, raised toilet seat, shower chair). They also evaluate and recommend appropriate home modifications.

Occupational therapy helps to improve strength, balance, coordination, and visual skills needed for daily activities (dressing, grooming, bathing); and thinking, including planning and managing a series of daily tasks.

Other activities that may be addressed include cooking, housekeeping, grocery shopping, and community outings when appropriate. These actually allow patients to work on cognitive skills such as divided attention, safety awareness, and problem solving in "real world" situations before leaving the hospital.

Speech Language Therapy (SLP)

SLP addresses language, cognition, speaking, and swallowing. Sometimes a video swallow test is used to assess swallowing problems. This is an X-ray taken during swallowing. A speech language pathologist will determine if exercises and/or dietary changes are needed.

Care Manager

Provides help planning for discharge including community resources, medical supplies, referrals for continued therapy, and follow up medical appointments. The Care Manager also provides information from team conferences on your weekly progress.

Clinical Dietitian

Assesses nutritional requirements, provides education, and answers any questions about nutrition.

Psychologist

Helps with emotional, cognitive and coping issues, and conducts neuropsychological testing when appropriate.

Some patients may also meet with these professionals: Recreational therapist, vocational therapist, prosthetist, orthotist, assistive technology specialist, respiratory therapist, and chaplain.

Planning for Discharge

The length of inpatient rehabilitation depends on progress in therapies, discharge destination, and insurance coverage.

The amount of help needed with daily personal care can be a factor in determining where a person will live after leaving the hospital. If little assistance is required, an individual could go home either alone, with family, with or without paid help. Another choice might be an assisted living facility where a minimal amount of assistance can be provided at different times throughout the day. If care needs are great and there is no one to assist at home, a skilled nursing facility may be the best discharge option. Skilled nursing facilities provide nursing care 24 hours a day and any therapy that may be required.

The majority of stroke patients continue with therapy after leaving the hospital. Day rehabilitation is a program for those who require more than one type of therapy (OT, PT, SLP). These are scheduled together in one site and transportation may be available. Individual outpatient therapies can also be obtained at a hospital or outpatient center, but transportation will not be provided. In-home therapy is an option for those who cannot easily get out. Finally, therapy is available at skilled nursing facilities for those who are residents.

Section 41.3

Day Rehabilitation for Stroke

Rehabilitation is a process that involves team of health care professionals working with a stroke survivor and family, using education and practical experiences to assist the patient in reaching the highest level of independence possible. Goals of rehabilitation are regaining previous skills, learning new skills to replace lost ones, and preventing future complications due to an injury or illness. This is an individualized treatment process in which each person sets specific goals, depending upon health status, life circumstances, personality, and interests.

Treatment Team

Several different types of rehabilitation specialists are part of the treatment team.

Physician

Physician specialists in Physical Medicine and Rehabilitation are called physiatrists. The physician is regularly updated on progress in therapy and makes changes when needed. Feel free to ask questions and express needs to your doctor at any time. Also, remember that it is important to continue with care from your primary physician.

Nurse

The nurse helps with medications and other medical issues, and educates each patient and family on the effects of stroke. The nurse can also help patients in scheduling a follow up appointment with a physiatrist and finding a primary care physician if needed.

Occupational Therapist (OT)

OT addresses activities necessary to function at home, work, school, or in the community. This includes all activities of daily living (ADL)—toileting, dressing, bathing, meal preparation, financial management, and leisure time. Therapists work with patients on developing strength, coordination, endurance, and other skills needed for these tasks.

Physical Therapist (PT)

PT improves mobility including walking, balance, coordination, strength, and endurance. The PT also helps decide if any special medical equipment is needed.

Speech and Language Pathologist (SLP)

Speech and language therapy improves communication. For those with swallowing problems, SLP also includes helpful eating methods or dietary changes.

Counselor/Psychologist/Social Worker

It is normal for patients and families to have many emotional issues related to the stroke. A supportive counselor helps with coping and emotional factors.

Other Team Members

Additional support may be provided by a vocational rehabilitation specialist, prosthetist, orthotist, or assistive technology specialist.

The treatment team is also responsible for:

- evaluating patients' home for safety, accessibility, and necessary modifications;
- ordering equipment;
- ensuring patient safety in the rehabilitation facility.

Having a secure environment and preventing falls are a priority. Patients and caregivers are requested to notify staff when leaving the premises.

Therapy Process—Physical and Occupational Therapy

There are two kinds of recovery following an injury to the brain. One is spontaneous—improvement based on brain ability to cleanse itself of dead cells and reduce swelling. The other is plasticity—the ability of new areas of the brain to take over function that the injured areas are no longer able to perform. Physical and occupational therapy promote recovery through both of these processes.

Some examples include [the following]:

- Strengthening muscles and areas that have become weak during hospitalization, or through damaging effects of the stroke

- Range of motion exercises to stretch tight or stiff joints which can occur due to pain, inactivity, decreased strength, or spasticity (an uncontrolled muscle tightness caused by a constant reflex with no relaxation)

- Improving balance for both sitting and standing; balance can be affected by weakness, decreased sensation, or the ability to feel one's body

- Improving hand coordination and strength to make tasks easier

- Weight bearing exercises to support body weight, strengthen weak muscles, and stretch tight muscles

Recovery and Support

Part of rehabilitation is learning how and when to return to life activities, such as living independently, driving, or working. The rehabilitation team will provide advice to each patient about these issues and make referrals to other programs if necessary, such as a driver training program.

Recovery after a stroke can take a long time. It is challenging for the stroke survivor to remain persistent and motivated for improvement. There is no magic formula for how to cope; each individual finds his or her own way. A few helpful tips:

- Connect with others for support.

- Stay flexible in expectations of one's self and others.

- Try to maintain a daily structure or schedule.

- Set small goals and look for even small signs of progress.

- Be positive and realistic.

The Rehabilitation Institute of Chicago (RIC), local hospitals, and the American Heart Association are also good resources. The RIC LIFE Center (312-238-5433) can help with locating a program or group.

Financial and Legal Issues

Medical Expenses

Coverage after a stroke varies depending on the insurance program.

- Private insurance (HMO/PPO) coverage is based on the type of policy. The clinical manager helps patients to verify benefits before rehabilitation begins.

- Medicare covers 80% of day rehabilitation therapy charges.

- Medicaid coverage is based individually on medical need.

When recovery is expected to be a long process, there may be other options for financial support through an employer or Social Security Disability. Employed patients should check benefit plans for long and short term disability coverage. The clinical manager can provide information on Social Security Disability requirements and application process. Medicaid can offer financial assistance for medicine refills, transportation, and other expenses, based on financial needs.

Medical insurance does not usually cover the cost of assistance with personal care at home. Some insurance policies offer a separate long term care option. Patients and families will need to work with employers and insurance carriers to determine what benefits are available.

In Illinois, two state agencies may be helpful. The Department of Rehabilitation Services (DORS) offers programs for individuals under age 60. These programs include help at home and vocational counseling. The Department of Aging (DOA) offers similar services for people age 60 and older, based on need.

Legal Concerns If a Patient Is Unable to Make Competent Decisions

A stroke survivor who is competent can name a family member or friend Power of Attorney for health care or financial matters. In situations where a person has become incapable of decision making and has not made Power of Attorney arrangements, Illinois law allows someone else to be designated. In order of priority, a guardian, spouse, adult children, parents, adult brothers or sisters, adult grandchildren, a close friend, or guardian of estate are listed as surrogate decision makers. In certain instances, a concerned family member or friend may also seek guardianship. Guardianship is a legal proceeding and involves time and expense.

454

For more information on stroke and reducing risk:

- National Stroke Association, 800-787-6537, www.stroke.org

- American Heart Association, 800-242-8721, www.strokeassocation.org

- National Heart, Lung and Blood Institute, 301-592-8573, www.nhlbi.nih.gov

- American Dietetic Association, www.eatright.org

Chapter 42

Cardiac Rehabilitation Programs Benefit Patients after Mini or Mild Stroke

Study Highlights

- Cardiac rehabilitation appears to benefit patients who have had a transient ischemic attack (TIA) or mild, non-disabling stroke by lowering risk factors that put them at risk for subsequent stroke.

- It is feasible, effective, and safe for patients who have had a TIA or mild stroke to participate in traditional cardiac rehabilitation programs.

Cardiac rehabilitation, traditionally used after heart attack to prevent future heart problems, seems similarly effective for people who have a transient ischemic attack (TIA) or mild stroke, according to research published in [the September 2011 issue of] *Stroke: Journal of the American Heart Association*.

TIA, also called mini-stroke, is a warning sign. While causing little or no permanent injury to the brain, patients are at high risk for subsequent, often debilitating strokes.

In the study, researchers defined a mild stroke as one that didn't cause significant disability. "Many of the risk factors that we worry about after a heart attack—high cholesterol, smoking, low exercise capacity, and high blood pressure—also concern us after a TIA," said Neville Suskin, MBChB, MSc, senior investigator of the study, medical director of the London Health Sciences Centre Cardiac Rehabilitation & Secondary Prevention Program and associate professor of medicine at the University of Western Ontario in London, Ontario, Canada. "We know that cardiac rehab addresses these risk factors in patients with heart conditions and wondered whether it was feasible, effective, and safe for patients after TIA or mild stroke."

Suskin and colleagues assessed cardiac risk factors in 100 patients who had experienced a TIA or mild stroke in the previous year. Patients participated in an outpatient cardiac rehab program for approximately 7 1/2 months and then were re-assessed for risk factors. Researchers assessed the effectiveness of the rehab process, which included exercise; drug management; nutrition education; smoking cessation; and addressing psychological issues such as stress, anxiety, or depression. Eighty patients completed the rehab process.

"Overall, following the cardiac rehab intervention, the TIA and mild stroke patients improved significantly in their risk profile," said Suskin who is also a scientist at Lawson Health Research Institute in London, Ontario, Canada.

Patients' peak exercise capacity improved by an average of about 31 percent by the end of cardiac rehabilitation.

Other findings include [the following]:

- Total cholesterol decreased by an average 11.6 milligrams per deciliter (mg/dl).

- Triglycerides decreased by 23.9 mg/dl.

- Low density lipoprotein (bad cholesterol) decreased by 9.3 mg/dl, while high density lipoprotein (good cholesterol) increased by 2.3 mg/dl (changes which were promising but statistically non-significant).

- Waist circumference decreased by 1 inch.

- Body mass index decreased by 0.5 kilograms per square meter (kg/m^2) and body weight decreased by 3.2 pounds.

- Systolic blood pressure dropped by 3 millimeters of mercury (mm Hg) and diastolic declined by 2 mm Hg (these represent promising but statistically non-significant changes in blood pressure).

- A significant number of patients became non-smokers.

The researchers also reported that 11 more patients, who at program entry were at moderate or high risk of dying during the next year, after cardiac rehab completion were recategorized to lowest risk of death.

"While a TIA or mild stroke may seem small, in reality these events are crucial warning signs of possible catastrophic stroke or heart attack," said Peter L. Prior, PhD, CPsych, lead author of the study, clinical psychologist in the London Health Sciences Centre Cardiac Rehabilitation & Secondary Prevention Program, and adjunct clinical professor in the Department of Psychology at the University of Western Ontario. "Our study is novel because it shows that cardiac rehabilitation, involving structured programs in exercise, nutrition, smoking cessation, and psychological services, is a feasible, potentially effective way for TIA or mild stroke patients to reduce their risk of strokes or heart attacks."

To confirm the results, the researchers are conducting a randomized controlled study, comparing the results of cardiac rehab in TIA or mild stroke patients, to a control group who receive only usual care.

Dr. Prior is also an associate scientist at Lawson Health Research Institute.

Other co-authors are Vladimir Hachinski, MD, DSc (co-principal investigator); Karen Unsworth, MSc; Richard Chan, MD; Sharon Mytka, BScN, MEd; and Christina O'Callaghan, BAppSc(PT). Author disclosures are on the manuscript.

The Ontario Ministry of Health and Long-term Care, through the Stroke Strategy of Ontario, funded the study.

Chapter 43

Recreational Therapy after Stroke

What Is Recreational Therapy?

Recreational therapy uses a holistic approach that involves assessment and intervention into the physical, social, cognitive, and emotional functioning of people with disabilities. Recreational therapists help clients improve their functional skills, adapt and teach recreational skills to enable full participation in activities that enhance quality of life, and provide community-based resources for independent functioning.

Recreational therapists use the arts, crafts, music, dance, drama, relaxation, horticulture, movement, volunteer activities, sports, and games that are specifically chosen to improve functional deficits in a safe, fun, and non-threatening environment. They focus on helping people with disabilities transfer their new skills to work, social relationships, and activities of daily living.

An underlying principle of recreational therapy is that when people with disabilities discover that they can continue to live a full and productive life, they will work hard to achieve their treatment goals.

An example of an intervention that a recreational therapist might use would be if a survivor has short-term memory deficits, fine motor deficits, and poor endurance, the therapist could play the card game Concentration and have the survivor use his or her affected hand to turn the cards while standing.

"Recreational Therapy: Healing Body and Spirit," reprinted with permission *Stroke Connection Magazine* September/October 2008, pp. 22–23 © 2008 American Heart Association, Inc.

Therapeutic recreation is provided by professionals who are trained, certified, and licensed to provide therapeutic recreation. For more information, visit the American Therapeutic Recreation Association website: www.atra-tr.org.

Healing Body and Spirit

Difficulty speaking or impaired memory and physical mobility can make stroke survivors feel like they can't participate in fulfilling activities. But finding ways to contribute to society can be an important part of surviving—and thriving.

In fall 2007, the recreational therapy students interning at The Center for Life Skills at Ithaca College (Longview), a retirement and independent living community, planned a community service project that engaged stroke survivors at Longview with students and faculty.

Community service projects offer many benefits, including learning computer skills, practicing speech and writing, developing fine motor skills, problem solving, and doing something useful for the community. Students discussed these at their first meeting with Longview survivors.

Participants brainstormed what types of community agencies would benefit from their work and decided to conduct a canned food and supplies drive for the local animal shelter.

Planning the Project

The survivors and student therapists made a list of essential jobs needed to complete the drive for the shelter.

Tasks included:

- asking the director for permission to proceed and inviting her to talk to the group about the shelter's needs;

- making a list of potential places where collection baskets could be placed and securing permission from managers to do so;

- creating posters that described the project;

- distributing and monitoring the collection baskets;

- developing public relations releases on the computer; and

- developing a speech to make when presenting the collected items to the agency.

Survivors were matched with tasks based on their need to practice certain skills. For example, those who had trouble speaking would call collection sites and the animal shelter. Participants who had difficulty writing made posters or collages that were placed with the baskets to explain the project. Those who wanted to learn to use the computer wrote letters and developed copy for the posters. Some survivors collected and cut out manufacturers' coupons to use their affected hands and practice cutting.

The Result—Everybody Wins

The project was a great success. The survivors stretched and grew, producing a meaningful result that they could each feel good about. And more than 10 laundry baskets of food and supplies were collected for the shelter.

As one participant reported, "It was a good idea to encourage us to be very active in this project because it made us feel useful. I really enjoyed making the collages. The speech I did was a bit scary, but I'm glad I had to do it."

In satisfaction surveys, survivors reported that they made the most significant gains in working together to make a difference and giving back to the community. They also became more comfortable communicating with people in the community and enjoyed the interaction with the students. Many shared the desire to do more projects; the Longview group embarked on a similar project the following semester.

Recreational therapists play a significant role in the rehabilitation process by using purposeful interventions to enhance the quality of life for survivors. These activities, matched to their functional disabilities, let survivors engage in meaningful activities that heal the body and the spirit.

Chapter 44

Transferring Skills Learned in Stroke Rehab to the Home Environment

Strokes are the No. 1 cause of disability—and the No. 3 cause of death—in the United States. Some of those disabilities could be prevented if stroke victims received better care, suggests new research. A study in *Stroke* (Vol. 34, No. 1), found that less than 10 percent of those who'd had a stroke within two years were receiving occupational or physical therapy—but patients who did get such care reported lower levels of disability and problems over time.

"Often, there's attention to the more obvious medical aspects, but as soon as the patient is able to walk, it's goodbye," says geropsychologist and stroke rehabilitation expert Robert Katz, PhD, director of psychology at the Peninsula Center for Extended Care in Far Rockaway, New York. "There are so many huge issues that aren't being addressed."

In addition, once patients return home, the skills they learned in the hospital aren't reinforced, says psychologist Tamara Bushnik, PhD, director of the Rehabilitation Research Center at the Rusk Institute for Rehabilitation in New York.

"While people might be quite independent in the inpatient facility, once they get home, the skills don't always transfer," she says.

And with the state of insurance reimbursement, she points out, in-home therapists can't always come in to help people during the crucial transition time.

These challenges have inspired a new wave of stroke research that aims at closing the gap between short- and long-term care and dramatically improving stroke survivors' long-term quality of life. Researchers are pinpointing the most successful components of already-proven treatments, developing therapy systems that patients can use at home, and testing treatments for patients with stroke-related problems that tend to go unnoticed and untreated, such as a subtle inability to attend to one side of one's visual space. Psychologists are also designing interventions based on new research that details how our brains recover from injury.

"It's an exciting time in stroke rehab because there's a lot of progress being made at the basic science level, in particular in our understanding of how malleable our nervous systems are," says psychologist Gitendra Uswatte, PhD, associate professor of psychology at the University of Alabama at Birmingham. "We're just starting to learn more about how you harness that neuroplasticity to the advantage of the patient."

Taking Gains Home

Research suggests that transferring skills from stroke survivors' hospital rooms to their homes is a crucial part of rehabilitation, says Uswatte, associate director of the lab headed by Edward Taub, PhD. For more than two decades, Taub's lab has been developing a behavioral intervention called Constraint-Induced Movement Therapy, or CI therapy, which trains people to better use their stroke-affected arms or lower limbs.

CI therapy has three components. One is a behavioral shaping component, in which therapists use verbal praise to encourage patients to engage in increasingly challenging daily tasks with their more affected arms, such as spooning beans into their mouth or drinking from a soda can. The second component is physical restraint of the better arm to force repeated use of the affected one. The third is a transfer package, a set of techniques that helps patients transfer gains from the lab into real world. These include elements like behavioral contracts, progress diaries, phone calls with their therapists, and physical restraint of the arm outside the training setting.

In a multisite randomized controlled trial reported in the *Journal of the American Medical Association* (Vol. 296, No. 17), the researchers showed the intervention was significantly superior to treatment as usual in helping people use their affected arms. Gains persisted even after two years.

The researchers have since attempted to tease out which elements make CI therapy so effective. In an unpublished study, stroke survivors received repetitive training of their affected arms and restraint of their other arms either with or without shaping elements. Within each group, half received transfer package elements and half did not.

To their surprise, treatment success didn't hinge on whether or not people received shaping: Only those who received transfer elements improved significantly in either training condition, Uswatte says.

"We didn't think about the transfer package as being something that was particularly interesting about the therapy," he says. "We just thought of it as something we automatically included when we did a behavioral intervention."

In a study published in May 2008 in *Stroke* (Vol. 39, No. 5), the team also analyzed structural magnetic resonance images of participants' brains before and after treatment. They found that only participants who received the transfer package showed a significant increase in gray matter. While it's unclear why the transfer package holds such power, it may be that it encourages and reinforces a person's attention or engagement, says Uswatte. Future studies will further parse elements of the package to see which might have the biggest effect, he adds.

Transferring the gains patients make through CI therapy might be even easier if the patients receive the initial therapy at home, Uswatte adds. Such therapy could be more convenient for patients and allow one therapist to work with four or more patients at a time, according to a preliminary study published in the *Journal of Rehabilitation Research and Development* (Vol. 43, No. 3). In that paper, Peter Lum, PhD, of the Catholic University of America in Washington, DC, Uswatte and Taub described a way to deliver CI therapy on automated, home-based work stations with therapy supervision provided by telehealth technology. The stations consist of arm-training devices, such as a pegboard and a tower with buttons, that are embedded with sensors wired to a personal computer. Computer software monitors patient progress using the information from these sensors and provides automated feedback and instruction. Meanwhile, a therapist at a base station observes how the patient is doing and overrides the automation depending on patient need, Uswatte explains.

In addition to potentially bringing a proven rehab technique to millions of homebound stroke survivors, the study shows how psychologists' expertise in learning can be applied directly to a physical problem, Uswatte adds. "While most rehab psychologists work on people's adjustment to a physical or cognitive disability or on cognitive rehabilitation," he says, "we work on the physical rehabilitation process itself."

Mysterious Symptoms

While a paralyzed arm is often the target of rehabilitation experts, up to half of stroke survivors suffer from a less visible disability: Spatial neglect. People with this condition may fail to see objects on one side of their body or even their own body parts. In one famous case, a woman only applied makeup to the right side of her face following a stroke.

For many patients, however, spatial neglect's symptoms are subtle and go undetected and untreated, says neurologist Anna Barrett, MD, who directs the Stroke Rehabilitation Research Laboratory at the Kessler Foundation Research Center in New Jersey. However, even mild cases of spatial neglect can lead to injury when people fail to notice steps on their left side, or oncoming traffic for instance.

"Failure to pay attention to this condition can be absolutely devastating," says Barrett's colleague Katz.

There are, however, few proven tests and treatments for spatial neglect, says Barrett, who closely studies the condition. To add to the arsenal of techniques that rehabilitation psychologists and other professionals can use, she's testing treatments for people with different types of spatial neglect. In a study of 80 right-hemisphere stroke patients, funded by the National Institute of Neurological Disorders and Stroke, Barrett's team is randomizing participants to one of two experimental treatments that they receive along with standard occupational therapy. Participants get two weeks of the intervention, then are assessed weekly for four weeks.

One intervention, a drug called bromocriptine, works to stimulate dopamine systems in the brain. Dopamine systems are thought to be dysfunctional in stroke patients with aiming problems—a type of spatial neglect characterized by trouble moving leftward. The other intervention, called prism adaptation therapy, uses special goggles that systematically shift patients' visual space to the right. Over time, researchers posit, the goggles might help people recalibrate their internal maps so that they orient more accurately to the left. In the study, participants wear the goggles for 15 minutes a day for two weeks and practice pointing at objects and marking the middle of a line.

In addition to testing participants using standard stroke-related measures, the team will observe how well subjects perform on daily tasks, such as dressing on their left side or paying attention to their caregivers on their left side, Barrett says.

Barrett's study is also training occupational and physical therapists to assess participants' daily functioning. It's a small but important step toward sharing what researchers are learning about stroke recovery with the larger medical community, she says.

"That's great for our study," she notes, "but it's even better for the purposes of giving these therapists more understanding of what is going on with patients and to help make care more standardized and research-based."

Part Six

Life after Stroke

Chapter 45

Regaining Cognitive Function after Stroke

Stroke can cause physical problems. It can also affect cognition. Cognition refers to thinking abilities. It's how people use their brains to talk, read, write, learn, understand, reason, and remember. Losing skills in this area may affect how you manage everyday tasks, take part in rehabilitation, and live on your own after stroke.

Stroke and Thinking Abilities

Every stroke is unique. The effect the stroke has on your thinking abilities depends on where and how the stroke injured the brain, and your overall health.

Each side of the brain controls different things. So, a stroke on one side of the brain will cause different problems than a stroke on the other side.

Damage to one side of the brain can cause loss of language skills (talking, reading, writing, understanding what people say). It can also cause verbal memory loss or the ability to remember things having to do with words.

Damage to the other side may cause attention, thinking, and behavior problems.

"Recovery after Stroke: Thinking and Cognition," © 2006 National Stroke Association (www.stroke.org). All rights reserved. Reprinted with permission. Reviewed by David A. Cooke, MD, FACP, January 24, 2013.

Stroke can also damage the front of the brain. In this case, you are more likely to lose your ability to control and organize thoughts and behavior. This makes it hard to think through the steps to complete a task. Front-brain strokes may not affect your ability to do or remember specific things.

Memory Loss

Memory loss after stroke is common, but not the same for everyone. There are many ways your memory can be affected by stroke.

- Verbal memory: Memory of names, stories, and information having to do with words.

- Visual memory: Memory of faces, shapes, routes, and things you see.

- If you have memory damage, you may have trouble learning new information or skills. Or you may be unable to remember and retrieve information.

- Stroke can cause vascular dementia (VaD), a greater decline in thinking abilities. Some experts believe that 10–20% of Americans over age 65 with dementia have VaD. This makes it second only to Alzheimer's disease as a leading cause of dementia.

- Therapies or medicines almost never fully restore memory after stroke. But, many people do recover at least some memory spontaneously after stroke. Others improve through rehabilitation.

What May Help

- Try to form a routine—doing certain tasks at regular times during the day.

- Try not to tackle too many things at once. Break tasks down into steps.

- If something needs to be done, make a note of it or do it right away.

- Make a habit of always putting things away in the same place where they can be easily seen or found.

Aphasia

After a stroke, one of the most common thinking problems is trouble with communication.

Aphasia is one of these problems. About 1 million people in the United States have aphasia. Most cases are the result of stroke.

Aphasia is a partial or total loss of ability to talk, understand what people say, read, or write. It may affect only one aspect of language.

For example, you may be unable to remember the names of objects or put words together into sentences. More often, many aspects are affected at the same time.

There are several types of aphasia. They differ by where the brain is damaged.

- Global aphasia is the most severe form. People with global aphasia can speak few familiar words and barely understand what people say. They cannot read or write.

- Another form is Broca's, or nonfluent, aphasia. People with this often omit certain kinds of words from sentences, speak slowly and with effort, and have a hard time with grammar. They mainly speak short statements of less than four words, like "walk dog." People with Wernicke's or fluent aphasia talk easily. But they use the wrong sounds in words, say the wrong words, or even make up words.

You may recover from aphasia without treatment. Most, however, benefit from therapy by a speech and language therapist. The goal is to improve your ability to communicate with other people.

This is done by helping you get back some of your language skills and learning new ways of getting your message across when needed.

Communication Tips

- Use props to make conversation easier (photos, maps).

- Draw or write things down on paper.

- Take your time. Make phone calls or try talking to people only when you have plenty of time.

- Show people what works best for you.

- Stay calm. Take one idea at a time.

- Create a communication book that includes words, pictures, and symbols that are helpful to you.

- The internet can be used to talk to people via email or to create a personal web page for yourself.

What Can Help

- Get information on stroke recovery from National Stroke Association. Visit www.stroke.org or call 800-STROKES (800-787-6537).

- Contact your local stroke association.

- Join a stroke support group. Other survivors will understand, validate your issues, and offer encouragement and ideas for dealing with memory loss.

Professionals Who Can Help

- Neuropsychologist: A doctor who can diagnose and treat changes in thinking, memory, and behavior after stroke. Ask your neurologist for a referral.

- Speech and language therapist: To find one in your area call the American Speech-Language Hearing Association at 800-638-8255.

Rehabilitation is a lifetime commitment and an important part of recovering from a stroke.

Through rehabilitation, you relearn basic skills such as talking, eating, dressing, and walking.

Rehabilitation can also improve your strength, flexibility, and endurance. The goal is to regain as much independence as possible.

Chapter 46

Adapting Your Home after Stroke

After a stroke, your loved one may fall or have trouble moving around. You can make changes to improve home safety. These types of changes are called home modification.

What You Need to Know

Some changes are easy and you can do them yourself. For bigger changes, you may need professional help. The changes you make depend on the needs of your loved one.

What You Can Do

Look around and find ways to make your home safe. Watch your loved one walk in the home to find areas that are unsafe.

Bathroom

- Buy non-slip bath mats, tub, or shower benches and toilet chairs.

- Install handrails beside the toilet and in the tub or shower.

- Install a hand-held shower head so your loved one can sit during a shower.

"Ways to Make the Home Safer (Home Modification)," by the U.S. Department of Veterans Affairs (VA), www.rorc.research.va.gov, 2008. Reviewed by David A. Cooke, MD, FACP, January 24, 2013.

Kitchen

- Buy a stove with controls in the front. Your loved one will be able to reach the controls when cooking.

- Lower counters to make them easier to reach while sitting.

- Keep oven mitts and heat-proof mats close to the stove. Leave areas near the stove clear to place hot dishes.

- Place a fire extinguisher in easy reach.

Bedroom

- Put bedrails on the bed for safety.

- Place a commode beside the bed so your loved one won't need to walk to the bathroom. This can prevent falls at night.

Changes for Stroke Survivors Who Use Wheelchairs

Remove the cabinet under the stove or sink so your loved one can roll under. Use heat-proof covering (insulation) on pipes in roll-under sinks and stoves to prevent burns.

Stroke survivors may have trouble moving wheelchairs on heavy carpet. Use non-slip flooring if you remove the carpet. Widen doorways to help stroke survivors get in and out of the home. Outdoor and indoor ramps can also be built.

General Home Changes

- Place pads on soft furniture to help with toileting accidents. Cover the pads so that other people will not notice.

- Remove throw rugs. Use double-sided tape to hold down carpets.

- Keep floors clear. Place large furniture far apart to help your loved one move around. Make sure furniture does not move if leaned on. Cover sharp corners of furniture.

- Place handrails on both sides of stairs for safety. Elevators or lifts for the home can help stroke survivors who cannot climb stairs.

- Replace door knobs and faucet knobs with lever handles. This will help stroke survivors who have trouble using their hands and arms.

Other Safety Changes

- Place a phone in each room or give your loved one a cell phone to call for help. Large-button phones are helpful for people who have trouble seeing.

- A medical alert system that the stroke survivor can carry may help.

- Lighting should be bright (use high wattage light bulbs) to prevent falls. Install overhead lights or nightlights in doorways, hallways, and bathrooms.

- Install and regularly check smoke detectors and carbon monoxide detectors.

- Move all cords out of the way. Make sure cords are in good repair to prevent shock or fires.

Helpful Tips

If possible, have your loved one visit the home before the last day in the hospital. Some hospitals and rehabilitation centers will let patients take weekend trips to visit family. This will help you learn how to make the house safe before your loved one comes home.

Occupational therapists, visiting nurses, and physical therapists can come to your house and help you make changes.

Purchase items for home safety at medical equipment stores and through catalogs.

Paying for Home Modification

Insurance and Medicaid

Some changes to the home may be covered by insurance. Talk to private insurance companies to see what can be covered. Medicaid may pay for some needed medical items.

Government Funding

The Veterans Association has some funding through its Home Loans program. Contact other government resources, such as the U.S. Department of Housing and Urban Development and the Social Security Administration to help with funding. You may also get information from Eldercare Locator. Talk to the social worker at your hospital to find out more about all of these programs.

Private Funding

Non-profit and volunteer groups may pay for some home changes. Contact groups like Rebuilding Together and NeighborWorks Network. You can find their contact information in the More Resources section.

Remember

The needs of your loved one should determine the changes you make. The healthcare team can help you make the right changes.

Home changes are often easy to make and you do not need a lot of money. Talk to a social worker if money is a problem. There are ways to obtain help in paying for home changes.

Look around and keep checking your home for ways to make it safe.

Chapter 47

Driving after Stroke

For most people, being able to drive is a sign of independence and freedom. Driving enables people to get to the places they want to go and do what they want to do. It is something that many of us have done for much, if not most, of our lives. Nevertheless, driving is a very complex skill. The ability to drive safely can be affected by changes in physical, emotional, and medical condition. The information in the following text describes:

*   how a stroke can affect driving ability; and
*   role of a driver's rehabilitation program.

How can having a stroke affect driving?

A stroke can affect strength, coordination, or ability to use or move different body parts. It can also affect thinking skills such as memory, concentration, or ability to make safe judgments and problem solve. In some instances, it may even affect your vision (double vision, blurry vision, or the inability to see out of the corners of your eyes). Due to these impairments, a stroke survivor may:

*   have trouble using the gas and brake pedals with one foot;

- have difficulty turning the steering wheel;
- become easily frustrated or confused when driving;
- not remember the location of familiar places;
- have difficulty seeing or being aware of traffic.

Is it possible to drive after having a stroke?

Most stroke survivors can return to independent and safe driving. As part of the rehabilitation process, it is important to discuss with your physician and other health care professionals your goals for returning to driving. Each state has medical and vision requirements for drivers. In Illinois, drivers must file a medical report form, completed by a physician, after experiencing any medical condition which could affect driving. Also, Illinois has specific visual requirements including on peripheral vision. For more information on driving requirements in Illinois, visit the Secretary of State website: http://www.cyberdriveillinois.com.

What is a driver rehabilitation program?

Depending on the severity of a stroke, your doctor may refer you to a driver rehabilitation program. A driver rehabilitation program provides a comprehensive driving evaluation that includes both clinical and behind the wheel (BTW) components. A driver rehabilitation specialist assesses the ability to return to safe driving and recommends the use of specific equipment if necessary.

In order to be seen in a driver rehabilitation program you will need a referral from your doctor, a valid driver's license (or permit) and payment.

During the clinical evaluation, an occupational therapist talks with you about your medical history, current condition, and goals for returning to driving. The therapist evaluates your vision, thinking skills, and overall strength, movement, and coordination. You may also be asked questions about your driving history and tested on your driving knowledge. If you need any special equipment for driving, it may also be introduced at this time. The clinical evaluation usually takes about one hour.

The behind the wheel evaluation consists of driving in a vehicle with a driving instructor in different types of traffic and driving situations. Adaptive equipment may also be introduced at this time. Certain types of driving equipment such as hand controls or left foot accelerators will require additional training sessions after your evaluation. The BTW evaluation takes about two hours.

What happens after the evaluation?

Results and any recommendations are given to both you and your doctor. These results will help you both to decide whether driving is a realistic option at that time.

Although everyone is eager to return to driving, it is important to deal with driving at the most appropriate time in the healing process. We often encourage patients to wait until they are at their highest level of functioning (physically, mentally, and emotionally) before addressing driving. Your doctor and your health care team can help you decide when this time might be.

Does insurance cover the driving evaluation?

Most insurance providers including private insurance companies and Medicare/Medicaid will cover the clinical evaluation but not any of the BTW cost, additional training, or equipment. Ask your health care team or call a driver rehabilitation program for more information about funding.

Chapter 48

Nutrition and Exercise Tips for Post-Stroke Patients

Chapter Contents

Section 48.1

Advice for People with Swallowing Difficulties

"Nutrition Tips for People with Swallowing Difficulties," March 2012, Copyright © Rehabilitation Institute of Chicago. All rights reserved. Reprinted with permission. For additional information, visit the website of the LIFE Center at the Rehabilitation Institute of Chicago, http:// lifecenter.ric.org.

Several types of health problems such as a stroke, brain injury, or cancer can result in difficulty with swallowing. As a result, it may be necessary to avoid certain foods in order to prevent aspiration (having food or liquids go the lungs), which can cause pneumonia.

Generally, a nutrition professional or nurse will provide instructions on foods to eat and those to avoid. Types of diets that are often used are listed in the following text.

Pureed Diet

Foods are mixed with liquid in a blender or food processor. To prepare pureed foods, chop any food into small pieces. Add one tablespoon liquid to every four tablespoons of food. Blend until smooth.

Foods that can be pureed:

- Cooked cereal
- Scrambled eggs
- Custard/pudding
- Cottage cheese
- Yogurt
- Mashed potatoes
- Fruit
- Vegetables
- Meat

Liquids to use:

- For beef: Beef broth or tomato sauce
- For chicken: Broth or gravy
- For vegetables: Tomato juice or cheese sauce
- Milk, water, or fruit juice

Ground Diet

Foods must be soft and moist:

- Cooked meat with sauce or dressing
- Well-cooked pasta
- Well-moistened pancakes
- Canned or cooked fruit
- Well-cooked vegetables that are mashable with a fork
- Soft, moist cakes with icing

Soft Diet

Foods must be soft and easy to chew:

- Breads/soft rolls—not toasted
- Most hot and cold cereals (milk must be added to cold cereal to achieve soft consistency)
- Cakes/pies/pudding
- Lean tender meats, poultry
- Cooked vegetables and fruits
- Soft cookies
- Potatoes, rice, and pasta
- Cooked or canned fish
- Cheese
- Avoid anything with a noticeable crunch, such as with raw or undercooked vegetables or fruit, nuts, pretzels, and toasted bread.

Thin Liquids

Thin liquids that are a similar consistency to water:

* Milk

* Juice

* Soft drinks

* Jell-O

* Coffee

* Hot cocoa

* Tea

* Broth

* Soups

* Ice cream (considered a thin liquid because it melts quickly)

Thick Liquids

Thick liquids include nectar-thick or honey-thick liquids. Any fluids can be thickened by adding thickener powders. These products are sold at most full service pharmacies, but may require a special order.

Malts and milk shakes are not suitable on a thick liquid diet because they melt quickly and become thin liquids. Ready-made nectar-thick or honey-thick liquids are preferable. However, if preparing your own thickened beverage using thickening powder, follow the instructions on the product to achieve desired consistency.

Section 48.2

Exercise after Stroke

Moving around safely and easily may not be something you think about, unless you've had a stroke.

Many stroke survivors have trouble moving around. These problems range from balance issues to arm or leg paralysis. As a result, about 40 percent of stroke survivors have serious falls within a year of their strokes. But, there is good news. Rehab and therapy may improve your balance and ability to move.

Movement

The most common physical effect of stroke is muscle weakness and having less control of an affected arm or leg. Survivors often work with therapists to restore strength and control through exercise programs. They also learn skills to deal with the loss of certain body movements.

Paralysis and Spasticity

Paralysis is the inability of muscle or group of muscles to move on their own. After stroke, signals from the brain to the muscles often don't work right. This is due to stroke damage to the brain. This damage can cause an arm or leg to become paralyzed and/or to develop spasticity

Spasticity is a condition where muscles are stiff and resist being stretched. It can be found throughout the body but may be most common in the arms, fingers, or legs. Depending on where it occurs, it can result in an arm being pressed against the chest, a stiff knee, or a pointed foot that interferes with walking. It can also be accompanied by painful muscle spasms.

Treatment Options for Spasticity

- Treatment for spasticity is often a combination of therapy and medicine. Therapy can include range-of-motion exercises, gentle stretching, and splinting or casting.

- Medicine can treat the general effects of spasticity and act on multiple muscle groups in the body.

- Injections of botulinum toxin can prevent the release of chemicals that cause muscle contraction.

- One form of treatment involves the delivery of a drug directly into the spinal fluid using a surgically placed pump.

- Surgery is the last option to treat spasticity. It can be done on the brain or the muscles and joints. Surgery may block pain and restore some movement.

Exercise

Walking, bending, and stretching are forms of exercise that can help strengthen your body and keep it flexible. Mild exercise, which should be undertaken every day, can take the form of a short walk or a simple activity like sweeping the floor. Stretching exercises, such as extending the arms or bending the torso, should be done regularly. Moving weakened or paralyzed body parts can be done while seated or lying down. Swimming is another beneficial exercise if the pool is accessible and a helper is available. Use an exercise program that is written down, with illustrations and guidelines for a helper if necessary.

Fatigue

Fatigue while exercising is to be expected. Like everyone else, you will have good and bad days.

You can modify these programs to accommodate for fatigue or other conditions. Avoid overexertion and pain. However, some discomfort may be necessary to make progress.

Sample Exercise Programs

There are two exercise programs in the following text. The first is for the person whose physical abilities have been mildly affected by the stroke. The second is for those with greater limitations. If you are not sure which one is appropriate, consult the profile that precedes each program.

All of the exercises may be performed alone if you are able to do so safely. However, for many stroke survivors, it is advisable for someone to stand nearby while an exercise session is in progress. Your caregiver should watch for errors in judgment that could affect safety. For instance, some stroke survivors are not aware that their balance is unsteady, nor can they tell left from right. Others may have lost the ability to read the exercise instructions, or may need assistance to remember a full sequence of movements.

In general, each exercise is performed five to 10 times daily, unless otherwise directed. The exercise session should be scheduled for a time of day when you feel alert and well. You might have these ups and downs frequently. If the exercises are too tiring, divide them into two sessions—perhaps once in the morning and again in the afternoon.

Because the effects of stroke vary, it is impossible to devise a single exercise program suitable for everyone. The two programs detailed here are general and are intended to serve as a guide.

You should consult an occupational therapist and/or physical therapist, who can help in selecting the specific exercises that will benefit you, and who will provide instruction for both you and your caregiver.

Resources

For referral to an occupational or physical therapist, consult your doctor or contact a home health agency, a family service agency, or the physical therapy department of your community hospital.

You may also try contacting the American Occupational Therapy Association at 301-652-2682 or the American Physical Therapy Association at 800-999-2782 for a referral in your area.

As with any exercise program, consult with your doctor and/or therapist before beginning this program. If any exercises are too difficult and cause pain or increased stiffness in your limbs, do not do them.

Exercise Program 1: For Those Mildly Affected by Stroke

Profile

If you were mildly affected by stroke, you may still have some degree of weakness in the affected arm and leg, but generally have some ability to control your movements. You may also have some obvious stiffness or muscle spasms, particularly with fatigue or stress.

You may be able to walk without someone's assistance, but may use a walker, cane, or brace.

For managing longer distances or uneven terrain, you may require some minimal assistance from another person, a more supportive walking aid, or a wheelchair.

Abnormalities may be present when you walk, but may be corrected by exercise and by fitting shoes with lifts or wedges. A prescription for these shoe modifications can be obtained from a doctor following evaluation by a physical therapist. You can usually use the stairs with or without handrails, with a helper close by or with very minimal assistance.

Clothing that does not restrict movement is appropriate for exercising. It is not necessary to wear shorts. Leisure clothing such as sweat suits or jogging suits is appropriate. Sturdy, well-constructed shoes with non-skid soles, such as athletic shoes, are recommended at all times. It is important that your foot on the affected side be checked periodically for reddened areas, pressure marks, swelling, or blisters—especially when there is poor sensation or a lack of sensation. Reddened areas and pressure marks should be reported to a doctor or physical therapist.

The following exercises can help you:

- require less assistance for stair climbing;

- move more steadily when you walk;

- improve balance and endurance;

- strengthen and refine movement patterns;

- improve the coordination and speed of movement necessary for fine motor skills, such as fastening buttons or tying shoelaces.

Note: In the instructions that follow, the word floor has been used to simplify the instructions; the exercises can be performed on the floor, on a firm mattress, or on any appropriate supportive surface.

Exercise 1

To strengthen the muscles that stabilize the shoulder:

- Lie on your back with your arms resting at your sides.

- Keep your elbow straight, lift your affected arm to shoulder level with your hand pointing to the ceiling.

- Raise your hand toward the ceiling, lifting your shoulder blade from the floor.

- Hold for three to five seconds, and then relax, allowing your shoulder blade to return to the floor.

- Slowly repeat the reaching motion several times.

- Lower your arm to rest by your side.

Exercise 2

To strengthen the shoulder muscles as well as those which straighten the elbow:

- Lying on your back, grasp one end of an elasticized band in each hand with enough tension to provide light resistance to the exercise, but without causing undue strain.

- To start, place both hands alongside the unaffected hip, keeping your elbows as straight as possible.

- Move your affected arm upward in a diagonal direction, reaching out to the side, above your head, keeping your elbow straight. Your unaffected arm should remain at your side throughout the exercise.

- During the exercise, stretch the band so that it provides resistance.

Notes: Elasticized bands are marketed as Thera-Band. They are available in varying strengths (color coded) to provide progressive resistance. Initially, a three or four foot length band—perhaps with the ends knotted together to improve grip—is sufficient for the exercise. To increase resistance as strength improves, the next density of Thera-Band can be purchased, or two or more bands of the original density can be used at once. Thera-Band can be obtained from a medical supply company. Similar elastic bands or cords are also available at many sporting goods stores where exercise equipment is sold. If it is too difficult to keep the elbow straight, the exercise can be done with the elbow bent. If you cannot grip with your hand, a loop can be tied at the end to slip your hand partially through the loop, leaving the thumb out to catch the loop during upward movement.

Exercise 3

To strengthen the muscles which straighten the elbow:

- Lie on your back with your arms resting at your sides and a rolled towel under the affected elbow.

- Bend affected elbow and move your hand up toward your shoulder. Keep your elbow resting on the towel.

493

- Hold for a few seconds.

- Straighten your elbow and hold.

- Slowly repeat several times.

Note: Try not to let the hand roll in towards your mid-section/stomach.

Exercise 4

To improve hip control in preparation for walking activities:

- Start with your unaffected leg flat on the floor and your affected leg bent.

- Lift your affected foot and cross your affected leg over the other leg.

- Lift your affected foot and un-cross, resuming the position of the second bullet point.

- Repeat the crossing and un-crossing motion several times.

Exercise 5

To enhance hip and knee control:

- Start with your knees bent, feet resting on the floor.

- Slowly slide the heel of your affected leg down so that the leg straightens.

- Slowly bring the heel of your affected leg along the floor, returning to the starting position. Keep your heel in contact with the floor throughout the exercise.

Note: Your foot will slide more smoothly if you do this exercise without shoes.

Exercise 6

To improve control of knee motions for walking:

- Lie on your unaffected side with the bottom knee bent for stability and your affected arm placed in front for support.

- Starting with your affected leg straight, bend your affected knee, bringing the heel toward your buttocks, then return to the straightened position.

494

- Concentrate on bending and straightening your knee while keeping your hip straight.

Exercise 7

To improve weight shift and control for proper walking technique:

- Start with your knees bent, feet flat on the floor and knees close together.
- Lift your hips from the floor and keep them raised in the air.
- Slowly twist your hips side to side. Return to center and lower your hips to the floor.
- Rest. Repeat motion.

Note: This exercise may be difficult for some stroke survivors and it may worsen back problems. Do not do it if you experience pain.

Exercise 8

To improve balance, weight shift, and control to prepare for walking activities:

- The starting position is on your hands and knees. Weight should be evenly distributed on both arms and both legs.
- Rock in a diagonal direction back toward your right heel as far as possible, then as far forward toward your left hand as possible.
- Repeat motion several times, slowly rocking as far as possible in each direction.
- Return to center.
- Rock in a diagonal direction toward your right hand. Move as far back as possible in each direction slowly.

Note: For safety, an assistant may be nearby to prevent loss of balance. This position may not be appropriate or safe for elderly stroke survivors. Consult your doctor and/or physical therapist before attempting this exercise.

Exercise 9

To simulate proper weight shift and knee control necessary for walking:

- Stand with your unaffected side next to a countertop or other firm surface. Rest your unaffected arm on the surface for support.

- Lift your unaffected foot from the floor so that you are standing on your affected leg.

- Slowly bend and straighten the leg on which you are standing through a small range of motion. Try to move smoothly, not allowing your knee to buckle when you bend, or to snap back when you straighten.

- Repeat the knee bending and straightening several times, slowly.

Exercise 10

To simulate proper weight shift while strengthening hip and pelvis muscles

- Stand facing a countertop or other firm surface for support.

- Shift your weight onto your right leg and lift your knee straight.

- Return to center with both feet on the floor.

- Shift your weight onto your left leg and lift your right leg out to the side keeping your back and knee straight.

- Repeat several times, alternating lifts.

Exercise Program II: For the Person Moderately Affected by Stroke

Profile

If you were moderately affected by your stroke, you may use a wheelchair most of the time. You are probably able to walk—at least around the house—with the aid of another person or by using a walking aid. A short leg brace may be needed to help control foot drop or inward turning of the foot. A sling may be used to help the arm and aid in shoulder positioning for controlling pain. Your affected arm and leg may be stiff or may assume a spastic posture that is difficult to control. The toe may turn inward or the foot may drag. When walking, you may lead with the unaffected side, leaving the other side behind. Often there are balance problems and difficulty shifting weight toward the affected side.

Clothing that does not restrict movement is appropriate for exercising. It is not necessary to wear shorts. Leisure clothing such as sweat suits or jogging suits is appropriate. Sturdy, well-constructed shoes with non-skid soles, such as athletic shoes, are recommended at all times. It is important that your foot on the affected side be checked periodically for reddened areas, pressure marks, swelling, or blisters—especially when there is poor sensation or a lack of sensation. Reddened areas and pressure marks should be reported to a doctor or physical therapist.

The purpose of this exercise program is to:

- promote flexibility and relaxation of muscles on the affected side;

- help return to more normal movement;

- improve balance and coordination;

- decrease pain and stiffness;

- maintain range of motion in the affected arm and leg.

For the Stroke Survivor

Begin with exercises done lying on your back, and then move on to those performed lying on your unaffected side, then sitting, and then standing. Make sure that the surface on which you lie is firm and provides good support. Take your time when you exercise. Don't rush the movements or strain to complete them.

Note: In the instructions that follow, the word floor has been used to simplify the instructions; the exercises can be performed on the floor, on a firm mattress, or on any appropriate supporting surface.

For the Helper

There may be no need to assist the stroke survivor in the exercises, but you should be nearby during the exercise session. If the survivor has difficulty reading or remembering the sequence of movements, you can repeat the instructions one by one. You can also offer physical assistance and encouragement when needed.

Exercise 1

To enhance shoulder motion and possibly prevent shoulder pain:

- Lie on your back on a firm bed. Interlace your fingers with your hands resting on your stomach.

- Slowly raise your arms to shoulder level, keeping your elbows straight.
- Return your hands to resting position on your stomach.

Note: If pain occurs, it may be reduced by working within the range of motion that is relatively pain-free, then going up to the point where pain is felt. The arm should not be forced if pain is excessive, but effort should be made to daily increase the range of pain-free motion.

Exercise 2

To maintain shoulder motion (may be useful for someone who has difficulty rolling over in bed):

- Lie on your back on a firm bed. Interlace your fingers, with your hands resting on your stomach.
- Slowly raise your hands directly over your chest, straightening your elbows.
- Slowly move your hands to one side and then the other.
- When all repetitions have been completed, bend your elbows and return your hands to resting position on your stomach.

Note: If shoulder pain occurs, move only to the point where it begins to hurt. If the pain continues, don't do this exercise.

Exercise 3

To promote motion in the pelvis, hip, and knee (can help to reduce stiffness and is also useful for rolling over and moving in bed):

- Lie on your back on a firm bed. Keep your interlaced fingers resting on your stomach.
- Bend your knees and put your feet flat on the bed.
- Holding your knees tightly together, slowly move them as far to the right as possible. Return to center.
- Slowly move your knees as far as possible to the left, still keeping them together. Return to center.

Note: The helper may provide assistance or verbal cues to help you keep your knees together during this exercise.

Exercise 4

To improve motion at the hip and knee, simulating the movements needed for walking (can be useful when moving toward the edge of the bed before coming to a sitting position):

- Lie on your unaffected side, with your legs together.

- Bend and move your affected knee as far as possible toward your chest. You may need your helper's assistance to support the leg you're exercising.

- Return to starting position.

Exercise 5

To strengthen the muscles that straighten the elbow (necessary for getting up from a lying position):

- Sitting on a firm mattress or sofa, put your affected forearm flat on the surface with your palm facing down if possible. You may want to place a firm pillow under your elbow.

- Slowly lean your weight onto your bent elbow. You may need your helper's assistance to maintain your balance.

- Push your hand down against the support surface, straightening your elbow and sitting more upright. (Assistance may be required to prevent sudden elbow collapse).

- Slowly allow your elbow to bend, returning your forearm to the support surface.

- Work back and forth between the two extremes (completely bent or completely straight) in a slow, rhythmical manner.

Note: This exercise should not be performed if your shoulder is not yet stable and/or will not support your upper body weight. Consult your doctor and/or physical therapist before attempting this exercise.

Exercise 6

To reduce stiffness in the trunk and promote the body rotation needed for walking:

- Sit on a firm straight chair with both feet flat on the floor. If necessary, a firm mattress, sofa, or wheelchair may be used.

- Interlace your fingers.

- Bend forward and reach with your hands toward the outside of your right foot, rotating your trunk.

- Move your hands upward in a diagonal direction toward your left shoulder, keeping your elbows as straight as possible.

- Repeat the motions, moving your hands from your left foot to your right shoulder.

Note: Only individuals with good balance who can sit fairly independently should do this exercise. If balance is impaired, an assistant may stand in front, guiding the arms through the motions.

Exercise 7

Movements needed to rise from a sitting position:

- Sit on a firm chair that has been placed against the wall to prevent slipping.

- Interlace your fingers. Reach forward with your hands.

- With your feet slightly apart and your hips at the edge of the seat, lean forward, lifting your hips up slightly from the seat.

- Slowly return to sitting.

Note: In a progression of the exercise, try to rise to a complete standing position (see the third bullet point) and return to sitting. However, this should only be done by someone with good balance who can come to a standing position safely.

Exercise 8

To maintain the ankle motion needed for walking (also maintains motion at the wrist and elbow):

- Stand at arm's length from the wall, knees straight, feet planted slightly apart and flat on the floor with equal weight on both feet.

- With your unaffected hand, hold your affected hand in place against the wall at chest level.

- Slowly bend your elbows, leaning into the wall. This places a stretch on the back of your lower legs. Keep your heels on the floor.

- Straighten your elbows, pushing your body away from the wall.

Note: If the stroke survivor's affected arm is very involved, he or she may find this exercise too difficult. Consult your doctor and/or physical therapist before attempting this exercise.

Getting up from a Fall

Before attempting to help a person stand up after a fall, make sure he/she has not been injured. If there are any cuts, bruises, or painful areas, make the person comfortable on the floor while you get help. Do not attempt to move the individual until help arrives.

Most falls, however, do not result in injury. The instructions that follow outline a recommended method for getting from the floor onto a chair. The individual who has fallen may need assistance, but should be able to rise using this technique.

Step 1

Assume a side-sitting position with the unaffected side close to a heavy chair or other object that will not move.

Step 2

Place the unaffected forearm on the seat of the chair and lean on the elbow or hand. Shift weight forward onto your knees and lift your hips until you are in a kneeling position.

Step 3

Supporting yourself with your unaffected arm, bring your unaffected foot forward, and place it flat on the floor. Some assistance may be required to keep the affected limb in the kneeling position while placing the unaffected one in the position illustrated.

Step 4

Lift yourself up by pushing with your unaffected arm and leg. Twist your hips toward the chair and sit on the seat.

Chapter 49

Skin Care after Stroke

Skin is an important part of the body that works in many ways to maintain health.

- Protects the body from outside injury, illness, and germs

- Prevents loss of fluids and nutrients

- Helps to control body temperature in hot and cold weather

Skin includes several layers of tissue. Some tissues are filled with tiny blood vessels that move oxygen and nutrients to the skin. The skin also has nerves which send messages from different parts of the body to the brain. These create awareness of touch, pain, and temperature. Other nerves provide information about where body parts (arms, legs) are positioned in space and whether you are lying on an object.

After experiencing a stroke, patients may be at risk for skin problems due to decreased movement and feeling. Several types of skin problems can occur:

- Sores, blisters, rashes, or skin color changes may develop if someone remains sitting or lying in one spot for long periods of time.

- Loss of feeling may affect ability to notice contact with something sharp or hot.

- Bladder or bowel accidents are special concerns because they can cause the skin to become irritated.

Older people tend to have greater skin problems after a stroke because skin becomes less elastic with age.

Keeping Skin Healthy

Healthy skin is intact, well lubricated with natural oils, and nourished by a good blood supply. Skin stays healthy with a balanced diet, good hygiene, regular skin checks and pressure relief. Relieving pressure and checking skin ensures a good blood supply. Skin problems can often be prevented. The following tips will help.

Hygiene

- Keep skin clean and dry. Urine, sweat, or stool can cause skin breakdown. Bathing every day in a tub or shower may not be necessary and may also wash away natural oils that lubricate the skin. A daily sponge bath, however, is good for exfoliation of dry skin and overall personal hygiene. Always try to keep palm side of affected hand and underarm clean.

- Dry well after bathing, but avoid hard rubbing with a towel—it can hurt the skin.

- Back rubs can be very relaxing, but should be done with lotion or oil, not alcohol, which is very drying to the skin.

- Trim nails regularly and avoid sharp edges or hang nails.

- Individuals with diabetes should do self-foot care examinations and see a podiatrist regularly.

Nutrition

- Eat a healthy diet. Protein, vitamins, and iron are especially important. Consult with a nutrition professional for help planning a diet that will meet your needs.

- Drink six to eight cups of fluid every day.

- Tube feedings are chosen to provide all necessary nutrients.

- Pureeing or chopping foods does not change the nutritional value.

Skin Inspection

- Check skin regularly to spot sores when they are just starting.

- Inspect entire body, especially bony areas.

- Check at least twice a day—morning and evening—when you change position. Check more often if increasing sitting or turning times.

- Check skin every hour when using new equipment.

- Do not depend on others to tell you how your skin looks. If you need help, however, clearly explain what warning signs to look for.

- Use a long handled mirror to help with hard to see areas.

- Be alert to areas that have been injured and healed. Scar tissue breaks down very easily.

- Look for red areas, blisters, openings in the skin, or rashes. In red areas, use the back of your stronger hand to feel for heat.

- Do not forget to check groin area. Men who wear an external catheter should check genital area for sores or other problems.

Chapter 50

Sleep and Sex after Stroke

Chapter Contents

Section 50.1

Sleep Disorders after Stroke

Getting a good night's sleep is an important part of stroke recovery.
And yet, sleep problems are common among stroke survivors.

When these sleep problems go on for a long time, they are considered sleep disorders.

Having a sleep disorder can be frustrating. It can make you tired
and irritable. It can affect your health and quality of life. It can also
pose serious dangers by increasing your risk for another stroke. The
good news is that there are things you can do to get a good night's sleep
again. Your sleepless nights are numbered.

Sleep Disorders Caused by Breathing Problems

About two-thirds (2/3) of stroke survivors have sleep-disordered
breathing (SDB). This type of sleep disorder is caused by abnormal
breathing patterns. With SDB, your sleep is interrupted several times
throughout the night.

So, during the day you may be really sleepy or have trouble thinking
or solving problems. SDB also poses dangerous health risks because it
can increase blood pressure, heart stress, and blood clotting.

There are several types of SDB. The most common is obstructive
sleep apnea (OSA). With OSA, you may stop breathing for 10 seconds
or more, many times during the night. You usually won't have breathing problems during the day when you are awake.

Symptoms

There are several tell-tale signs that you have sleep-disordered
breathing. Some are seen at night and others during the day.

Symptoms you might see at night include:

- loud snoring;

- waking up frequently during the night, gasping for breath;
- increased sweating;
- shortness of breath;
- insomnia, or being unable to fall asleep or remain asleep throughout the night.

Sleeping problems at night can cause problems the next day, including:

- excessive daytime sleepiness;
- memory or attention problems;
- headaches;
- fatigue (low energy level);
- irritability;
- depression or extreme sadness.

Diagnosing a Sleep Disorder

Most often, your bed partner is the first to notice the symptoms. Or you may notice them yourself.

Either way, you should talk to your doctor if you think you may have a sleeping disorder. To officially diagnose the problem, your doctor may arrange a sleep test called a polysomnogram (PSG). This painless, all-night test will study your sleep patterns. It is typically done in a special sleep center.

Treating Your Sleep Disorder

Treatments vary, depending on whether your case is mild or more serious.

- You may be able to improve mild cases by losing weight, staying away from alcohol and avoiding sleep medicines.

- For mild to moderate cases, your doctor may prescribe a special dental appliance. Worn at night while you sleep (like a retainer), this tool can open up your airways and improve your breathing.

- In some cases, the problem is caused by your sleeping position and can be treated by keeping you from turning onto your back at night. This can be done by sewing an object such as a tennis ball to your pajamas, making it uncomfortable for you to turn over.

- The most successful treatment is usually continuous positive airway pressure (CPAP), a form of breathing assistance during sleep. CPAP uses air pressure to open up your airways. The CPAP machine is a little larger than an average toaster. It blows heated, humidified air through a short tube to a mask that you wear. The mask must fit snugly to prevent air from leaking. The CPAP machine is portable and can be taken on trips. People using CPAP report having higher energy levels, better thinking abilities, and improved well-being during the day. They also say they are less sleepy.

- Severe cases may require surgery.

Other Sleep Disorders

There are a few other sleep disorders commonly seen in stroke survivors.

- About 20–40% of survivors have circadian disturbances or sleep-wake cycle disorders (SWDs). With this sleep problem, your sleep schedule is no longer determined by day and night. Bright light therapy may help you get your sleep-wake schedule back on track.

- Another frequent sleeping problem after stroke is insomnia, or trouble falling asleep or staying asleep throughout the night.

Treating this often complex problem may involve behavioral or medical intervention.

Professionals Who Can Help

- A doctor or sleep medicine specialist
- Health psychologist or behavioral sleep medicine specialist
- Certified sleep center

Section 50.2

Sexuality after Stroke

A stroke can change many aspects of life including the ability to walk, talk, think, and care for oneself. It can also affect the ability to have sex and how you and your partner feel about sex. Sex is an important aspect of life and is a very reasonable activity to want to return to following a stroke. The following are some practical points for stroke patients, and their partners.

A common fear is that having sex can cause another stroke. However, there are many other activities that can cause one's heart rate and breathing to increase without causing another stroke. Talk to your physician if you are concerned about whether it is safe for you to engage in sexual activity.

Often times, people experience a decreased sex drive following a stroke. It is normal to lack interest in sex right after a stroke. It may take a lot of energy just to get through the day, leaving little energy for anything else. Sometimes people feel down or depressed which can affect the desire for sex. Decreased sex drive may also be a side effect of medications. However, do not change any of your medications without talking to your doctor. Following a stroke, communication is important. Talk to your partner, choose a quiet, familiar place, take your time, and share your feelings and concerns to ensure that you are physically and emotionally ready to engage in sexual behavior.

Stroke can often cause decreased strength, movement, or feeling (sensation) on one or both sides of the body. If your stroke affected movement or feeling on one side of your body, it may be necessary to use new positions for safety and support. Some suggestions include using pillows to support a weak arm or leg. Other positions include sitting in a wheelchair, sitting on a shower seat, or lying on your side. Try touching, caressing, and kissing on the stronger side or increasing the touch on your weaker side. Again, communication is important and

511

describing what you are doing may also help. If you are experiencing muscle spasms that interfere with your sexual activity, talk to your doctor as some medications may be used to control the spasms.

Sexual experience can be affected due to problems with memory and concentration. Let your partner help you through short familiar steps. Your ability to understand what is being said and your ability to communicate your wants and needs can also be affected if you have any changes in cognition and language. If you are having difficulty with verbal communication, both partners should focus on facial expressions and gestures to exchange thoughts and feelings.

Following a stroke, your bowel and bladder function may be affected and you may have less control. Prior to engaging in sexual activity, it may be a good idea to try and go to the bathroom. Indwelling catheters can be taped out of the way or removed for a short time during sexual activity. However, speak with your physician regarding any catheter removal, as this may put you at a higher risk for urinary tract infections. If an accident happens, be prepared and have clean-up items nearby just in case.

In order to keep you and your partner safe and healthy, it is important to practice safe sex including the use of condoms to prevent the spread of sexually transmitted diseases. If you plan on becoming pregnant or are a woman and able to become pregnant, discuss appropriate birth control methods with your physician prior to engaging in sexual activity. Some oral contraceptives may interfere with other medications and you should never change medications without consulting your physician.

Returning to sexual activity is an important life activity and a stroke should not stop your ability to engage in this meaningful activity. Communication, respect, consultation with your physician, and patience are all key factors when resuming sexual activity and expanding your relationships.

Chapter 51

Dealing with Depression after Stroke

A Stroke Can Trigger Depression

For most people, the word stroke brings to mind a constellation of problems, including paralysis and difficulty with speech. But if someone has recently had a stroke, you're probably well aware that the effects go well beyond the physical. The emotional aftermath can be just as overwhelming and far more difficult to sort out.

Although depression can strike anyone, those who've suffered a catastrophic illness may be more susceptible than other people. And when you throw a brain injury into the mix, the risk of developing a mood disorder becomes even greater. As many as half of stroke survivors will become depressed, according to James Castle, a neurologist at Stanford University.

Depression isn't just miserable, it may also make a stoke survivor more susceptible to pain and fatigue and may even delay his recovery.

In a study published in the journal *Stroke*, researchers reported that stroke survivors who were treated for depression demonstrated improved recovery in regular daily activities compared with those whose depression went untreated.

People who are depressed also tend to be less compliant with rehabilitation and more resistant to making lifestyle changes to prevent a second stroke.

Fortunately, depression can be treated. With the appropriate care, a patient will lead a happier life—and life will be easier for you, too. Here are some practical things you can do if you think the person you're caring for is depressed after a stroke.

Be Alert to Warning Signs of Depression after a Stroke

It's not always easy to recognize depression. In the case of someone who's had a stroke, the situation can be even more complicated. If a patient has trouble talking or understanding language, it might be especially difficult to recognize depression. Increased emotional lability—sudden and extreme mood swings, common after a stroke—may also hide symptoms of depression.

You may also think he has good reason to feel depressed. After all, he's just had a stroke and can't do the things he used to be able to do. But there's a difference between the normal grieving process and depression. The warning signs of depression include:

- frequent crying episodes;
- feelings of hopelessness or worthlessness;
- poor appetite or increased appetite;
- sleeping too much or not enough;
- increased agitation and restlessness;
- loss of interest in life;
- expressing thoughts of dying or suicide.

A stroke survivor should be evaluated for depression if he has had several of these symptoms for more than two weeks.

Encourage a Stroke Survivor to Be Tested for Depression

If you believe a patient is depressed, the first step is to talk to him about his feelings. This isn't always easy, especially if he isn't used to expressing emotions. Ask him if he's feeling sad or hopeless. Try to get an idea if it's really depression or just a temporary case of the blues.

The next step is to schedule an evaluation. His primary care physician may want to talk to him first, or she may refer him to a psychiatrist or counselor. In any case, the evaluating doctor will talk to him and assess his mood. She may also order screening tests to rule out other medical conditions that can mimic depression, such as a thyroid disorder or infection.

If he resists the idea of testing because he's embarrassed or afraid, help him understand that a diagnosis of depression isn't the shameful secret it once may have been. It doesn't mean he's crazy or is going to be taken away to a nursing home. And his test results are private, so no one but he and his doctor needs to know.

If he absolutely refuses to see a doctor, there's not a whole lot you can do. "There's no way to force the issue unless there are severe circumstances," says Castle. If he has become psychotic or suicidal, or if his depression has progressed to the point where he can no longer care for himself, Castle recommends that you notify his doctor or emergency medical services immediately. Otherwise, your best bet is to enlist family members and friends to try to persuade him to seek help.

Support a Stroke Survivor during Treatment for Depression

If a patient is diagnosed with depression, the doctor may prescribe antidepressant medications and/or recommend psychotherapy. "Most doctors take a multidirected approach toward battling depression," says Castle. "Medicines can be highly effective, but often there's a role for psychotherapy and lifestyle changes."

Even if a primary care doctor diagnosed depression, a patient may still benefit from seeing a mental health professional, says Castle. "Some primary care physicians feel comfortable treating this disorder, but many would prefer the assistance of a psychiatrist or psychologist." Castle says this can be difficult for people who associate a stigma with mental health treatment. "It's important for the family to support the patient over that barrier."

The person in your care may also be nervous about taking antidepressants, but Castle points out that they present very little risk: "If anything, there's some evidence to suggest that these medicines might actually decrease the chance of having another stroke." Some of the common side effects, such as loss of libido or excessive sweating, can be annoying, but they're nothing compared to the misery of depression. And the doctor can work with the patient to find the most effective medication with the fewest side effects.

Other Ways You Can Help a Stroke Survivor with Depression

Simply supporting the patient as he struggles with depression can help him a great deal. Here are some other things you can do:

- Help him stay as physically active as possible. Talk to the doctor and rehabilitation team about what exercises are appropriate. Find activities you can do together, such as a morning walk around the neighborhood.

- Depressed people often want to sleep during the day. "As much as possible, don't allow a patient to slip into a depressed routine," says Castle. "Break the cycle by encouraging him to be awake during the day with exposure to sunlight." A simple walk outdoors or some time in the garden can really help.

- Structure the day around activities that give him pleasure and a sense of purpose. For example, meet friends for lunch or enjoy a leisurely walk through the mall.

- Try to stay positive and upbeat, but don't foster unrealistic expectations. Instead of saying, "You'll be hiking again in no time," you might say, "If we keep walking together every day, you'll notice that it gets a lot easier."

- Join a support group—for either or both of you. Talking to other people who're struggling with similar issues can be enormously comforting and helpful. It's also a great way to connect with other stroke survivors and caregivers. Remember that it's not all up to you.

In the end, it's really up to the stroke survivor to get help for depression. If he won't talk to his doctor or comply with treatment, you can't make him—and you shouldn't blame yourself. Keep offering support and provide positive reinforcement when he takes those difficult steps toward recovery.

But there's only so much you can do. If feelings of guilt and sadness overwhelm you, you may need help coming to terms with the fact that he isn't going to get help. Ask his doctor for information about support groups and other resources to help you manage your own feelings.

Chapter 52

Tips for Caregivers of Stroke Patients

Dealing with Emotional Distress

It is not unusual for a family member to experience emotional distress at any phase of the rehabilitation process. Often, the family member is unaware of the distress because the primary focus is always on the survivor's needs. You, the caregiver, are also in need of professional help during this family crisis.

During and immediately after the aneurysm, the family of the survivor experiences a broad range of intense emotions, such as shock, fear, worry, anger, frustration, and hopelessness. As the rehabilitation process unfolds, these emotions may continue to prey on you and further add to your already suffering. Depression, worry, anger, and grief may pile on top of your own fragile emotions. You might feel guilty and brush this feeling aside because you are so anxious to take proper care of your loved one. You may find it difficult to fully express and explore your feelings if the survivor is present.

Others in your situation probably undergo the same feelings and you are not alone. The emotional distress that you may experience is a natural part of the rehabilitation process and you must realize that self-care is just as important as survivor care. Your emotional well-being is necessary for a positive outcome for both you and the brain aneurysm survivor.

"Family & Friends: For Caregivers," reprinted with permission from the Brain Aneurysm Foundation, © 2012. All rights reserved. For additional information, visit www.bafound.org.

517

There are many forms of emotional distress. You, the caregiver, should not view these depressed, anxious, or hopeless moods as a sign of weakness. When you realize the gamut of emotions that you have experienced from the beginning of the aneurysm episode until the present, you will begin to appreciate how stressful life has been for you as well as for your loved one. It is important to release your emotions and understand the commonality of your feelings amongst caregivers.

It will be important for you to maintain a positive outlook throughout your care giving, which will help you develop patience with the survivor and the process. You will learn that personality and behavior changes after an aneurysm are generally not intentional, but reflect changes in brain function.

The way any family member interprets the survivor's behavior and progress plays a major role in his/her emotional condition. Consider the family of a survivor who has an aneurysm that affected the function of her frontal lobes. The frontal lobe has a great deal to do with initiation and motivation, and survivors with damage to this area may not take obvious steps toward recovery, and seem lazy or uncaring. The family of a survivor with poor motivation may become upset if they believe that the survivor has lost interest and given up. If you, as the caregiver, think that the patient is deliberately avoiding recovery work, you may become quite frustrated or angry with that survivor. If, on the other hand, you understand the neurological basis for the survivor's poor motivation, you will deal much more effectively with the problem. You will have the patience to structure the survivor's activities, and actively encourage him/her to work toward rehabilitation goals.

As the caregiver, you must remember that your emotional wellbeing is crucial to the progress of your survivor's health. You must recognize and tend to your own emotional struggles in order to be successful. If you are the primary caregiver, consider the benefits of an aneurysm support group or a caregiver support group or private therapy. It will be a safe harbor to moor your emotions during this turbulent time.

Ten Tips for Caregivers

1. Caregiving is a job and respite is your earned right. Reward yourself with respite breaks often.

2. Watch out for signs of depression, and don't delay in getting professional help when you need it.

3. When people offer to help, accept the offer and suggest specific things that they can do.

4.   Educate yourself about your loved one's condition and how to communicate effectively with doctors.

5.   There's a difference between caring and doing. Be open to technologies and ideas that promote your loved one's independence.

6.   Trust your instincts. Most of the time, they'll lead you in the right direction.

7.   Caregivers often do the lifting, pushing, and pulling. Be good to your back.

8.   Grieve for your losses and then allow yourself to dream new dreams.

9.   Seek support from other caregivers. There is great strength in knowing you are not alone.

10. Stand up for your rights as a caregiver and a citizen.

Chapter 53

How to Organize a Successful Stroke Support Group

Living with Stroke: An Adjustment for the Family

Relationships often change drastically after someone has a stroke. Physical difficulties and the emotional problems a stroke can cause may quickly change how stroke survivors, their families, and others get along.

Survivors often say friends and family members feel uncomfortable around them. "He just is not himself," people say. Or, "She is not like she used to be." The old circle of family and friends begins to disappear, and survivors say it's hard to fit in like they did before.

After a stroke, even simple things like shopping, talking on the telephone or taking a walk may seem impossible. Talking or writing a letter may be too difficult for a stroke survivor who has problems using or understanding language. Something as common as going out to eat can be a major challenge.

Survivors also may not be able to drive a car or use public transportation. Other day-to-day activities may become major obstacles to survivors.

Stroke affects more than the survivor. Family members can also be confused, frustrated, and feel isolated. Relationships may become strained, especially when a family member becomes a caregiver. And the caregivers may get angry or feel guilty about their feelings toward

Excerpted from *Successful Stroke Support Groups*, reprinted with permission from the American Stroke Association, www.strokeassociation.org, a division of the American Heart Association. © 2012 American Heart Association, Inc.

the survivor, who is taking so much of their time and energy. Individual family members may have to adjust how they feel about themselves and others as responsibilities shift and family relationships change.

There are no easy answers to the problems a stroke can create. These changes can negatively affect the survivor's rehabilitation and recovery after getting out of the hospital. The longer a stroke survivor is not in society, the harder it is to rejoin society again.

The Need for Peer Support, Hope, and Encouragement

Stroke survivors and their family caregivers need help adjusting to the changes in their lives. That's why many stroke survivors join support groups.

Sharing similar problems helps survivors learn to live with the changes. Stroke support groups offer survivors, their caregivers, and other family members' chances to share concerns and support each other.

They unite around their common experiences and find positive solutions.

Stroke support groups allow stroke survivors to help themselves and other survivors create meaningful lives after stroke. Coming together in an atmosphere of caring and cooperation, survivors, their family caregivers, and friends can forge a new sense of community. New goals and friendships are started, renewing hope and encouraging independence.

A sense of empowerment is at the heart of a self-help or mutual-help group. It can motivate passive patients to become thriving survivors and create active new roles for themselves. Stroke creates many physical and emotional challenges. Each stroke survivor faces a unique set of disabilities and losses, and each copes with them in his or her own way. However, the warmth, acceptance, and emotional support that a stroke support group offers can often be the key to uncovering the hidden strengths in many survivors.

Discovering the Value of Support

Social support is important in stroke recovery. Social isolation has been called a risk factor for a poor outcome after stroke. Family and friends provide important support for many survivors, but stroke support groups can also play a vital role in stroke recovery. They can decrease the isolation of both survivors and family, and introduce new friends to replace those often lost after the stroke.

Stroke survivors not only face new disabilities, but also possible medical complications and the need to prevent recurrent strokes. A stroke support group that empowers members with information and provides emotional support can promote both good health and a good quality of life.

Finding a Way to Help

Stroke families can't benefit from belonging to a support group if none exist in their community. You can help by organizing a new stroke support group in your community or strengthening an existing one.

There are many ways to start and sustain a stroke support group. What works for one group may not work for others, since members are unique. The purpose of these guidelines is to help you plan a group that fits the needs of your members.

Setting Goals

The purpose of a stroke support group is to provide stroke survivors and their family caregivers an opportunity to support each other as they strive to rebuild their lives and promote health, independence, and well-being. Goals clarify what the group wants to accomplish. Consider these items as you develop the goals for your group:

- To provide accurate information for group education that promotes a better understanding of stroke recovery, rehabilitation, and prevention of recurrent stroke

- To offer a way for stroke survivors to meet others with similar challenges and experiences and provide mutual positive support

- To renew hope and promote independence by offering opportunities for survivors to challenge themselves and continue to improve their performance of daily living activities.

- To provide caregivers and family members a structured way to share and support each other

- To offer stroke families the resources and support they need to live an active and satisfying life while coping with their losses and disabilities due to stroke

The goals of a stroke group should change as the group's membership and focus changes. Review the goals regularly and adapt or add to them. Here are some more ideas:

- To encourage and strengthen dignity and self-esteem by providing volunteer opportunities within the stroke group and the community

- To educate people in the local community about stroke prevention and stroke disabilities

- To reach out to new stroke survivors and their families by providing a support service such as the American Stroke Association's Peer Visitor Program

- To improve communication and understanding among stroke families

- To offer support uniquely designed to help stroke family caregivers

- To encourage the active involvement of survivors with aphasia who have difficulty communicating in the group

- To reach out to stroke survivors in communities without active stroke support groups

Getting Organized

Starting a stroke support group takes a lot of work but can be very rewarding. It's extremely satisfying to help stroke families rebuild their lives. Sharing responsibilities makes getting organized easier and gives others a sense of ownership. Laying a strong foundation now will also have long-term benefits such as dedicated members, widespread publicity, and committed leaders.

Contact stroke survivors, family members, and stroke healthcare professionals for more guidance. When you talk to individuals or groups, tell them how group members can benefit from friendly, supportive, informal meetings. Once you find two or three interested people, you're ready to take the next steps for starting your group.

Organizing a new stroke group will be easier if you include these components:

- A key person (or two)

- An advisor, group facilitator, or healthcare professional

- A sponsoring agency

- A planning committee

Finding Leaders and Facilitators

A key person (or two) is someone who has a prime interest in organizing a new stroke group. This person may be a stroke survivor, the caregiver of a stroke survivor, or a social worker or other healthcare professional from a rehabilitation center or community services agency. It's important for this person to be able to commit the time and effort needed. Whether the key person or the sponsoring agency comes first varies with the community.

Typically, a need surfaces and the order follows logically. Direction may be needed, but a stroke support group will emerge.

The role of an advisor or group facilitator will vary with individual groups and as groups pass through different stages of development. An advisor can act as an advocate and consultant, especially while the group is forming. That role may shift to facilitator or guide as leaders emerge and the support aspects of the group become focused.

Both lay and healthcare professional facilitators can share their unique perspectives. However, the collective experience and knowledge of the group is more important than that of the facilitator. A good facilitator must be able to empower the members to support each other. That allows the internal leadership to thrive.

An advisor or facilitator should have a strong interest and ability to empathize with the problems resulting from a stroke, and have good group facilitating skills.

Enlisting a qualified healthcare professional in this role can enrich the group with additional knowledge of stroke, rehabilitation, and group process. A professional's contacts in the healthcare community can help members generate support and referrals for the new group, and find speakers and other helpful resources.

If a sponsoring agency is found first, its staff may be able to recommend an advisor. The advisor's main duties are:

- to provide or be the liaison with the sponsoring agency;

- to help manage the group;

- to facilitate the process as the group develops programs, defines function, promotes leadership among members, and helps establish and carry out the group's goals.

Obtaining the commitment of a recognized organization can be very useful in helping the group reach its goals. A sponsoring agency can also help provide continuity as the group evolves and its membership changes. The agency could be the local office of a national organization, a hospital or rehabilitation center, or a community service group. Some possible organizations that may be interested in sponsoring a stroke support group include [the following]:

- American Stroke Association, a division of the American Heart Association

- Nursing homes

- Easter Seal Society

- Nurses associations

- Hospital rehabilitation departments

- YMCA and YWCA

- Community rehabilitation centers

- Outpatient clinic

- Speech and hearing associations

- Family service agencies

- Senior citizens' agencies

- Mental health groups

When you contact these organizations, ask if they sponsor a stroke support group or plan to start one.

If there's an existing group, you may want to visit and ask them to partner with you to start a new group. A partnership like this lets you share valuable member resources.

A sponsoring agency may be able to provide some needed services— such as meeting space—and help with funds for refreshments and mailings. In addition, many services and staff of the sponsoring agency may be available to help the group. Social workers, speech/language pathologists, occupational or physical therapists, and other healthcare specialists can advise or facilitate, or be involved occasionally as guest speakers.

Forming a planning committee of three to five members to plan the initial meeting and establish some basic ground rules and an organizational structure isn't necessary but can be very helpful. A planning committee can share responsibility and help prevent leader burnout. This fosters a sense of ownership among group members.

Forming a committee to guide your support group provides a way for members to be actively involved.

It also establishes the group as a stronger entity in the community. Involving stroke survivors and caregivers on the committee is essential to assessing the needs accurately and setting appropriate goals.

Recruiting healthcare professionals for your committee can strengthen its credibility and also increase its visibility. Healthcare professionals are valuable to you for three reasons:

1. They know people who can present educational programs on stroke rehabilitation and mental health.

2. They meet stroke survivors daily who are potential group members.

3. Their knowledge of the community and stroke recovery and rehabilitation benefits your stroke support group.

A committee may also be helpful if your group plans to partner with community organizations, such as the local American Heart Association office.

How long should your committee serve? That's up to you. Some groups never disband their committee.

Others use the committee until their support group has become stable.

Next Steps

Once you have commitments from one or two key people, the next steps are to locate a sponsoring agency, a planning committee, and an advisor or facilitator. Your nearest American Heart Association/American Stroke Association office may be able to help.

Here are some steps adapted from those used by the American Heart Association/American Stroke Association Texas Affiliate office. You can adapt these ideas to fit your group's needs.

• Review advantages of developing a stroke support group in your community with the stroke program committee of your nearest American Heart Association/American Stroke Association office.

• Ask the American Heart Association/American Stroke Association program committee about helping to organize a stroke support group and whether it would be a sponsoring organization. Review the advantages of involving other organizations to co-sponsor the group.

- Ask the American Heart Association/American Stroke Association program committee to help organize a stroke group planning committee made up of healthcare professionals (such as physicians, physical therapists, speech therapists, occupational therapists, rehab nurses, etc.); two or more stroke survivors and caregivers; and one or two other interested persons.

- Ask the planning committee to help locate a suitable advisor or facilitator for the stroke support group.

- The committee creates a list of sources for new members with the planning committee, including physicians, public health nurses, Visiting Nurses Association, rehabilitation hospitals and centers, VA hospitals, etc. Committee members will ask these individuals and organizations for stroke survivor referrals.

- The committee sends invitations announcing the first meeting of the stroke support group and publicizes the group.

- The committee may set the date and time for meetings, choose a stroke survivor to lead the meeting along with an advisor, and suggest a meeting location, types of programs, and frequency of meetings.

- Before the first meeting, the temporary group leader and advisor will meet with the committee to develop a detailed meeting agenda. This group can also identify potential support group leaders.

- At the first meeting, the stroke support group leader and committee will present their ideas to the group. The members present at the initial meetings will decide how often to meet, the kinds of activities the support group will sponsor and where the group will meet. An acting stroke support group leader will be chosen if one hasn't been selected and how long the term leaders will serve will be decided.

- File a list of members and guidelines governing your group with your nearest American Heart Association/American Stroke Association. The local office may want to submit this list to the American Heart Association/American Stroke Association affiliate stroke group coordinator or the person at the state level with stroke responsibilities.

- Review your group's activities after six months and make any changes necessary.

Finding Members

Stroke support groups use different criteria for membership. In addition to stroke survivors, some groups include individuals with other medical conditions, such as head injury and other disabling conditions. Restricting membership to survivors of stroke or perhaps other types of brain injury keeps problems and challenges similar. This allows group members to more strongly identify with one another.

Advocates of a broader membership believe that added diversity makes for a more interesting group.

Broad membership often attracts more members to the support group. Your group can include family members and friends of stroke survivors, or you can create a separate group for caregivers. You may want to experiment with your membership.

You'll probably attract enough people to your first few meetings. Over time you'll want to involve more people to keep attendance high. Aside from your personal contacts, some reliable sources for new support group members are physician referrals, healthcare professionals, public health agencies, social services, and the ministry. Community publicity is another way to attract interested members and their families.

The first meeting is very important. Allow enough lead time for extensive publicity so information can be circulated. The first program should be well planned, constructive, and purposeful. It could feature a healthcare professional speaker on a topic dealing with the psychosocial aspects of stroke as it affects survivors and families. The speaker should be well-qualified and understand the goals of the group. Another option is to feature a stroke survivor who has made a successful adjustment to a changed lifestyle after stroke and can give an inspiring presentation. The first program should also highlight these items:

- Purpose and goals of the stroke group

- Possible organizational structure

- Possible future programs

- Role of sponsoring agency, committee members, and leaders

- Introductions of those attending with brief background information

Be sure that everyone who attends feels welcome.

Use nametags and designate some committee members as hosts. Serving refreshments is a must.

Identifying a Meeting Place

How often and when you hold meetings is up to you. Groups meet weekly, every other week, monthly, and even every other month. Monthly meetings are the most common. Afternoon and evening meetings are more popular than morning meetings, although some groups do host morning meetings. Most support groups meet on weekdays.

- Choose a convenient time for you and the two or three people working with you. Later, if members prefer, schedule meetings that are more convenient for the group.

- Most meetings last 1 1/2 to 2 hours and offer programs and social time. Your meetings should be long enough to offer value and short enough to avoid being tiresome.

- Meeting in the same place eliminates confusion, so scout around to find a convenient location.

- Many meeting rooms are free. Personally inspect meeting facilities before you accept or reject them.

- Choose a safe, easily accessible location with ample parking. Notice restroom availability, noise level, lighting and ease of entry in the facility you're considering. Policies regarding building hours, janitorial services, and refreshments will play a big part in your choice. For instance, if you want to serve refreshments at your meetings, consider a meeting facility with a kitchen.

- A clean, cheerful meeting place with plenty of room to seat everyone will enhance the quality of your meetings. Possible locations include [the following]:
  - Your local American Heart Association office
  - Hospitals
  - Rehabilitation centers
  - Nursing homes
  - Easter Seal centers
  - Adult day care centers
  - Speech/hearing centers
  - Senior citizen centers
  - Civic centers

- Churches

- Community halls

- Libraries

- Schools

- YMCA and YWCA

- Shopping centers or malls (some malls offer unoccupied space to nonprofit groups)

Elderly members are often reluctant to drive during evening hours, on busy highways, or if there is bad weather. Some groups don't meet during the winter months because of weather, while others take a break in the summer when members may be too busy. Transportation can challenge your stroke support group, no matter when you schedule your meetings. Check your community services and public bus service for vans and special transportation for members who are unable to drive.

Carpooling may be another solution.

Acquiring Funds for Activities and Other Expenses

Funding for stroke groups can vary greatly depending on whether a local organization has agreed to sponsor the group and its activities.

Consider working with an organization or collaborating with your local American Heart Association for meeting space, use of equipment, refreshments, and postage in exchange for the members' commitment of their time to volunteer when help is needed for local stroke outreach events.

Support groups report these main expenses:

- Publicity-related: Printing, copying, postage, advertisements

- Group bulletin or newsletter

- Refreshments

The group should make the decision to collect or not collect fees. Some groups collect $1.00 annually, quarterly or monthly. Stroke groups report that the money is used mostly for refreshments. If you charge any fees, remember that some members may not be able to pay. You may consider fundraising projects once your group is strong enough.

These projects can finance events that build bonds among members.

Chapter 54

Health Insurance and Disability Concerns after Stroke

Chapter Contents

Section 54.1

Health Insurance Information for Stroke Patients

Stroke recovery can require lots of time and medical attention. Ideally, some of that medical care is covered by health insurance. Dealing with health insurance companies, however, can be a challenge. But, taking the time to understand the specific benefits of your health care plan will help you manage your stroke recovery.

Dealing with Insurance Companies

Rehab programs can be costly. So it is important to know what portion of the bill your health insurance will pay and what you will have to pay out of pocket. It is also good to know if you can choose any doctor you want.

Some plans require that you choose a doctor or specialist in a particular network.

There are two main types of health plans: Indemnity plans and managed care plans.

Traditional Indemnity Insurance

This type of health insurance usually:

- involves a deductible, or amount you must pay toward your medical expenses before the insurance company will pay anything at all on your behalf;

- pays part of your expense (usually 80%), once your deductible is met;

- pays only for covered services listed in material sent by the insurance company;

- allows you the flexibility to go to any doctor or rehab facility you choose;

- requires more paperwork than other plans because you have to fill out and submit claim forms to receive your insurance benefits;

- involves higher payments by you.

Managed Care

Managed care plans provide complete health services at reduced prices for their members, who agree to use doctors and facilities that belong to their plan. Under managed care plans:

- all medical costs are covered except for a small co-payment that you have to pay each time you are seen by a doctor or therapist;

- your out-of-pocket expenses are often less;

- your choice of providers, facilities, and services is usually limited to those within the network of health care providers. If you see a doctor or therapist that is not in the network you may have to pay full price.

There are different kinds of managed care plans. The two most common are [the following]:

- Health maintenance organization (HMO): With an HMO, you usually have to get a referral from your doctor in order to see a specialist.

- Preferred provider organization (PPO): With a PPO, no referrals are necessary. You can go to any specialist in the network or pay more to go to a specialist that is not in the network.

Settings and Services

Stroke recovery may require extensive rehabilitation. This may include many services in different settings. Check with your health insurance company to make sure you are covered under the following settings and services.

- Acute care (inpatient) and rehab hospitals: Provide 24-hour medical care and a full range of rehab services in a hospital setting.

- Sub-acute facilities: Provide daily nursing care and a fairly wide range of rehab services.

- Long term care facilities or skilled nursing homes: Provide rehab services several times per week to long-term and short-term residents.

- Outpatient facilities: Provide a wide range of rehab services for people who live at home and can come to the center for treatment several times a week.

- Home health agencies: Provide rehab services to stroke survivors in their own homes.

It is important to remember that there are inpatient and outpatient settings and services.

Inpatient services are those that are given to hospital residents who get treatments while they are staying in the hospital. Outpatient services are those given to patients who live in their own homes. These patients come into an office to see a doctor or therapist. Insurance companies sometimes pay different rates/benefits for these two types of services.

Key Questions on Coverage

Figuring out what your insurance plan pays for requires that you ask a lot of questions. Examples include [the following]:

- Does the plan cover rehabilitation services? Which services?

- Does the plan require me to pay more for rehab services than for regular doctor visits?

- Are my doctors and facilities in the provider network?

- Does the plan require my primary care doctor to give me a referral to see a specialist?

- Does the plan provide coverage for prescription drugs?

- What medical equipment is covered by the plan (power wheelchair, adaptive equipment, braces, equipment to continue therapy at home)?

- How much of the equipment cost is paid by health insurance? How much do I pay?

- Does the plan limit the number of days for rehab program visits (either inpatient days in a facility or outpatient days/doctor visits, or combined)?

- If days are limited, are they renewed from year to year?

- Does the plan limit coverage, or require special referrals for treatment of a pre-existing condition or a repeat experience, such as a stroke? Note that under the 2010 Affordable Care Act (often called the Health Reform Bill or Obamacare), insurers will not be able to exclude or treat pre-existing conditions differently, starting in 2014.

- Does the plan require me to have speech therapy in order to receive occupational therapy (help with performing daily activities)?

- Does the plan cover outpatient speech therapy?

- Does the plan limit the dollar amount it will pay for a particular setting or service?

- Can the plan suddenly remove my doctor or therapist from the network, leaving me without coverage to continue with them? Can the plan decide I will no longer be covered? In either situation, how much advance notice would I receive?

- What are the procedures to appeal a decision made by the health insurance plan? Does the insurance company or an independent reviewer handle an appeal?

- Does the plan exclude cognitive therapy (a form of treatment used to change patterns of thinking, such as depression)?

- What type of home care is covered? What do I pay for home care?

Disability Benefits

If you are working in a place where you are covered by the Family Medical Leave Act (FMLA), you must apply as soon as possible. For one, FMLA will protect your job. Also, you often have to apply for FMLA before you can apply for short-term and long-term disability from an employer-sponsored plan.

It is important that you apply for disability benefits shortly after your stroke. These benefits can assist you financially until you are able to go back to work.

There are several types of disability benefits that may apply to you, including private disability insurance or government disability benefits.

Private disability insurance benefits are provided by an employer or through a disability insurance plan you purchased on your own. If you have private disability insurance, take these steps to apply:

- If your disability insurance is through your employer, contact human resources to assist you in applying for benefits.

- Check with your employer to see if you will have to pay taxes on the money received.

- If you have your own disability insurance policy, call your insurance agent to help you apply for benefits.

- Not all disability plans are the same. Some will pay if you cannot do your current job. Others will only pay if you cannot do any job at all. Check to see which applies to your situation.

- Check your life insurance policies because they may pay your premiums while you are disabled.

Government Disability Benefits

The Social Security Administration (SSA) has two programs that provide money to people who are disabled and unable to work.

- Social Security Disability Insurance (SSDI)
- Supplemental Security Income (SSI)

You can learn more about Social Security programs on the web at www.ssa.gov or by calling 800-772-1213. There are a few things to consider:

- If you are already retired and receive a Social Security benefit, you will not be eligible to receive additional benefits.

- SSA's definition of disability is a physical or mental condition that lasts for at least 12 months and keeps you from working.

- Apply for benefits even if you plan to go back to work.

- You will need to describe to them the impact the stroke has had on you physically—they need to know why you can't work.

Because of the time needed to process the paperwork, be sure to contact them as soon as possible.

Also, make and keep copies of all the documents you send to them and letters they have sent to you. Keep track of the names of all the people you talked to, dates, and what they told you.

Changes in Your Abilities

After stroke, what you are able to do may change many times. For example, you may start walking after years of using a wheelchair. Or you may regain sensation in an arm or leg. You may even lose the ability to do something that you once could do.

Changes may happen shortly after stroke or take place years later. Either way, they generally require new rehab treatments.

Under Medicare and many private health plans, you are entitled to reenter the system at any time if you experience a change in your abilities.

This means that you can reapply for added rehab benefits based on the change.

What Can Help

Every health insurance plan has coverage limitations. But you may have options for getting the rehab services you need.

- Try contacting the exceptions department of your health plan.

- Ask to work with a case manager for chronic or catastrophic illness.

- Seek help from your employer in dealing with the plan.

- Trade inpatient rehab days for outpatient days. Some plans have short inpatient coverage but longer home care/outpatient coverage.

- File an appeal if you feel you are being denied payment or a medical service to which you are entitled. The Affordable Care Act provides additional specific consumer protections and rights to appeal service denials by insurers.

- If you need help talking to your insurance company about your health care and recovery, consider contacting resources in your community, including vocational rehabilitation services, aging agencies, disability law/elder law projects, and the Social Security Administration Office of Disability (www.ssa.gov/disability).

- For more information on Medicare coverage for stroke rehab, call 800-MEDICARE or visit www.medicare.gov.

- For information on your specific private health insurance plan, contact your insurance company or your employer's benefits administrator.

Section 54.2

Social Security Disability

Stroke is a leading cause of adult long-term disability. Between 50 and 70 percent of stroke survivors regain functional independence, but 15 to 30 percent are permanently disabled.

Some disability types include:

• paralysis or movement problems;

• sensory disturbances (e.g., pain);

• language problems;

• thinking and memory problems;

• emotional disturbances.

Post-stroke disability may leave survivors unable to work, which can lead to serious financial issues for survivors and their families. Survivors unable to work due to a physical or mental impairment may be eligible for Social Security Disability Insurance (SSDI) benefits.

What Is SSDI?

SSDI is a payroll tax-funded, federal insurance program. It provides income to individuals unable to work due to a disability and guarantees income if their condition does not improve. Once retirement age is met—65 or older—recipients move from SSDI to Social Security retirement income.

Regardless of age, survivors are eligible for Medicare benefits 24 months after the date of entitlement to SSDI cash benefits.

SSDI Eligibility

An individual is defined as disabled if a physical or mental impairment prevents that person from engaging in any substantial gainful work and the condition is expected to last at least 12 months or result in death.

Medical proof is required. You must have been disabled before reaching full retirement age (65 to 67). In addition, you must have worked and paid into the program (payroll taxes) for five of the past 10 years.

Benefits of SSDI

SSDI benefits include [the following]:

- **Regular monthly income:** Receive a regular monthly payment with annual cost-of-living increases. A portion may be tax free.

- **Medicare benefits:** Regardless of age, recipients are eligible for Medicare benefits 24 months after the date of entitlement to SSDI cash benefits. Medicare includes Part A (hospital benefits), Part B (medical benefits), and Part D (prescription drug plan).

- **COBRA extension:** If you receive SSDI, you may be able to extend COBRA benefits by an additional 11 months.

- **Long-term disability (LTD) benefits:** Private LTD insurance providers often require individuals to apply for SSDI, and doing so can help protect the ability to receive LTD income.

- **Protected retirement benefits:** SSDI recipients' Social Security earnings records are frozen during the period of disability, potentially increasing future Social Security retirement benefits.

- **Dependent benefits:** Dependents under age 18 may be eligible for benefits.

- **Return-to-work incentives:** Receive return-to-work opportunities while still receiving disability benefits.

Getting Started

The SSDI application process can be challenging. It can take from two to four years to receive benefits, but professional representation is available to help. On average, individuals with professional representation are approved at higher rates than those applying on their own.

When selecting representation, ask the following questions:

- Will they represent you at the application stage? Look for someone with experience at all stages of the SSDI process, including the initial application stage. The early application process can be very detailed and lead a person to abandon the application.

- What is the organization's success rate? Will the organization handle all of your paperwork and filing, including retrieval of medical records from your healthcare professional? Will they charge you extra for records?

- Does the organization charge extra for miscellaneous items such as photocopying, travel, and postage?

- How will the organization monitor your claim status and upcoming deadlines, such as a scheduled hearing?

- How long has the organization been providing SSDI representation?

Visit www.stroke.org/ssdi for more information about the application process.

Allsup offers free SSDI eligibility screening and evaluation (NSA. Allsup.com, 888-841-2126).

Allsup Medicare Advisor® offers Medicare plan selection services (NSA-AMA.Allsup.com, 888-271-1173).

SSDI Myths Exposed

Myths exist about filing for SSDI benefits, often deterring individuals from applying as soon as they are eligible.

Myth: SSDI is only available to poor or low-income individuals.

Truth: Income is not a factor. Applicants must have enough credits based on taxes they paid and work history.

Typically, if you worked five of the past 10 years you will have enough credits.

Myth: There is a 12-month waiting period after disability onset or leaving a job to apply for SSDI.

Truth: You can and should apply as soon as possible to receive and protect all benefits for which you are eligible.

Myth: You need an attorney to file for SSDI.

Truth: You do not need an attorney to file for SSDI or to appeal SSDI denials at the initial, reconsideration, or hearing levels. There are many advantages to using a non-attorney representative.

Post-Stroke Financial Planning

The following are tips for adjusting to new financial demands after a stroke:

- Create a financial plan. Establish a budget to spend down assets in the least harmful way. Use savings or other resources before withdrawing from retirement accounts.

- Maintain health insurance. This is critical to help pay for post-stroke care.

- Contact your mortgage company or landlord. If you see yourself having difficulty paying your mortgage or rent, be proactive and begin discussing your options. Research local and federal housing assistance programs. [Find local resources by calling 211 or visiting www.resources.allsup.com.]

- Seek assistance with utilities, food, and other necessities. There are hundreds of federal, local, and private resources available in most communities, including neighborhood food pantries and federally funded programs.

Warning Signs of Stroke

Learn the many warning signs of a stroke. Act fast and call 911 immediately at any sign of a stroke.

Use FAST to remember warning signs:

- **F—Face:** Ask the person to smile. Does one side of the face droop?

- **A—Arms:** Ask the person to raise both arms. Does one arm drift downward?

- **S—Speech:** Ask the person to repeat a simple phrase. Is their speech slurred or strange?

- **T—Time:** If you observe any of these signs, call 911 immediately.

Note the time when any symptoms first appear. If given within three hours of the first symptom, there is an FDA [U.S. Food and Drug Administration]-approved clot-buster medication that may reduce long-term disability for the most common type of stroke.

Chapter 55

Choosing Long-Term Care for Those Disabled by Stroke

Chapter Contents

Section 55.1

What Is Long-Term Care?

"Long-Term Care," by the Centers for Medicare and Medicaid Services
(CMS, www.medicare.gov), August 3, 2012.

Long-term care is a variety of services that includes medical and
non-medical care to people who have a chronic illness or disability.
Long-term care helps meet health or personal needs. Most long-term
care is to assist people with support services such as activities of daily
living like dressing, bathing, and using the bathroom. Long-term care
can be provided at home, in the community, in assisted living, or in
nursing homes. It is important to remember that you may need long-
term care at any age.

You may never need long-term care. This year, about nine million
men and women over the age of 65 will need long-term care. By 2020,
12 million older Americans will need long-term care. Most will be cared
for at home; family and friends are the sole caregivers for 70 percent
of the elderly. A study by the U.S. Department of Health and Human
Services says that people who reach age 65 will likely have a 40 percent
chance of entering a nursing home. About 10 percent of the people who
enter a nursing home will stay there five years or more.

While there are a variety of ways to pay for long-term care, it is
important to think ahead about how you will fund the care you get.
Generally, Medicare doesn't pay for long-term care. Medicare pays
only for medically necessary skilled nursing facility or home health
care. However, you must meet certain conditions for Medicare to pay
for these types of care. Most long-term care is to assist people with
support services such as activities of daily living like dressing, bathing, and using the bathroom. Medicare doesn't pay for this type of
care called custodial care. Custodial care (non-skilled care) is care
that helps you with activities of daily living. It may also include care
that most people do for themselves, for example, diabetes monitoring. Some Medicare Advantage Plans (formerly Medicare + Choice)
may offer limited skilled nursing facility and home care (skilled care)
coverage if the care is medically necessary. You may have to pay some
of the costs.

Medicaid is a State and Federal Government program that pays for certain health services and nursing home care for older people with low incomes and limited assets. In most states, Medicaid also pays for some long-term care services at home and in the community. Who is eligible and what services are covered vary from state to state. Most often, eligibility is based on your income and personal resources.

Choosing Long-Term Care

Choosing long-term care is an important decision. Planning for long-term care requires you to think about possible future health care needs. It is important to look at all of your choices. You will have more control over decisions and be able to stay independent. It is important to think about long-term care before you may need care or before a crisis occurs. Even if you plan ahead, making long-term care decisions can be hard.

Long-term care is made up of many different services and may include help with activities of daily living like dressing, bathing, eating, and using the bathroom, as well as help with care most people do themselves like taking medications. Long-term care can take place at home, in senior centers, at community centers, in special retirement or assisted living facilities, or in nursing homes. Someone with a long-term physical illness, a disability, or a memory or thought problem (such as Alzheimer disease) often needs long-term care.

Choosing long-term care is a very important decision. You should plan and think about long-term care before you need care or before a crisis occurs. Planning ahead allows you the time to talk with your doctor about your health and any problems you may be having. It is also very important to talk with your family about the kind of long-term care services you think you might need someday, how much they would cost, and how you would pay for them. The best time to talk about long-term care is before you need services.

Section 55.2

Assisted Living

What Is Assisted Living?

The Assisted Living Federation of America (ALFA) defines assisted living as a long-term care option that combines housing, support services, and health care, as needed. Assisted living is designed for individuals who require assistance with everyday activities such as meals, medication management or assistance, bathing, dressing and transportation. Some residents may have memory disorders including Alzheimer's, or they may need help with mobility, incontinence, or other challenges. Residents are assessed upon move in, or any time there is a change in condition. The assessment is used to develop an Individualized Service Plan.

Overview of Assisted Living

Assisted living is a residential alternative to nursing home care. According to the National Investment Center Investment Guide 2010, there are 6,315 professionally managed assisted living communities nationwide with approximately 475,500 apartments. A relatively new concept 25 years ago, today assisted living is the most preferred and fastest growing long-term care option for seniors.

Based on the varied preferences and needs of the elderly, there are a variety of settings from which to choose. These choices range from high-rise buildings to one-story Victorian mansions to large multi-acre campuses.

Assisted Living Resident Demographics

The average assisted living resident is an 87 year old female widow who requires assistance with two or more activities of daily living. The average resident stays in assisted living for 28 months and has an average annual income of $27,260.

Assisted Living Philosophy

The philosophy of assisted living is to provide personalized, resident centered care in order to meet individual preferences and needs. Assisted living treats all residents with dignity, provides privacy, and encourages independence and freedom of choice. Residents' family members and friends are encouraged to get involved in the assisted living community. Encourage your loved ones to learn about the care provider philosophy.

Freedom of Choice

The most progressive state regulations take cues from consumers and focus on protecting consumers in a way that provides the most choice and independence possible. ALFA supports certain principles and public policy positions that should be included in every state's assisted living legislative and regulatory framework.

Typical Services Offered in Assisted Living Communities

Assisted living communities provide more personal care services than an independent living retirement community. They offer a less-expensive, residential approach to delivering many of the same services available in skilled nursing, either by employing personal care staff or contracting with home health agencies and other outside professionals. Learn more about assisted living services and amenities.

Amenities in assisted living typically include [the following]:

- Three meals a day served in a common dining area
- Housekeeping services
- Transportation
- 24-hour security
- Exercise and wellness programs
- Personal laundry services
- Social and recreational activities

Personal care in assisted living typically includes [the following]:

- Staff available to respond to both scheduled and unscheduled needs
- Assistance with eating, bathing, dressing, toileting, and walking

- Access to health and medical services, such as physical therapy and hospice
- Emergency call systems for each resident's apartment
- Medication management
- Care for residents with cognitive impairments

What Is the Cost of Assisted Living?

Assisted living costs vary with the residence, apartment size, and types of services needed. The basic rate may cover all services or there may be additional charges for special services. Most assisted living residences charge on a month-to-month lease arrangement, but a few require long-term arrangements. Assisted living is of often less expensive than home health or nursing home care in the same geographic area.

According to the National Investment Center Investment Guide 2010, the median rate for a monthly rental rates in an assisted living community is $3,326 per month. In comparison, the NIC *Investment Guide 2010* also indicates the median rate of Nursing Care at $7,001 per month. The median is the midpoint, which means half of residences participating in the research have lower fees and half have higher fees. The rental rate includes the base rent and service fees charged by the assisted living community.

While 86.2% of assisted living residents today pay for long-term care from their personal financial resources, 41 states offer "home and community-based waivers" that allow low-income residents to live in assisted living. More seniors are purchasing long-term care insurance to help plan for and finance their long-term care needs.

Is Assisted Living Regulated?

Assisted living is regulated in all 50 states. State regulations generally address the mandatory services a senior living residence must provide. All settings offer 24-hour care and supervision for those who need assistance. Care is provided with dignity and respect.

Finding a Senior Living Community That's Right for You

Before you start your search for senior living options, ask yourself key questions about what you are looking for, what you need to know, what your ideal outcome would be a year after move-in, how you will cover the cost of living in a senior living community, and how you will make the distinction between price and value.

Chapter 56

Advance Care Planning

Advance care planning is not just about old age. At any age, a medical crisis could leave someone too ill to make his or her own healthcare decisions. Even if you are not sick now, making healthcare plans for the future is an important step toward making sure you get the medical care you would want, even when doctors and family members are making the decisions for you.

More than one out of four older Americans face questions about medical treatment near the end of life but are not capable of making those decisions. This text will discuss some questions you can think about now and describe ways to share your wishes with others. Write them down or at least talk about them with someone who would make the decisions for you. Knowing how you would decide might take some of the burden off family and friends.

What Is Advance Care Planning?

Advance care planning involves learning about the types of decisions that might need to be made, considering those decisions ahead of time, and then letting others know about your preferences, often by putting them into an advance directive. An advance directive is a legal document that goes into effect only if you are incapacitated and unable to speak for yourself. This could be the result of disease

"Advance Care Planning," by the National Institute on Aging (NIA, www.nia .nih.gov), part of the National Institutes of Health, March 28, 2012.

or severe injury—no matter how old you are. It helps others know what type of medical care you want. It also allows you to express your values and desires related to end-of-life care. You might think of an advance directive as a living document—one that you can adjust as your situation changes because of new information or a change in your health.

Decisions That Could Come up near Death

Sometimes when doctors believe a cure is no longer possible and you are dying, decisions must be made about the use of emergency treatments to keep you alive. Doctors can use several artificial or mechanical ways to try to do this. Decisions that might come up at this time relate to:

- CPR (cardiopulmonary resuscitation);
- ventilator use;
- artificial nutrition (tube feeding) or artificial hydration (intravenous fluids);
- comfort care.

CPR: CPR (cardiopulmonary resuscitation) might restore your heartbeat if your heart stops or is in a life-threatening abnormal rhythm. The heart of a young, otherwise healthy person might resume beating normally after CPR. An otherwise healthy older person, whose heart is beating erratically or not beating at all, might also be helped by CPR. But for an older person who is ill, can't be successfully treated, and is already close to death, CPR is less likely to work. It involves repeatedly pushing on the chest with force, while putting air into the lungs. This force has to be quite strong, and sometimes ribs are broken or a lung collapses. Electric shocks known as defibrillation and medicines might also be used as part of the process.

Ventilator use: Ventilators are machines that help you breathe. A tube connected to the ventilator is put through the throat into the trachea (windpipe) so the machine can force air into the lungs. Putting the tube down the throat is called intubation. Because the tube is uncomfortable, medicines are used to keep you sedated (unconscious) while on a ventilator. If you can't breathe on your own after a few days, a doctor may perform a tracheotomy or trach (rhymes with make). During this bedside surgery, the tube is inserted directly into the trachea through a hole in the neck. For long-term help with breathing, a trach is more comfortable, and sedation is not needed. People using such a breathing tube aren't able to speak without special help because exhaled air goes out of the trach rather than past their vocal cords.

Artificial nutrition or artificial hydration: A feeding tube and/or intravenous (IV) liquids are sometimes used to provide nutrition when a person is not able to eat or drink. These measures can be helpful if you are recovering from an illness. However, if you are near death, these could actually make you more uncomfortable. For example, IV liquids, which are given through a plastic tube put into a vein, can increase the burden on failing kidneys. Or if the body is shutting down near death, it is not able to digest food properly, even when provided through a feeding tube. At first, the feeding tube is threaded through the nose down to the stomach. In time, if tube feeding is still needed, the tube is surgically inserted into the stomach.

Comfort care: Comfort care is anything that can be done to soothe you and relieve suffering while staying in line with your wishes. Comfort care includes managing shortness of breath, offering ice chips for dry mouth, limiting medical testing, providing spiritual and emotional counseling, and giving medication for pain, anxiety, nausea, or constipation. Often this is done through hospice, which may be offered in the home, in a hospice facility, in a skilled nursing facility, or in a hospital. With hospice, a team of healthcare providers works together to provide the best possible quality of life in a patient's final days, weeks, or months. After death, the hospice team continues to offer support to the family.

Getting Started

Start by thinking about what kind of treatment you do or do not want in a medical emergency. It might help to talk with your doctor about how your present health conditions might influence your health in the future. For example, what decisions would you or your family face if your high blood pressure leads to a stroke?

If you don't have any medical issues now, your family medical history might be a clue to thinking about the future. Talk to your doctor about decisions that might come up if you develop health problems similar to those of other family members.

In considering treatment decisions, your personal values are key. Is your main desire to have the most days of life, or to have the most life in your days? What if an illness leaves you paralyzed or in a permanent coma and you need to be on a ventilator? Would you want that?

What makes life meaningful to you? You might want doctors to try CPR if your heart stops or to try using a ventilator for a short time if you've had trouble breathing, if that means that, in the future, you could be well enough to spend time with your family. Even if the emergency leaves you simply able to spend your days listening to books on tape or gazing out the window watching the birds and squirrels compete for seeds in the bird feeder, you might be content with that.

But in some cases, other scenarios could arise. Here are a few. What would you decide?

If a stroke leaves you paralyzed and then your heart stops, would you want CPR? What if you were also mentally impaired by the stroke? Does your decision change?

What if you develop dementia, don't recognize family and friends, and, in time, cannot feed yourself? Would you want a feeding tube used to give you nutrition?

What if you are permanently unconscious and then develop pneumonia? Would you want antibiotics and a ventilator used?

For some people, staying alive as long as medically possible is the most important thing. An advance directive can help make sure that happens.

Your decisions about how to handle any of these situations could be different at age 40 than at age 85. Or they could be different if you have an incurable condition as opposed to being generally healthy. An advance directive allows you to provide instructions for these types of situations and then to change the instructions as you get older or if your viewpoint changes.

Making Your Wishes Known

There are two elements in an advance directive—a living will and a durable power of attorney for health care. There are also other documents that can supplement your advance directive or stand alone. You can choose which documents to create, depending on how you want decisions to be made. These documents include:

- living will;

- durable power of attorney for health care;

- other documents discussing DNR (do not resuscitate) orders, organ and tissue donation, dialysis, and blood transfusions.

Living will: A living will is a written document that helps you tell doctors how you want to be treated if you are dying or permanently unconscious and cannot make decisions about emergency treatment. In a living will, you can say which of the procedures described in the preceding text you would want, which ones you wouldn't want, and under which conditions each of your choices applies.

Durable power of attorney for health care: A durable power of attorney for health care is a legal document naming a healthcare proxy, someone to make medical decisions for you at times when you might not be able to do so. Your proxy, also known as a surrogate or agent, should be familiar with your values and wishes. This means that he or she will be able to decide as you would when treatment decisions need to be made. A proxy can be chosen in addition to or instead of a living will. Having a healthcare proxy helps you plan for situations that cannot be foreseen, like a serious auto accident.

A durable power of attorney for health care enables you to be more specific about your medical treatment than a living will.

Some people are reluctant to put specific health decisions in writing. For them, naming a healthcare agent might be a good approach, especially if there is someone they feel comfortable talking with about their values and preferences.

Other advance care planning documents: You might also want to prepare separate documents to express your wishes about a single medical issue or something not already covered in your advance directive. A living will usually covers only the specific life-sustaining treatments discussed earlier. You might want to give your healthcare proxy specific instructions about other issues, such as blood transfusion or kidney dialysis. This is especially important if your doctor suggests that, given your health condition, such treatments might be needed in the future.

Two medical issues that might arise at the end of life are DNR orders and organ and tissue donation.

A DNR (do not resuscitate) order tells medical staff in a hospital or nursing facility that you do not want them to try to return your heart to a normal rhythm if it stops or is beating unevenly. Even though a living will might say CPR is not wanted, it is helpful to have a DNR order as part of your medical file if you go to a hospital. And posting a DNR next to your bed might avoid confusion in an emergency situation. Without a DNR order, medical staff will make every effort to restore the normal rhythm of your heart. A non-hospital DNR will alert emergency medical personnel to your wishes regarding CPR and other measures to restore your heartbeat if you are not in the hospital. A similar document that is less familiar is called a DNI (do not intubate) order. A DNI tells medical staff in a hospital or nursing facility that you do not want to be put on a breathing machine.

Organ and tissue donation allows organs or body parts from a generally healthy person who has died to be transplanted into people who need them. Commonly, the heart, lungs, pancreas, kidneys, corneas, liver, and skin are donated. There is no age limit for organ and tissue donation. You can carry a donation card in your wallet. Some states allow you to add this decision to your driver's license. Some people also include organ donation in their advance care planning documents. At the time of death, family may be asked about organ donation. If those close to you, especially your proxy, know how you feel about organ donation, they will be ready to respond.

Selecting Your Healthcare Proxy

If you decide to choose a proxy, think about people you know who share your views and values about life and medical decisions. Your proxy might be a family member, a friend, your lawyer, or someone with whom you worship. It's a good idea to also name an alternate proxy. It is especially important to have a detailed living will if you choose not to name a proxy.

You can decide how much authority your proxy has over your medical care—whether he or she is entitled to make a wide range of decisions or only a few specific ones. Try not to include guidelines that make it impossible for the proxy to fulfill his or her duties. For example, it's probably not unusual for someone to say in conversation, "I don't want to go to a nursing home," but think carefully about whether you want a restriction like that in your advance directive. Sometimes, for financial or medical reasons, that may be the best choice for you.

Of course, check with those you choose as your healthcare proxy and alternate before you name them officially. Make sure they are comfortable with this responsibility.

Making It Official

Once you have talked with your doctor and have an idea of the types of decisions that could come up in the future and whom you would like as a proxy, if you want one at all, the next step is to fill out the legal forms detailing your wishes. A lawyer can help but is not required. If you decide to use a lawyer, don't depend on him or her to help you understand different medical treatments. That's why you should start the planning process by talking with your doctor.

Many states have their own advance directive forms. Your local Area Agency on Aging can help you locate the right forms. You can find your area agency phone number by calling the Eldercare Locator toll-free at 800-677-1116 or going online at www.eldercare.gov.

Some states want your advance directive to be witnessed; some want your signature notarized. A notary is a person licensed by the state to witness signatures. You might find a notary at your bank, post office, or local library, or call your insurance agent. Some notaries charge a fee.

Some people spend a lot of time in more than one state—for example, visiting children and grandchildren. If that's your situation also, you might consider preparing an advance directive using forms for each state—and keep a copy in each place, too.

After You Set up Your Advance Directive

There are key people who should be told that you have an advance directive. Give copies to your healthcare proxy and alternate proxy. Give your doctor a copy for your medical records. Tell key family members and friends where you keep a copy. If you have to go to the hospital, give staff there a copy to include in your records. Because you might change your advance directive in the future, it's a good idea to keep track of who receives a copy.

Review your advance care planning decisions from time to time—for example, every 10 years, if not more often. You might want to revise your preferences for care if your situation or your health changes. Or, you might want to make adjustments if you receive a serious diagnosis; if you get married, separated, or divorced; if your spouse dies; or if something happens to your proxy or alternate. If your preferences change, you will want to make sure your doctor, proxy, and family know about them.

Still Not Sure?

What happens if you have no advance directive or have made no plans and you become unable to speak for yourself? In such cases, the state where you live will assign someone to make medical decisions on your behalf. This will probably be your spouse, your parents if they are available, or your children if they are adults. If you have no family members, the state will choose someone to represent your best interests.

Remember, an advance directive will only be used to make healthcare decisions if you are in danger of dying and cannot make your wishes known.

Looking Toward the Future

Nobody can predict the future. You may never face a medical situation where you are unable to speak for yourself and make your wishes known. But having an advance directive may give you and those close to you some peace of mind.

Part Seven

Additional Help
and Information

Chapter 57

Glossary of Terms Related to Stroke

acute stroke: A stage of stroke starting at the onset of symptoms and lasting for a few hours thereafter.

agnosia: A cognitive disability characterized by ignorance of or inability to acknowledge one side of the body or one side of the visual field.

aneurysm: A weak or thin spot on an artery wall that has stretched or ballooned out from the wall and filled with blood, or damage to an artery leading to pooling of blood between the layers of the blood vessel walls.

anoxia: A state of almost no oxygen delivery to a cell, resulting in low energy production and possible death of the cell; see hypoxia.

anticoagulants: A drug therapy used to prevent the formation of blood clots that can become lodged in cerebral arteries and cause strokes.

antiplatelet agents: A type of anticoagulant drug therapy that prevents the formation of blood clots by preventing the accumulation of platelets that form the basis of blood clots; some common antiplatelets include aspirin and ticlopidine.

antithrombotics: A type of anticoagulant drug therapy that prevents the formation of blood clots by inhibiting the coagulating actions of

Definitions in this chapter are excerpted from "Stroke: Hope Through Research," published by the National Institute of Neurological Disorders and Stroke (NINDS, www.ninds.nih.gov), part of the National Institutes of Health, October 15, 2012.

the blood protein thrombin; some common antithrombotics include warfarin and heparin.

aphasia: The inability to understand or create speech, writing, or language in general due to damage to the speech centers of the brain.

apoptosis: A form of cell death involving shrinking of the cell and eventual disposal of the internal elements of the cell by the body's immune system. Apoptosis is an active, non-toxic form of cell suicide that does not induce an inflammatory response. It is often called programmed cell death because it is triggered by a genetic signal, involves specific cell mechanisms, and is irreversible once initiated.

apraxia: A movement disorder characterized by the inability to perform skilled or purposeful voluntary movements, generally caused by damage to the areas of the brain responsible for voluntary movement.

arteriography: An X-ray of the carotid artery taken when a special dye is injected into the artery.

arteriovenous malformation (AVM): A congenital disorder characterized by a complex tangled web of arteries and veins.

atherosclerosis: A blood vessel disease characterized by deposits of lipid material on the inside of the walls of large to medium-sized arteries which make the artery walls thick, hard, brittle, and prone to breaking.

atrial fibrillation: Irregular beating of the left atrium, or left upper chamber, of the heart.

blood-brain barrier: An elaborate network of supportive brain cells, called glia, that surrounds blood vessels and protects neurons from the toxic effects of direct exposure to blood.

carotid artery: An artery, located on either side of the neck, that supplies the brain with blood.

carotid endarterectomy: Surgery used to remove fatty deposits from the carotid arteries.

central stroke pain (central pain syndrome): Pain caused by damage to an area in the thalamus. The pain is a mixture of sensations, including heat and cold, burning, tingling, numbness, and sharp stabbing and underlying aching pain.

cerebral blood flow (CBF): The flow of blood through the arteries that lead to the brain, called the cerebrovascular system.

cerebrospinal fluid (CSF): Clear fluid that bathes the brain and spinal cord.

cerebrovascular disease: A reduction in the supply of blood to the brain either by narrowing of the arteries through the buildup of plaque on the inside walls of the arteries, called stenosis, or through blockage of an artery due to a blood clot.

cholesterol: A waxy substance, produced naturally by the liver and also found in foods, that circulates in the blood and helps maintain tissues and cell membranes. Excess cholesterol in the body can contribute to atherosclerosis and high blood pressure.

clipping: Surgical procedure for treatment of brain aneurysms, involving clamping an aneurysm from a blood vessel, surgically removing this ballooned part of the blood vessel, and closing the opening in the artery wall.

computed tomography (CT) scan: A series of cross-sectional X-rays of the brain and head; also called computerized axial tomography or CAT scan.

Coumadin: A commonly used anticoagulant, also known as warfarin.

detachable coil: A platinum coil that is inserted into an artery in the thigh and strung through the arteries to the site of an aneurysm. The coil is released into the aneurysm creating an immune response from the body. The body produces a blood clot inside the aneurysm, strengthening the artery walls and reducing the risk of rupture.

duplex Doppler ultrasound: A diagnostic imaging technique in which an image of an artery can be formed by bouncing sound waves off the moving blood in the artery and measuring the frequency changes of the echoes.

dysarthria: A disorder characterized by slurred speech due to weakness or incoordination of the muscles involved in speaking.

dysphagia: Trouble swallowing.

edema: The swelling of a cell that results from the influx of large amounts of water or fluid into the cell.

embolic stroke: A stroke caused by an embolus.

embolus: A free-roaming clot that usually forms in the heart.

endothelial wall: A flat layer of cells that make up the innermost lining of a blood vessel.

extracranial/intracranial (EC/IC) bypass: A type of surgery that restores blood flow to a blood-deprived area of brain tissue by rerouting a healthy artery in the scalp to the area of brain tissue affected by a blocked artery.

functional magnetic resonance imaging (fMRI): A type of imaging that measures increases in blood flow within the brain.

hemiparesis: Weakness on one side of the body.

hemiplegia: Complete paralysis on one side of the body.

hemorrhagic stroke: Sudden bleeding into or around the brain.

heparin: A type of anticoagulant.

high-density lipoprotein (HDL): Also known as the good cholesterol; a compound consisting of a lipid and a protein that carries a small percentage of the total cholesterol in the blood and deposits it in the liver.

homeostasis: A state of equilibrium or balance among various fluids and chemicals in a cell, in tissues, or in the body as a whole.

hypertension (high blood pressure): Characterized by persistently high arterial blood pressure defined as a measurement greater than or equal to 140 mm/Hg systolic pressure over 90 mm/Hg diastolic pressure.

hypoxia: A state of decreased oxygen delivery to a cell so that the oxygen falls below normal levels.

incidence: The extent or frequency of an occurrence; the number of specific new events in a given period of time.

infarct: An area of tissue that is dead or dying because of a loss of blood supply.

infarction: A sudden loss of blood supply to tissue, causing the formation of an infarct.

intracerebral hemorrhage: Occurs when a vessel within the brain leaks blood into the brain.

ischemia: A loss of blood flow to tissue, caused by an obstruction of the blood vessel, usually in the form of plaque stenosis or a blood clot.

ischemic stroke: Ischemia in the tissues of the brain.

lacunar infarction: Occlusion of a small artery in the brain resulting in a small area of dead brain tissue, called a lacunar infarct; often caused by stenosis of the small arteries, called small vessel disease.

large vessel disease: Stenosis in large arteries of the cerebrovascular system.

lipoprotein: Small globules of cholesterol covered by a layer of protein; produced by the liver.

low-density lipoprotein (LDL): Also known as the bad cholesterol; a compound consisting of a lipid and a protein that carries the majority of the total cholesterol in the blood and deposits the excess along the inside of arterial walls.

magnetic resonance angiography (MRA): An imaging technique involving injection of a contrast dye into a blood vessel and using magnetic resonance techniques to create an image of the flowing blood through the vessel; often used to detect stenosis of the brain arteries inside the skull.

magnetic resonance imaging (MRI) scan: A type of imaging involving the use of magnetic fields to detect subtle changes in the water content of tissues.

mitochondria: The energy producing organelles of the cell.

mitral valve stenosis: A disease of the mitral heart valve involving the buildup of plaque-like material on and around the valve.

necrosis: A form of cell death resulting from anoxia, trauma, or any other form of irreversible damage to the cell; involves the release of toxic cellular material into the intercellular space, poisoning surrounding cells.

neuron: The main functional cell of the brain and nervous system, consisting of a cell body, an axon, and dendrites.

neuroprotective agents: Medications that protect the brain from secondary injury caused by stroke.

oxygen-free radicals: Toxic chemicals released during the process of cellular respiration and released in excessive amounts during necrosis of a cell; involved in secondary cell death associated with the ischemic cascade.

plaque: Fatty cholesterol deposits found along the inside of artery walls that lead to atherosclerosis and stenosis of the arteries.

plasticity: The ability to be formed or molded; in reference to the brain, the ability to adapt to deficits and injury.

platelets: Structures found in blood that are known primarily for their role in blood coagulation.

prevalence: The number of cases of a disease in a population at any given point in time.

recombinant tissue plasminogen activator (r-tPA): A genetically engineered form of tPA, a thrombolytic, anti-clotting substance made naturally by the body.

small vessel disease: A cerebrovascular disease defined by stenosis in small arteries of the brain.

stenosis: Narrowing of an artery due to the buildup of plaque on the inside wall of the artery.

stroke belt: An area of the southeastern United States with the highest stroke mortality rate in the country.

stroke buckle: Three southeastern states, North Carolina, South Carolina, and Georgia, that have an extremely high stroke mortality rate.

subarachnoid hemorrhage: Bleeding within the meninges, or outer membranes, of the brain into the clear fluid that surrounds the brain.

thrombolytics: Drugs used to treat an ongoing, acute ischemic stroke by dissolving the blood clot causing the stroke and thereby restoring blood flow through the artery.

thrombosis: The formation of a blood clot in one of the cerebral arteries of the head or neck that stays attached to the artery wall until it grows large enough to block blood flow.

thrombotic stroke: A stroke caused by thrombosis.

tissue necrosis factors: Chemicals released by leukocytes and other cells that cause secondary cell death during the inflammatory immune response associated with the ischemic cascade.

total serum cholesterol: A combined measurement of a person's high-density lipoprotein (HDL) and low-density lipoprotein (LDL).

tPA: See recombinant tissue plasminogen activator.

transcranial magnetic stimulation (TMS): A small magnetic current delivered to an area of the brain to promote plasticity and healing.

transient ischemic attack (TIA): A short-lived stroke that lasts from a few minutes up to 24 hours; often called a mini-stroke.

vasodilators: Medications that increase blood flow to the brain by expanding or dilating blood vessels.

vasospasm: A dangerous side effect of subarachnoid hemorrhage in which the blood vessels in the subarachnoid space constrict erratically, cutting off blood flow.

vertebral artery: An artery on either side of the neck; see carotid artery.

warfarin: A commonly used anticoagulant, also known as Coumadin.

Chapter 58

Directory of Organizations That Help Stroke Patients and Their Families

Government Agencies That Provide Information about Stroke

Administration on Aging
Washington, DC 20201
Toll-Free: 800-677-1116
(Eldercare Locator)
Phone: 202-619-0724
Fax: 202-357-3555
Website: www.aoa.gov
E-mail: aoainfo@aoa.hhs.gov

Agency for Healthcare Research and Quality
Office of Communications and Knowledge Transfer
540 Gaither Road
Suite 2000
Rockville, MD 20850
Phone: 301-427-1104
Website: www.ahrq.gov

Centers for Medicare and Medicaid Services
7500 Security Boulevard
Baltimore, MD 21244
Toll-Free: 800-MEDICARE
(800-633-4227)
(Medicare Service Center)
Toll-Free TTY: 877-486-2048
(Medicare Service Center)
Toll-Free: 877-267-2323
(Employee directory available)
Toll-Free TTY: 866-226-1819
Phone: 410-786-3000
TTY: 410-786-0727
Website: www.cms.hhs.gov

Resources in this chapter were compiled from several sources deemed reliable; all contact information was verified and updated in January 2013.

Centers for Disease Control and Prevention
1600 Clifton Road
Atlanta, GA 30333
Toll-Free: 800-CDC-INFO
(800-232-4636)
Toll-Free TTY: 888-232-6348
Phone: 404-639-3311
Websites: www.cdc.gov;
www.cdcnpin.org; www.cdc.gov/
nchhstp; www.hivtest.org/
stdtesting.aspx
E-mail: cdcinfo@cdc.gov

Equal Employment Opportunity Commission
1801 L Street NW
Washington, DC 20507
Toll-Free: 800-669-4000
Toll-Free TTY: 800-669-6820
Phone: 202-663-4900
TTY: 202-663-4494
Website: www.eeoc.gov
E-mail: info@eeoc.gov

Healthfinder®
National Health Information
Center
PO Box 1133
Washington, DC 20013-1133
Toll-Free: 800-336-4797
Phone: 301-565-4167
Fax: 301-984-4256
Website: www.healthfinder.gov
E-mail: healthfinder@nhic.org

National Cancer Institute
NCI Office of Communications
and Education
Public Inquiries Office
6116 Executive Boulevard
Suite 300
Bethesda, MD 20892-8322
Toll-Free: 800-4-CANCER
(800-422-6237)
Toll-Free TTY: 800-332-8615
Website: www.cancer.gov
E-mail:
cancergovstaff@mail.nih.gov

National Center for Complementary and Alternative Medicine
National Institutes of Health
NCCAM Clearinghouse
PO Box 7923
Gaithersburg, MD 20898-7923
Toll-Free: 888-644-6226
Toll-Free TTY: 866-464-3615
Toll-Free Fax: 866-464-3616
Website: www.nccam.nih.gov
E-mail: info@nccam.nih.gov

National Center for Health Statistics
3311 Toledo Road
Hyattsville, MD 20782
Toll-Free: 800-CDC-INFO
(800-232-4636)
Website: www.cdc.gov/nchs
E-mail: cdcinfo@cdc.gov

National Heart, Lung, and Blood Institute

NHLBI Health
Information Center
PO Box 30105
Bethesda, MD 20824-0105
Phone: 301-592-8573
TTY: 240-629-3255
Fax: 240-629-3246
Website: www.nhlbi.nih.gov
E-mail: nhlbiinfo@nhlbi.nih.gov

National Institute of Neurological Disorders and Stroke

PO Box 5801
Bethesda, MD 20824
Toll-Free: 800-352-9424
Phone: 301-496-5751
TTY: 301-468-5981
Websites: www.ninds.nih.gov;
www.stroke-site.org

National Institute on Aging

Building 31, Room 5C27
31 Center Drive, MSC 2292
Bethesda, MD 20892
Toll-Free: 800-222-2225
Toll-Free TTY: 800-222-4225
Phone: 301-496-1752
Fax: 301-496-1072
Website: www.nia.nih.gov
E-mail: niaic@nia.nih.gov

National Institutes of Health

9000 Rockville Pike
Bethesda, MD 20892
Phone: 301-496-4000
TTY: 301-402-9612
Website: www.nih.gov
E-mail: NIHinfo@od.nih.gov

National Women's Health Information Center

Office on Women's Health
200 Independence Avenue SW
Room 712E
Washington, DC 20201
Toll-Free: 800-994-9662
Toll-Free TDD: 888-220-5446
Phone: 202-690-7650
Fax: 202-205-2631
Website: www.womenshealth.gov

Office of Minority Health Resource Center

PO Box 37337
Washington, DC 20013-7337
Toll-Free: 800-444-6472
Phone: 240-453-2882
TDD: 301-251-1432
Fax: 240-453-2883
Website: minorityhealth.hhs.gov
E-mail: info@minorityhealth.hhs.gov

Social Security Administration

Office of Public Inquiries
Windsor Park Building
6401 Security Boulevard
Baltimore, MD 21235
Toll-Free: 800-772-1213
Website: www.socialsecurity.gov

U.S. Department of Health and Human Services

Room 443 H
200 Independence Avenue SW
Washington, DC 20201
Toll-Free: 877-696-6775
Website: www.hhs.gov;
www.HeartHealthyWomen.org

U.S. Department of Veterans Affairs
Resources and Education
for Stroke Caregivers'
Understanding and
Empowerment (RESCUE)
810 Vermont Avenue NW
Washington, DC 20420
Toll-Free: 855-260-3274
(Caregiver Support)
Website: www.rorc.research
.va.gov/rescue

U.S. National Library of Medicine
References and Web Services
8600 Rockville Pike
Bethesda, MD 20894
Toll-Free: 888-FIND-NLM
(888-346-3656)
Toll-Free TDD: 800-735-2258
Phone: 301-594-5983
Fax: 301-402-1384
Website: www.nlm.nih.gov
E-mail: custserv@nlm.nih.gov

Private Agencies That Provide Information about Stroke

American Academy of Family Physicians
PO Box 11210
Shawnee Mission, KS
66207-1210
Toll-Free: 800-274-2237
Phone: 913-906-6000
Fax: 913-906-6075
Website: www.aafp.org
E-mail: fp@aafp.org

American Academy of Neurology
201 Chicago Avenue
Minneapolis, MN 55415
Toll-Free: 800-879-1960
Phone: 612-928-6000
Fax: 612-454-2746
Website: www.aan.com
E-mail: memberservices@aan.com

American Academy of Pediatrics
141 Northwest Point Boulevard
Elk Grove Village, IL
60007-1098
Toll-Free: 800-433-9016
Phone: 847-434-4000
Fax: 847-434-8000
Website: www.aap.org
E-mail: kidsdocs@aap.org

American Academy of Physical Medicine and Rehabilitation
9700 West Bryn Mawr Avenue
Suite 200
Rosemont, IL 60018-5701
Phone: 847-737-6000
Fax: 847-737-6001
Website: www.aapmr.org
E-mail: info@aapmr.org

American Association of Neurological Surgeons
5550 Meadowbrook Drive
Rolling Meadows, IL 60008-3852
Toll-Free: 888-566-AANS
(888-566-2267)
Phone: 847-378-0500
Fax: 847-378-0600
Website: www.aans.org
E-mail: info@aans.org

American Congress of Obstetricians and Gynecologists
PO Box 70620
Washington, DC 20024-9998
Toll-Free: 800-673-8444
Phone: 202-638-5577
Website: www.acog.org
E-mail: resources@acog.org

American College of Radiology
1891 Preston White Drive
Reston, VA 20191
Phone: 703-648-8900
Website: www.acr.org
E-mail: info@acr.org

American Congress of Rehabilitation Medicine
11654 Plaza America Drive
Suite 535
Reston, VA 20190
Phone: 703-435-5335
Toll-Free Fax: 866-692-1619
Website: www.acrm.org

American Heart Association/American Stroke Association
National Center
7272 Greenville Avenue
Dallas, TX 75231
Toll-Free: 800-AHA-USA-1
(800-242-8721)
Toll-Free: 888-4-STROKE
(888-478-7653)
Websites:
www.americanheart.org;
www.strokeassociation.org

American Medical Association
515 North State Street
Chicago, IL 60654
Toll-Free: 800-621-8335
Website: www.ama-assn.org

American Occupational Therapy Association
4720 Montgomery Lane
Suite 200
Bethesda, MD 20814-3449
Toll-Free: 800-377-8555
Phone: 301-652-2682
Fax: 301-652-7711
Website: www.aota.org

American Physical Therapy Association
1111 North Fairfax Street
Alexandria, VA 22314-1488
Toll-Free: 800-999-2782
Phone: 703-684-2782
TDD: 703-683-6748
Fax: 703-684-7343
Website: www.apta.org

American Society of Neurorehabilitation
5841 Cedar Lake Road
Suite 204
Minneapolis, MN 55416
Phone: 952-545-6324
Fax: 952-545-6073
Website: www.asnr.com
E-mail: asnr@llmsi.com

American Speech-Language-Hearing Association (ASHA)
2200 Research Boulevard
Rockville, MD 20850-3289
Toll-Free: 800-638-8255
Fax: 301-296-8580
Website: www.asha.org
E-mail: actioncenter@asha.org

Brain Aneurysm Foundation, Inc.
269 Hanover Street
Building 3
Hanover, MA 02339
Toll-Free: 888-272-4602
Phone: 781-826-5556
Fax: 781-826-5566
Website: www.bafound.org
E-mail: office@bafound.org

Brain Injury Association of America
1608 Spring Hill Road
Suite 110
Vienna, VA 22182
Toll-Free: 800-444-6443
Phone: 703-761-0750
Fax: 703-761-0755
Website: www.biausa.org

Brain Injury Recovery Network
840 Central Avenue
Carlisle, OH 45005
Toll-Free: 877-810-2100
Fax: 877-810-2100
Website: www.tbirecovery.org
E-mail: help@tbirecovery.org

Caregiver Action Network
(Formerly the National Family Caregivers Association)
10400 Connecticut Ave., Suite 500
Kensington, MD 20895-3944
Toll-Free: 800-896-3650
Phone: 301-942-6430
Fax: 301-942-2302
Website: www.caregiveraction.com
E-mail: info@caregiveraction.com

Caring.com
2600 S. El Camino Real, Suite 300
San Mateo, CA 94403
Website: www.caring.com

Children's Hemiplegia and Stroke Association (CHASA)
4101 West Green Oaks
Suite 305, #149
Arlington, TX 76016
Websites: www.chasa.org;
www.pediatricstroke.org

Cleveland Clinic
9500 Euclid Avenue
Cleveland, OH 44195
Toll-Free: 800-223-CARE
(800-223-2273)
Info Line: 866-588-2264
Info Line: 216-636-5860
TTY: 216-444-0261
Website: my.clevelandclinic.org

Family Caregiver Alliance
785 Market Street, Suite 750
San Francisco, CA 94103
Toll-Free: 800-445-8106
Phone: 415-434-3388
Fax: 415-434-3508
Website: www.caregiver.org
E-mail: info@caregiver.org

Hazel K. Goddess Fund for Stroke Research in Women
1217 S. Flagler Drive, Suite 302
West Palm Beach, FL 33401
Phone: 561-623-0504
Fax: 561-623-0502
Website: www.thegoddessfund.org

Internet Stroke Center
UT Southwestern Medical Center
Department of Neurology
and Neurotherapeutics
5323 Harry Hines Boulevard
Dallas, TX 75390
Phone: 214-648-3111
Website: www.strokecenter.org

Job Accommodation Network (JAN)
PO Box 6080, 224 Spruce Street
Morgantown, WV 26506-6080
Toll-Free: 800-526-7234
Toll-Free TTY: 877-781-9403
Website: www.jan.wvu.edu
E-mail: jan@askjan.org

National Alliance for Caregiving
4720 Montgomery Ln., 2nd Floor
Bethesda, MD 20814
Phone: 301-718-8444
Fax: 301-951-9067
Website: www.caregiving.org
E-mail: info@caregiving.org

National Aphasia Association
350 Seventh Avenue, Suite 902
New York, NY 10001
Toll-Free: 800-922-4622
Website: www.aphasia.org
E-mail:
responsecenter@aphasia.org

National Brain Tumor Society
124 Watertown Street, Suite 2D
Watertown, MA 02472
Phone: 617-924-9997
Fax: 617-924-9998
Website: www.braintumor.org
E-mail: nbtf@braintumor.org

National Center for Learning Disabilities
381 Park Ave. South, Suite 1401
New York, NY 10016
Toll-Free: 888-575-7373
Phone: 212-545-7510
Fax: 212-545-9665
Website: www.ncld.org

National Information Center for Children and Youth with Disabilities (NICHCY)
1825 Connecticut Avenue NW
Washington, DC 20009
Toll-Free: 800-695-0285
(Voice and TTY)
Phone: 202-884-8200
(Voice and TTY)
Fax: 202-884-8441
Website: www.nichcy.org
E-mail: nichcy@fhi360.org

National Rehabilitation Information Center
8400 Corporate Drive, Suite 500
Landover, MD 20785
Toll-Free: 800-346-2742
Phone: 301-459-5900
TTY: 301-459-5984
Fax: 301-459-4263
Website: www.naric.com
E-mail: naricinfo
@heitechservices.com

National Stroke Association
9707 East Easter Lane, Suite B
Centennial, CO 80112
Toll-Free: 800-STROKES
(800-787-6537)
Fax: 303-649-1328
Website: www.stroke.org
E-mail: info@stroke.org

Neuro-Patient Resource Center
Montreal Neurological Institute
and Hospital
McGill University
Health Center
3801 University, Room 354
Montreal, Quebec
Canada H3A 2B4
Phone: 514-398-5358
Website: infoneuro.mcgill.ca/
index.php?option=com_
resources&Itemid=122&task=
disres&id=276
E-mail:
infoneuro@muhc.mcgill.ca

Rehabilitation Institute of Chicago
LIFE Center
345 E. Superior St., First Floor
Chicago, IL 60611
Toll-Free: 800-354-REHAB
(800-354-7342)
Phone: 312-238-LIFE
(312-238-5433)
Fax: 312-238-2860
Website: lifecenter.ric.org
E-mail: lifecenter@ric.org

Society for Vascular Surgery
633 North Saint Clair Street
22nd Floor
Chicago, IL 60611
Toll-Free: 800-258-7188
Phone: 312-334-2300
Fax: 312-334-2320
Website: www.vascularweb.org
E-mail:
vascular@vascularsociety.org

Stroke Association UK
Stroke House, 240 City Road
London, EC1V 2PR
United Kingdom
Phone: 020 7566 0300
Website: www.stroke.org.uk
E-mail: info@stroke.org.uk

Stroke Awareness Foundation
1400 Parkmoor Avenue
Suite 230
San Jose, CA 95126
Phone: 408-961-9815
Fax: 408-961-9856
Website: www.strokeinfo.org

Well Spouse Association
63 West Main Street, Suite H
Freehold, NJ 07728
Toll-Free: 800-838-0879
Phone: 732-577-8899
Fax: 732-577-8644
Website: www.wellspouse.org
E-mail: info@wellspouse.org

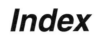

Index

Index

Page numbers followed by 'n' indicate a footnote. Page numbers in *italics* indicate a table or illustration.

Health Reference Series